The Atypical Pneumonias

Guest Editor

BURKE A. CUNHA, MD, MACP

INFECTIOUS DISEASE CLINICS OF NORTH AMERICA

www.id.theclinics.com

Consulting Editor
ROBERT C. MOELLERING Jr, MD

March 2010 • Volume 24 • Number 1

SAUNDERS an imprint of ELSEVIER, Inc.

W.B. SAUNDERS COMPANY
A Division of Elsevier Inc.
1600 John F. Kennedy Blvd., Suite 1800, Philadelphia, PA 19103-2899.
http://www.theclinics.com
INFECTIOUS DISEASE CLINICS OF NORTH AMERICA Volume 24, Number 1
March 2010 ISSN 0891–5520, ISBN-13: 978-1-4377-1830-0
Editor: Barbara Cohen-Kligerman

Infectious Disease Clinics of North America (ISSN 0891–5520) is published in March, June, September, and December by Elsevier Inc., 360 Park Avenue South, New York, NY 10010-1710. Periodicals postage paid at New York, NY and additional mailing offices. Subscription prices are $235.00 per year for US individuals, $395.00 per year for US institutions, $118.00 per year for US students, $278.00 per year for Canadian individuals, $489.00 per year for Canadian institutions, $332.00 per year for international individuals, $489.00 per year for international institutions, and $163.00 per year for Canadian and international students. To receive student rate, orders must be accompained by name of affiliated institution, date of term, and the *signature* of program/residency coordinator on institution letterhead. Orders will be billed at individual rate until proof of status is received. Foreign air speed delivery is included in all *Clinics* subscription prices. All prices are subject to change without notice. **POSTMASTER**: Send address changes to *Infectious Disease Clinics of North America,* Elsevier Health Sciences Division, Subcription Customer Service, 3251 Riverport Lane, Maryland Heights, MO 63043. **Customer Service: 1-800-654-2452 (US). From outside of the US and Canada, call 1-314-447-8871. Fax: 1-314-447-8029. E-mail: JournalsCustomerService-usa@elsevier.com (print support) or JournalsOnlineSupport-usa@elsevier.com (online support).**

Infectious Disease Clinics of North America is also published in Spanish by Editorial Inter-Médica, Junin 917, 1er A 1113, Buenos Aires, Argentina.

Reprints. For copies of 100 or more of articles in this publication, please contact the Commercial Reprints Department, Elsevier Inc., 360 Park Avenue South, New York, New York 10010-1710. Tel. (212) 633-3812, Fax: (212) 462-1935, E-mail: reprints@elsevier.com.

Infectious Disease Clinics of North America is covered in *MEDLINE/PubMed (Index Medicus), Current Contents/Clinical Medicine, Science Citation Alert, SCISEARCH,* and *Research Alert.*

Printed and bound by CPI Group (UK) Ltd, Croydon, CR0 4YY

Transferred to Digital Print 2011

Contributors

CONSULTING EDITOR

ROBERT C. MOELLERING JR, MD
Shields Warren-Mallinckrodt Professor of Medical Research, Harvard Medical School; Department of Medicine, Beth Israel Deaconess Medical Center, Boston, Massachusetts

GUEST EDITOR

BURKE A. CUNHA, MD, MACP
Chief, Infectious Disease Division, Winthrop-University Hospital, Mineola, Long Island, New York; Professor of Medicine, State University of New York School of Medicine, Stony Brook, New York

AUTHORS

MARIE-ELISABETH BOUGNOUX, MD, PhD
Université Paris Descartes, Hôpital Necker-Enfants Malades, Service de Microbiologie, Paris, France

EMILIO BOUZA, MD, PhD
Professor, Microbiology Department, Universidad Complutense; Clinical Microbiology and Infectious Diseases Department, Hospital General Universitario Gregorio Marañón, Madrid, Spain; CIBER de Enfermedades Respiratorias (CIBERES), Majorca, Spain

ALMUDENA BURILLO, MD, PhD
Clinical Microbiology Department, Hospital Universitario de Móstoles, Móstoles, Madrid, Spain

EMILIE CATHERINOT, MD, PhD
Université Paris Descartes, Service de Maladies Infectieuses et Tropicales, Centre d'Infectiologie Necker-Pasteur, Hôpital Necker-Enfants Malades, Paris, France; Université Versailles-Saint Quentin, Hôpital Foch, Service de Pneumologie, Suresnes, France

DENNIS J. CLERI, MD, FACP, FAAM, FIDSA
Program Director, Internal Medicine Residency Program, St Francis Medical Center, Trenton, New Jersey; Professor of Medicine, Seton Hall University School of Graduate Medical Education, South Orange, New Jersey; Department of Medicine, St Francis Medical Center, Trenton, New Jersey

LOUIS-JEAN COUDERC, MD, PhD
Université Versailles-Saint Quentin, Hôpital Foch, Service de Pneumologie, Suresnes, France

BURKE A. CUNHA, MD, MACP
Chief, Infectious Disease Division, Winthrop-University Hospital, Mineola, Long Island, New York; Professor of Medicine, State University of New York School of Medicine, Stony Brook, New York

CHESTON B. CUNHA, MD
Department of Medicine, Brown University, Alpert School of Medicine, Rhode Island Hospital & The Miriam Hospital, Providence, Rhode Island

IBRAHIM FARUQI, MD, MPH
Fellow, Division of Pulmonary and Critical Care Medicine, University of Kansas, Kansas City, Kansas

M. LINDSAY GRAYSON, MBBS, MD, MSc, FRACP, FAFPHM
Director, Department of Infectious Diseases, Austin Health, Heidelberg; Professor, Department of Epidemiology and Preventive Medicine, Monash University; Professor, Department of Medicine, University of Melbourne, Melbourne, Australia

FANNY LANTERNIER, MD, MSc
Université Paris Descartes, Service de Maladies Infectieuses et Tropicales, Centre d'Infectiologie Necker-Pasteur, Hôpital Necker-Enfants Malades, Paris, France

MARC LECUIT, MD, PhD
Université Paris Descartes, Service de Maladies Infectieuses et Tropicales, Centre d'Infectiologie Necker-Pasteur, Hôpital Necker-Enfants Malades, Paris, France

OLIVIER LORTHOLARY, MD, PhD
Université Paris Descartes, Service de Maladies Infectieuses et Tropicales, Centre d'Infectiologie Necker-Pasteur, Hôpital Necker-Enfants Malades; Institut Pasteur, Centre National de Référence Mycologie et antifongiques, Paris, France

THOMAS J. MARRIE, MD
Dean, Faculty of Medicine, Clinical Research Centre, Dalhousie University, Halifax, Nova Scotia, Canada

SAURIN PATEL, MD
Fellow, Division of Pulmonary and Critical Care Medicine, University of Kansas, Kansas City, Kansas

ANTHONY J. RICKETTI, MD, FCCP
Chairman, Department of Medicine, Head, Section of Allergy and Immunology, and Associate Program Director, Internal Medicine Residency, St. Francis Medical Center, Trenton, New Jersey; Associate Professor of Medicine, Seton Hall University School of Graduate Medical Education, South Orange, New Jersey

WILLIAM SCHAFFNER, MD
Chairman, Department of Preventive Medicine, Professor of Medicine (Infectious Diseases), Vanderbilt University Medical Center, Nashville, Tennessee

DAVID SCHLOSSBERG, MD, FACP
Professor of Medicine, Temple University School of Medicine; Adjunct Professor of Medicine, University of Pennsylvania School of Medicine; Medical Director, Tuberculosis Control Program, Philadelphia Department of Public Health, Philadelphia, Pennsylvania

STEVEN Q. SIMPSON, MD
Associate Professor of Medicine, Division of Pulmonary and Critical Care Medicine, University of Kansas, Kansas City, Kansas

LEON G. SMITH, MD, MACP
Chairman, Infectious Disease Foundation of Saint Michael's Medical Center; Professor of Medicine and Preventive Medicine, Department of Preventive Medicine, New Jersey Medical School, Newark, New Jersey

LESLIE SPIKES, MD
Fellow, Division of Pulmonary and Critical Care Medicine, University of Kansas, Kansas City, Kansas

ANDREW J. STEWARDSON, MBBS
Infectious Diseases Registrar, Department of Infectious Diseases, Austin Health, Heidelberg, Melbourne, Victoria, Australia

RENÉ TE WITT, BSc
PhD student, Department of Medical Microbiology and Infectious Diseases, Unit Research and Development, Erasmus MC, Rotterdam, The Netherlands

LORA D. THOMAS, MD, MPH
Assistant Professor, Division of Infectious Diseases, Department of Medicine, Vanderbilt University Medical Center; Chief, Division of Infectious Diseases, VA Medical Center, Nashville, Tennessee

ALEX VAN BELKUM, PhD
Professor of Molecular Microbiology, Department of Medical Microbiology and Infectious Diseases, Unit Research and Development, Erasmus MC, Rotterdam, The Netherlands

WILLEM B. VAN LEEUWEN, PhD
Molecular Microbiologist, Department of Medical Microbiology and Infectious Diseases, Unit Research and Development, Erasmus MC, Rotterdam, The Netherlands

JOHN R. VERNALEO, MD, FACP
Chief, Division of Infectious Diseases, Wyckoff Heights Medical Center, Brooklyn, New York

Contents

Preface xiii

Burke A. Cunha

Historic Aspects

The First Atypical Pneumonia: The History of the Discovery of *Mycoplasma pneumoniae* 1

Cheston B. Cunha

The subject of atypical pneumonias is of great medical and historical interest to modern physicians. Although these diseases have no doubt affected humans throughout our history, it is not until the mid-twentieth century that physicians first began to differentiate certain atypical pulmonary infectious processes from typical pneumonia. Physicians at the time were unclear as to the precise etiology of these infections. As time progressed and study of these organisms continued, physicians were better able to identify the causative agent and devise tests with which to detect the disease. This article focuses on the description and ultimate identification of *Mycoplasma pneumoniae*.

Zoonotic Atypical Pneumonias

Psittacosis 7

Andrew J. Stewardson and M. Lindsay Grayson

Psittacosis is a systemic zoonotic infection with protean clinical features. The major risk factor is exposure to birds; bird owners, veterinarians, those involved with breeding and selling birds, and commercial poultry processors are most at risk. Patients typically present with 1 week of fevers, headache, myalgias, and a nonproductive cough. Although pneumonia is the most common manifestation, all organ systems can be involved. Serology remains the mainstay of diagnosis; however, polymerase chain reaction techniques offer a rapid and specific alternative. Doxycycline is the treatment of choice.

Q Fever Pneumonia 27

Thomas J. Marrie

Q fever is a disease found in both humans and animals, caused by the bacterium *Coxiella burnetii.* The epidemiology of Q fever is that of the animal reservoirs of the infection including both direct and indirect contact and use of a variety of products from such animals as cattle, sheep, and goats. Pneumonia is the major manifestation of Q fever in some countries. It is

mild to moderate in severity, and mortality is unusual. It can occur as sporadic or outbreak cases.

Tularemia Pneumonia 43

Lora D. Thomas and William Schaffner

Francisella tularensis is a zoonotic infection that can be acquired in multiple ways, including a bite from an arthropod, the handling of animal carcasses, consumption of contaminated food and water, or inhalation of infected particles. The most virulent subspecies of *F tularensis* is type A, which is almost exclusively seen in North America. Pneumonia can occur in tularemia, as either a primary process from direct inhalation, or as a secondary manifestation of ulceroglandular or typhoidal disease. This article describes the history of this infection, epidemiology, methods of diagnosis and treatment, and its potential as a bioterrorism weapon.

Non-Zoonotic Atypical Pneumonias

Mycoplasma Pneumonia and Its Complications 57

Leon G. Smith

Mycoplasma pneumoniae continues to be the most frequent cause of atypical pneumonia. Fortunately, the antibiotics listed in this article are generally very effective. Major skills are needed to detect *M pneumoniae* extrapulmonary diseases, which require a special heightened awareness and sensitivity. It is not known whether early therapy prevents dreaded complications.

Chlamydophila pneumoniae 61

Almudena Burillo and Emilio Bouza

Chlamydophila pneumoniae is estimated to cause about 10% of community-acquired pneumonia (CAP) cases and 5% of bronchitis cases, although most patients with *C pneumoniae* infection are asymptomatic, and the course of respiratory illness is relatively mild. The incubation period of *C pneumoniae* infection is around 21 days, and such symptoms as cough and malaise show a gradual onset, yet may persist for several weeks or months despite appropriate antibiotic therapy. Diagnosis by nasopharyngeal specimen culture, serum antibody titers, or molecular techniques is usually delayed with respect to the onset of symptoms, antibiotic treatment, or disease resolution and there is no accurate, standardized, commercial US Food and Drug Administration–cleared diagnostic method available. Erythromycin, tetracycline, and doxycycline are used as first-line therapy, although some investigators report no clinical or survival benefits from treating CAP caused by atypical pathogens. Meanwhile, adequate prospective studies have met with ethical and logistic barriers. Despite these limitations, North American guidelines recommend the antimicrobial treatment of patients with acute *C pneumoniae* respiratory infection.

Legionnaires' Disease: Clinical Differentiation from Typical and Other Atypical Pneumonias 73

Burke A. Cunha

This article describes the clinical differentiation of legionnaires' disease from typical and other atypical pneumonias, with reference to the history, microbiology, epidemiology, clinical presentation (including radiologic manifestations, clinical extrapulmonary features, nonspecific laboratory findings, clinical syndromic diagnosis, and differential diagnosis), therapy, complications, and prognosis of the disease.

Non-Classic Atypical Pneumonias

***Pneumocystis jirovecii* Pneumonia** 107

Emilie Catherinot, Fanny Lanternier, Marie-Elisabeth Bougnoux, Marc Lecuit, Louis-Jean Couderc, and Olivier Lortholary

Pneumocystis jirovecii has gained attention during the last decade in the context of the AIDS epidemic and the increasing use of cytotoxic and immunosuppressive therapies. This article summarizes current knowledge on biology, pathophysiology, epidemiology, diagnosis, prevention, and treatment of pulmonary *P jirovecii* infection, with a particular focus on the evolving pathophysiology and epidemiology. *Pneumocystis* pneumonia still remains a severe opportunistic infection, associated with a high mortality rate.

Acute Tuberculosis 139

David Schlossberg

Both primary and reactivation tuberculosis may present as an acute process and mimic community-acquired pneumonia. Tuberculosis should always be included in the initial differential diagnosis, and suspicion should be heightened by a variety of clinical and epidemiologic clues, as well as by multiple underlying conditions. This article reviews the pathophysiology, risk factors, and clinical manifestations of acute presentations of tuberculosis.

Cytomegalovirus Pneumonia: Community-Acquired Pneumonia in Immunocompetent Hosts 147

Burke A. Cunha

Cytomegaloviruses (CMVs) are DNA viruses and are members of the Herpesviridae family. Morphologically, CMV resembles other herpes viruses, particularly herpes simplex viruses, with important cytopathic differences. CMVs are recognized pathogens that cause community-acquired pneumonia (CAP) in compromised hosts, such as, those who undergo transplants and those on immunosuppressive drugs or steroids. This article discusses the clinical presentation, diagnosis, and therapy for this viral CAP.

FORTHCOMING ISSUES

June 2010

Infections in Transplant and Oncology Patients

Kieren A. Marr, MD, and
Aruna Subramanian, MD, *Guest Editors*

September 2010

Emerging Respiratory Infections in the 21st Century

Alimuddin Zumla, MBChB, MSc, PhD,
Wing-Wai Yew, MBBS, MD, and
David SC Hui, MBBS, *Guest Editors*

December 2010

Diseases of the Gastrointestinal Tract and Associated Infections

Guy D. Eslick, PhD, *Guest Editor*

RECENT ISSUES

December 2009

Antibacterial Therapy and Newer Agents

Keith S. Kaye, MD, MPH, and
Donald Kaye, MD, *Guest Editors*

September 2009

Infections in the Intensive Care Unit

Marin H. Kollef, MD, and
Scott T. Micek, PharmD, *Guest Editors*

June 2009

Meta-analysis in Infectious Diseases

Matthew E. Falagas, MD, MSc, DSc,
Guest Editor

ISSUES OF RELATED INTEREST

Emergency Medicine Clinics of North America May 2008 (Vol. 26, No. 2)
Infectious Diseases in Emergency Medicine
Daniel R. Martin, MD, *Guest Editor*
Available at: http://www.emed.theclinics.com/

Clinics in Laboratory Medicine December 2009 (Vol. 29, No. 4)
Respiratory Viruses in Pediatric and Adult Populations
Alexander J. McAdam, MD, PhD, *Guest Editor*
Available at: http://www.labmed.theclinics.com/

Preface

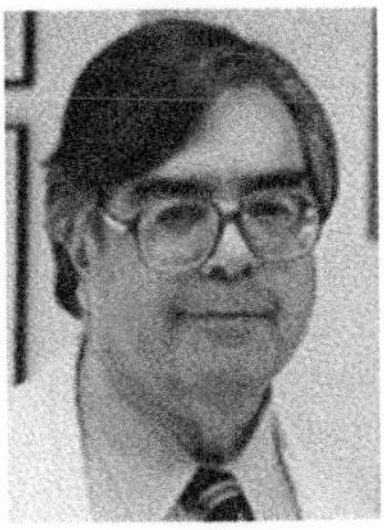

Burke A. Cunha, MD, MACP
Guest Editor

The term "atypical pneumonia" was first used by Reimann in 1941 to describe community-acquired pneumonias (CAP) caused by an atypical organism subsequently identified as *Mycoplasma pneumoniae*. The term atypical pneumonia was used because, unlike the typical bacterial pneumonias (eg, *S pneumoniae, H influenzae, M catarrhalis*), *M pneumoniae*, CAP was not only characterized by a different radiographic presentation but was also accompanied by a variety of extrapulmonary manifestations. To this day, the main distinguishing characteristic that clinically separates the typical bacterial from atypical CAPs is the presence or absence of extrapulmonary findings. Typical bacterial CAP has findings confined to the lungs and no extrapulmonary findings, whereas in CAP patients the presence of otherwise unexplained extrapulmonary features is indicative of an atypical CAP. As the usually prototype atypical pneumonia pathogen, *M pneumoniae*, unlike typical CAPs, presents with unilateral patchy infiltrates without consolidation or cavitation. In contrast, radiographically, the hallmark of typical bacterial CAPs is focal segmental/lobar infiltrates usually with consolidation and/or pleural effusion. In addition to lung findings, the extrapulmonary features of *M pneumoniae* CAP include meningoencephalitis (central nervous system), *E multiforme*/Stevens-Johnson syndrome (skin), bullous myringitis/otitis media (ears, nose, throat [ENT]), non-exudative pharyngitis (ENT), loose stools/watery diarrhea (gastrointestinal), and so forth. *M pneumoniae* CAP may also be accompanied by different nonspecific laboratory abnormalities compared to typical CAP pathogens (ie, elevated cold agglutinin titers). For this reason, *M pneumoniae* originally was described as "cold agglutinin" pneumonia.

Since *M pneumoniae* CAP, other atypical pathogens have been described that are now well-recognized causes of atypical CAP (ie, Legionnaires' disease and *Chlamydophila (Chlamydia) pneumoniae*). As with *M pneumoniae*, Legionnaires' disease and *C pneumoniae* CAPs are systemic infectious diseases with pulmonary manifestations. The key to the clinical recognition and differentiation of atypical CAPs is based upon their characteristic patterns of extrapulmonary organ involvement.

Before *M pneumoniae* was described, the term atypical pneumonia was an accepted and widely used term. Infectious disease clinicians recognized that the zoonotic pulmonary pathogens causing CAP were, in fact, the original atypical

Infect Dis Clin N Am 24 (2010) xiii–xvii
doi:10.1016/j.idc.2009.10.015

pneumonias. The most common causes of zoonotic atypical CAPs include tularemia (*F tularensis*), psittacosis (*C psittaci*), and Q fever (*C burnetti*). Like the non-zoonotic atypical CAPs, in addition to pneumonia, each zoonotic atypical pneumonia is characterized by its own particular pattern of extrapulmonary organ involvement. For clinicians approaching patients with CAP, the first diagnostic consideration is to determine whether pneumonia is present alone or if there are also extrapulmonary findings. If CAP with extrapulmonary features is present, by definition patients have an atypical CAP. The next diagnostic consideration is to differentiate zoonotic from non-zoonotic atypical CAP. Because the acquisition of zoonotic atypical pathogens is not random, there must be a recent/close contact with the appropriate zoonotic vector. A negative recent/close zoonotic contact history effectively eliminates zoonotic atypical pathogens from further diagnostic consideration. If a recent/close contact zoonotic history is positive, specific tests for each zoonotic vector determine the pathogen. Contact should prompt fewer tests. The next diagnostic consideration in patients who have a zoonotic or non-zoonotic atypical CAP is to determine the pattern of extrapulmonary organ involvement. Although some individual features of extrapulmonary organ involvement overlap, the pattern of organ involvement, which is variable with each of these infectious diseases, nevertheless has sufficient distinguishing features for accurate presumptive clinical diagnosis. Using this approach in patients who have CAP with extrapulmonary findings, clinicians should easily be able to generate an accurate presumptive diagnosis. The benefit of this diagnostic approach is to eliminate unlikely diagnostic possibilities and to prompt the physician to order appropriate diagnostic tests to confirm or rule out the working diagnosis.

Knowledge of key differential diagnostic features is of great clinical usefulness and is the basis of differential diagnosis in the common non-zoonotic atypical CAP (ie, Legionnaires' disease vs *Mycoplasma pneumoniae*). Although *Legionella sp* and *M pneumoniae* CAP may be accompanied by loose stools/watery diarrhea, dry cough, and headache, a few key clinical findings will rapidly differentiate these two entities irrespective of their chest X ray appearance. Legionnaires' disease, regardless of *Legionella sp* is accompanied by a pulse temperature deficit (ie, relative bradycardia) but *M pneumoniae* CAP is not. Liver involvement manifested by mildly transiently elevated serum transaminases aspartate aminotransferase/alanine aminotransferase is common in Legionnaires' disease but is not a feature of *M pneumoniae* CAP. Otherwise unexplained hypophosphatemia is the hallmark nonspecific laboratory abnormality associated with Legionnaires' disease. Hypophosphatemia is not a feature of *M pneumoniae* CAP or any other typical or atypical CAP. In patients who have CAP with extrapulmonary findings and a negative zoonotic contact history, relative bradycardia, slightly increased serum transaminases, and hypophosphatemia tests makes Legionnaires' disease likely. Legionella titers and Legionella urinary antigen tests should be obtained to confirm the diagnosis. With this approach, *M pneumoniae* is so unlikely that there is no need to order cold agglutinin or *M pneumoniae* titers.

The continued clinical usefulness of the term atypical pneumonia is based on the original description of the common zoonotic atypical CAP (psittacosis, Q fever, tularemia) and the common non-zoonotic atypical CAP (*M pneumoniae,* Legionnaires' disease, *C pneumoniae*). Since the classic atypical CAP pathogens were described, other causes of CAP with extrapulmonary features have been recognized (ie, hantavirus pulmonary syndrome [HPS], avian influenza [H5N1] pneumonia, swine influenza [H1N1] pneumonia, cytomegalovirus [CMV] and adenovirus).

This issue of *Infectious Disease Clinics of North America* includes articles on these "nonclassical" causes of atypical CAP. Also included are other pneumonias that are often in the differential diagnosis of atypical CAP. However, because they are not usually accompanied by extrapulmonary findings (ie, *M tuberculosis* and *Pneumocystic* [carinii] *jirovecii*) they should not be termed atypical CAP. The designation of atypical pneumonia caused by either classic or newly described atypical pathogens remains clinically useful. A benefit of the clinical diagnostic syndromic approach is that it emphasizes the characteristic pattern of extrapulmonary involvement associated with each atypical pathogen that, unlike chest film findings, is the key to the presumptive diagnosis.

Some have criticized the continued use of the term atypical pneumonia based on the notion that many of these pathogens are no longer uncommon or unusual. The term atypical pneumonia is based on the presence of extrapulmonary findings in patients who have CAP and not the frequencies of these pathogens in clinical practice. The term atypical pneumonia remains useful because it reminds the clinician that the atypical pathogens are systemic infectious diseases with extrapulmonary findings. Atypical pneumonia remains a useful designation clinically and conceptually.

The lead article in this issue of *Infectious Disease Clinics of North America* on Atypical Pneumonias is by Cheston B. Cunha, who reviews historical aspects of *M. pneumoniae*, the original atypical pneumonia. Other articles included are reviews of psittacosis by M. Lindsay Grayson and Andrew J. Stewardson; Thomas Marrie on Q fever; and William Schaffner and Lora D. Thomas on tularemia. Leon Smith reviews *M pneumoniae* and Emilio Bouza and Almudena Burillo review *C pneumoniae*. Dennis Cleri and colleagues give us their clinical perspective on SARS as do Steven Simpson and colleagues on HPS. Articles on Legionnaires' disease, swine influenza, and CMV were written by me. Alex von Belkum and colleagues reviewed specific laboratory tests for atypical pathogens. Although not atypical CAP pathogens, other pathogens that may mimic atypical CAPs are included in the contributions of Olivier Lortholary and colleagues on *Pneumocystis (carinii) jiroveci* and David Schlossberg on acute tuberculosis.

This issue of *Infectious Disease Clinics of North America* on the Atypical Pneumonias is the only current, in-depth compilation of its kind from a clinical perspective. Physicians should benefit greatly from the practical clinical points in each article. The newly described atypical pneumonias (ie, HPS, H5N1, and H1N1) will certainly be followed in the future by other atypical pneumonias that are yet to be described. The hallmark of these atypical CAP pathogens will also be their unique pattern of extrapulmonary organ involvement linking them to the traditional classic and more recently described atypical pulmonary pathogens causing CAP.

Burke A. Cunha, MD, MACP
Infectious Disease Division
Winthrop-University Hospital
259 First Street
Mineola, Long Island, NY 11501, USA

FURTHER READINGS

Boermsa WG, Daniels JM, Lowernberg A, et al. Reliability of radiographic findings and the relation to etiologic agents in community-acquired pneumonia. Respir Med 2006;100:926–32.

Buescher EL. Respiratory disease and the adenoviruses. Med Clin North Am 1967;51:769–79.

Chanock RM. Mycoplasma infections of man. N Engl J Med 1965;273:1199–206, 1257–64.

Cunha BA, Quintiliani R. The atypical pneumonias, a diagnostic and therapeutic approach. Postgrad Med 1979;66:95–102.
Cunha BA. Atypical pneumonias. In: Conn RD, Borer WZ, Snyder JW, editors. Current diagnosis 9. Philadelphia: WB Saunders; 1996.
Cunha BA. Ortega AM Atypical pneumonia. Extrapulmonary clues guide the way to diagnosis. Postgrad Med 1996;99:123–8.
Cunha BA. Clinical diagnosis of Legionnaires' Disease. Semin Respir Infect 1998;13: 116–27.
Cunha BA. Diagnostic Significance of relative bradycardia. Clin Microbiol Infect 2000; 6:633–4.
Cunha BA. Community-acquired pneumonia: diagnostic and therapeutic considerations. Med Clin North Am 2001;85:43–77.
Cunha BA. Ambulatory community acquired pneumonia: the predominance of atypical pathogens. Eur J Clin Microbiol Infect Dis 2003;2:579–83.
Cunha BA. Hypophosphatemia: diagnostic significance in legionnaires' disease. Am J Med 2006;119:5–6.
Cunha BA. The atypical pneumonias: clinical diagnosis and importance. Clin Microbiol Infect 2006;12:12–24.
Cunha BA, Syed U, Stroll S, et al. Winthrop-University Hospital Infectious Disease Division's swine influenza (H1N1) pneumonia diagnostic weighted point score system for hospitalized adults with influenza-like illnesses (ILIs) and negative rapid influenza diagnostic tests (RIDTs). Heart & Lung; 2009;38(6):534–8.
Cunha BA, editor. Pneumonia essentials. 3rd edition. Sudbury (MA): Jones & Bartlett; 2010.
Cutler SJ, Bouzid M, Cutler RR. Q fever. J Infect 2007;54:313–8.
Duchin JS, Koster FT, Peters CJ, et al. Hantavirus pulmonary syndrome: a clinical description of 17 patients with a newly recognized disease. N Engl J Med 1994;330:949–55.
File TH Jr, Tan JS, Plouffe JF. The role of atypical pathogens: *Mycoplasma pneumoniae, Chlamydia pneumoniae*, and *Legionella pneumophilia* in respiratory infection. Infect Dis Clin North Am 1998;12:569–92.
Forgie S, Marrie TJ. Healthcare-associated atypical pneumonia. Semin Respir Crit Care Med 2009;30:67–85.
Fraser DW, Tsai TR, Orenstein W, et al. Legionnaire's disease: description of an epidemic of pneumonia. N Engl J Med 1977;297:1189–97.
Gregory DW, Schaffner W. Psittacosis. Semin Respir Infect 1997;12:7–11.
Kirby BD, Snyder KM, Meyer RD, et al. Legionnaire's disease: report of 65 nosocomially acquired cases and review of the literature. Medicine 1980;59:188–205.
Kirchner JT. Psittacosis. Is contact with birds causing your patient's pneumonia? Postgrad Med 1997;102:181–2.
Ksiazek TG, Erdman D, Goldsmith CS, et al. A novel coronavirus associated with severe acute respiratory syndrome. N Engl J Med 2003;348:1953–66.
Liles WC, Burger RJ. Tularemia from domestic cats. West J Med 1993;158:619–22.
McDade JE, Shepard CC, Fraser DW, et al. Legionnaire's disease: isolation of a bacterium and demonstration of its role in other respiratory diseases. N Engl J Med 1977;297:1197–203.
Marrie TJ, Haldane D, Bezanson G, et al. Nosocomial Legionnaire's disease: clinical and radiographic patterns. Can J Infect Dis 1992;3:253–60.
Marlow E, Whelan C. Legionella pneumonia and use of the Legionella urinary antigen test. J Hosp Med 2009;4(3):E1–2.
Marrie TJ. Q fever pneumonia. Curr Opin Infect Dis 2004;17:137–42.

Masiá M, Gutiérrez F, Padilla S, et al. Clinical characterisation of pneumonia caused by atypical pathogens combining classic and novel predictors. Clin Microbiol Infect 2007;13:153–61.

Miyashita N, Fukano H, Yoshida K, et al. Is is possible to distinguish between atypical pneumonia and bacterial pneumonia? Evaluation of the guidelines for community acquired pneumonia in Japan. Respir Med 2004;98:952–60.

Nakashima K, Tanaka T, Kramer MH, et al. Outbreak of Chlamydia pneumoniae infection in a Japanese nursing home, 1999–2000. Infect Control Hosp Epidemiol 2006;27:1171–7.

Parker NR, Barralet JH, Bell AM. Q fever. Lancet 2006;367:679–88.

Pedro-Botet ML, Yu VL. Treatment strategies for Legionella infection. Expert Opin Pharmacother 2009;10(7):1109–21.

Peters CJ, Hkan AS. Hantavirus pulmonary syndrome: the new American hemorrhagic fever. Clin Infect Dis 2002;34:1224–31.

Phares CR, Russell E, Thigpen MC, et al. Legionnaires' disease among residents of a long-term care facility: the sentinel event in a community outbreak. Am J Infect Control 2007;5:319–23.

Reimann HA. An acute infection of the respiratory tract with atypical pneumonia. JAMA 1938;111:2377–84.

Sanford JP. Tularemia. JAMA 1983;3225–6.

Schneeberger PM, Dorigo-Zetsma JW, van der Zee A, et al. Diagnosis of atypical pathogens in patients hospitalized with community-acquired respiratory infection. Scand J Infect Dis 2004;36:269–73.

Sopena N, Sabria-Leal M, Pedro-Botet ML, et al. Comparative study of the clinical presentation of Legionella pneumonia and other community-acquired pneumonias. Chest 1998;113:1195–200.

Sopena N, Pedro-Botet ML, Sabria M, et al. Comparative study of community-acquired pneumonia caused by *Streptococcus pneumoniae, Legionella pneumophila* or *Chlamydia pneumoniae*. Scand J Infect Dis 2004;36:330–4.

Teutsch SM, Martone WJ, Brink EW, et al. Pneumonic tularemia on Martha's Vineyard. N Engl J Med 1979;301:826–8.

Troy CJ, Peeling RW, Ellis AG, et al. *Chlamydia pneumoniae* as a new source of infectious outbreaks in nursing homes. JAMA 1997;277:1214–8.

Tsai TF, Finn DR, Plikaytis BD, et al. Legionnaire's disease: clinical features of the epidemic in Philadelphia. Ann Intern Med 1979;90:509–17.

The First Atypical Pneumonia: The History of the Discovery of *Mycoplasma pneumoniae*

Cheston B. Cunha, MD

KEYWORDS

- Atypical pneumonia • *Mycoplasma pneumoniae*
- Mycoplasma pneumonia • Pulmonary infections

The subject of atypical pneumonias is of great medical and historical interest to modern physicians. Although these diseases have no doubt affected humans throughout our history, it is not until the mid-twentieth century that physicians first began to differentiate certain atypical pulmonary infectious processes from typical pneumonia. Physicians at the time were unclear as to the precise etiology of these infections. As time progressed and study of these organisms continued, physicians were better able to identify the causative agent and devise tests with which to detect the disease. For the purpose of this article, I will focus on the description and ultimate identification of *Mycoplasma pneumoniae*.

Although physicians such as Hobert and Bryman[1] in 1938 initially described an acute infection within the respiratory tract most likely caused by a nonfilterable virus, the first attempt to isolate this organism came during the Second World War among US Army troops who were suffering from a poorly defined febrile respiratory illness. It was clear to the physicians at that time that this respiratory syndrome was clinically isolated from that of psittacosis and Q fever. Despite being clinically different, there was no laboratory study that could be used to confirm the diagnosis. In 1942, serum samples from individuals infected with what was then termed primary atypical pneumonia were used to infect animals in an attempt to isolate the organism responsible for this syndrome. They found that, despite the best isolation techniques available at the

Department of Medicine, Brown University, Alpert School of Medicine, Rhode Island Hospital & The Miriam Hospital, 593 Eddy Street, Providence, RI 02903, USA
E-mail address: cheston.cunha@gmail.com

Infect Dis Clin N Am 24 (2010) 1–5
doi:10.1016/j.idc.2009.10.007

time, the causative agent was too small to be filtered. Typical culture techniques demonstrated no growth using the standard medium or agar.

In 1943, Peterson and colleagues[1] first noted an increase in cold agglutination titers in individuals exhibiting symptoms consistent with primary atypical pneumonia. It was this finding that first prompted him to suggest the use of the cold agglutination study as a diagnostic test.

Meiklejohn and Eaton[1] began collecting serum samples in the mid 1940s from patients who had symptoms of primary atypical pneumonia (a total of 74 individuals) and compared them with serum from patients with other respiratory diseases. Primary atypical pneumonia was diagnosed primarily through clinical presentation along with chest x-ray findings and sputum without a causative organism. They analyzed the serum of both populations, which were drawn at various stages of the patients' illness. Their goal was to determine how frequently cold agglutinin titers were found in primary atypical pneumonia in comparison with other respiratory diseases (including influenza, tuberculosis, pneumococcal pneumonia, and febrile urinary tract infections [URIs]) and healthy individuals. Serum samples were tested for cold agglutinins at the onset of disease, throughout the course of disease, and during convalescence.

Meiklejohn[1] found that there was a definite difference between titers in individuals with clinically diagnosed primary atypical pneumonia and the control group. Sixty of the 74 individuals demonstrated a titer above 1:20, and 45 of those had a titer above 1:40. Five of the 74 had a titer of 0 on presentation, which rose during the course of disease but always remained less than 1:20. In comparison, none of the control group demonstrated an elevated cold agglutinin level greater than 1:20 during the entire course of their disease.

Meiklejohn[1] realized that during the first 8 days of illness, cold agglutinins would not commonly be elevated. Indeed, only 20% of individuals had a positive cold agglutinin at time of disease onset. There would typically be a sharp increase in titer levels on days 8 to 10, with a titer peak between days 12 and 25 and a rapid decrease in titer during the convalescent phase of the disease. There did not seem to be a correlation between titer levels and the severity of disease, but there was a retrospectively observed correspondence between transmissibility and the degree to which the titers were elevated.

Meiklejohn[1] was also able to determine that testing of serum samples was confounded by the fact that, if stored improperly or for a prolonged period of time, the detected titer level could be erroneously low. Despite that fact, this was the first time that a specific test was identified as directly aiding in the diagnosis of this clinical syndrome. Meiklejohn[1] himself said that this was a "roundabout way" of testing for the disease, but was quite a milestone at the time considering the causative agent was still unknown. Obviously, as the titer is often negative at the onset of disease, the positive test may develop after the patient is already in the midst of illness or even in the beginning of the convalescent stage.

Later that year, Eaton[2] began experiments injecting serum of infected individuals into cotton rats to further study the agent responsible for this pneumonia, as laboratories were unable to culture it using their standard techniques. He used various isolation techniques and tested antibiotic effectiveness in an effort to better understand the organism. He states "The exact nature of the agent causing primary atypical pneumonia has not been established but filtration data indicate that it may be representative of a class of agents sensitive to aureomycin but somewhat smaller than viruses of the psittacosis-lymphogranuloma group which are also inhibited by this drug."[2] Although Eaton never specifically commits to the nature of the organism, because of his work, the disease is widely accepted as being caused by a nonfilterable virus for the next decade. As a result of his efforts to isolate and identify the organism, it is given the name "Eaton agent."[2]

In 1954, Watson[3] developed an indirect fluorescent antibody test for the Eaton agent, which was then used by Liu[3] in 1957 to test the original Eaton and Meiklejohn serum samples in addition to serum from new cases of Eaton agent pneumonia for evidence of the Eaton agent. His testing revealed that among cases of clinically diagnosed primary atypical pneumonia with positive cold agglutinin titers, 67% to 90% had a positive fluorescent antibody study, confirming Eaton agent as the causative organism.

By 1960, Cook and colleagues[3] at Walter Reed again sought to prove the link between cold agglutinin and the Liu antibody test. They performed a study where all serum samples available from prior research on Eaton agent pneumonia were found to be antigenically similar, suggesting one common etiology. Cook and colleagues were able to inoculate cotton rats intranasally with isolates from these samples, as Eaton had before him, in an attempt to better understand the disease. The serum samples that were obtained from these atypical pneumonia patients were retested and found that most had either a positive cold agglutinin test or a positive streptococcus MG test. Cook and colleagues set out to confirm that these positive results were indicative of the same causative agent responsible for causing Eaton agent pneumonia. Using the indirect antibody test, they tested the serum they were able to obtain from the National Institutes of Health from Eaton's work and samples from Liu's study, as well as serum from individuals with newly diagnosed atypical pneumonia, against a control group of individuals who had cold agglutinin and streptococcus MG–negative serum. This was done to ensure that Eaton agent was indeed the causative organism for the syndrome of atypical pneumonia.

Cook and colleagues inoculated chick embryos with all strains available to them, and subsequently inoculated into an animal model, in which they could perform further studies. First they attempted to detect levels of cold agglutinin and streptococcus MG in these samples. They also used the indirect fluorescent antibody test to confirm the presence of Eaton agent. Last, Cook and colleagues analyzed lung tissue from the infected animals, and then performed complement fixation studies on their samples, searching for the presence of Q fever, psittacosis, lymphogranuloma venereum, adenovirus, coxsackie B, and respiratory syncytial virus to ensure that these were not the causative agent of this syndrome of atypical pneumonia. This also allowed them to see that these other organisms could not give a false positive cold agglutinin, streptococcus MG titer, or indirect Ab test that might confound testing for suspected Eaton agent pneumonia. Cook and colleagues also used a technique of hemaglutination inhibition study on all samples to detect influenza in all cold agglutinin–negative samples. This laboratory technique was used to study addition serum samples that Cook and colleagues obtained from across the United States and even parts of Europe.

Cook and colleagues were able to demonstrate that Eaton agent was fluorescent antibody–positive in 85% of cold agglutinin– or streptococcus MG–positive samples, and the antibody was often positive before the serum titers of cold or streptococcus agglutinins became positive. Indeed, 26% of patients without an initially positive cold agglutinin or streptococcus MG demonstrated Eaton agent antigen. This demonstrated that the indirect antibody testing for Eaton agent had a relatively high specificity for primary atypical pneumonia, as it would not be positive in cases of psittacosis, Q fever, or the other diseases mentioned previously.

By reviewing the reports of disease that accompanied these serum samples, Cook and colleagues were able to make some epidemiologic conclusions about the Eaton agent pneumonia. Specifically, he found that the pneumonia principally affected younger individuals, and rather than occurring in large outbreaks, could occur sporadically at any time of the year. This set it apart from the other typical and atypical pneumonias known at that time.[3]

Also in 1960, Chanock and colleagues[4] published an article noting similar findings in children using the same technique as Cook and colleagues. In fact, this study showed that the indirect antibody test may have been even more specific that the adult study had proven. Chanock and colleagues[4] attempted to, but were unable to isolate the Eaton agent itself through filtration techniques, and could only prove its presence through indirect testing.

Around that time, Evans and Brobst[5] released an article confirming the importance of Eaton agent as the causative organism in primary atypical pneumonia. Wisconsin students between 1953 and 1960 who presented to physician with symptoms of bronchitis, pneumonitis, or pneumonia had their serum tested using Liu's Eaton antibody technique. They found that Eaton agent antigen was rarely positive in cases of psittacosis and parainfluenza, something that prior studies had failed to show. Although this study did not find the same degree of correlation between cold agglutinin and antibody testing as the prior studies had, a clear link between the two testing modalities was again demonstrated. That being said, the authors admit that their study suffered from technical difficulty, stating, "The correlation between Eaton agent antibody and cold agglutinin elevations may thus be much better than our data indicate." This error may have been because they were not always able to test for cold agglutinins at the time in the disease when they were at their peak level, ie, the second to third week of disease. Evans and Brobst go on to explain that "Questions have been raised about the specificity of the Eaton agent antibody response in view of the appearance of nonspecific substances like the cold agglutinins and Str. MG agglutinins in serums from many of the patients with viral pneumonitis. These doubts have largely been dispelled through the work of Chanock and his associates who have isolated Eaton agent from the throat washings in such cases and have shown the almost exclusive occurrence of Eaton agent antibody in patients with respiratory disease not associated with influenza, parainfluenza, or adenovirus."[5]

In 1961, Chanock and colleagues[6,7] studied a population of 238 Marine Corps recruits who developed the signs and symptoms of primary atypical pneumonia, a febrile URI, or an afebrile URI. The one thing that these subjects had in common was that they all demonstrated an elevated cold agglutinin titer. They were again searching for a correlation between the clinical syndrome of primary atypical pneumonia, and the presence of Eaton agent. They were able to find that 68% of these subjects were Eaton agent positive on antibody testing, suggesting a more varied manifestation of Eaton agent pneumonia than originally thought. It was also noted that "The Eaton agent was not highly communicable, an attribute which favored its persistence in the recruits."[6,7]

Eaton and Liu had never confirmed, one way or another, their thoughts on the precise nature of the organism responsible for the clinical syndrome of primary atypical pneumonia. Up to this time it had been referred to almost exclusively as a nonfilterable virus. It was not until 1963 when Goodburn and his associates[8] in Leeds decided to reconsider the nature of the organism that further progress was made. For years, Goodburn and colleagues had been experimenting with Giemsa staining tissue cultures and chick embryos (which had been the only method of growing the organism) for evidence of Eaton agent. They were finally able to visualize coccobacillary bodies on staining. They were not able to specifically identify the organism, but felt that owing to the organism's size, clinical manifestations, Giemsa staining evidence, and the sensitivity of the organism to antibiotics and some organic gold compounds, that rather than being a virus, it was a pleuropneumonia-like organism (PPLO) of the mycoplasma group.[8]

Further progress was made, again by Chanock,[9] by taking tissue cultures from chicken embryos previously studied were able to grow the Eaton agent organism in special Difco PPLO media and agar. With the new ability to readily grow the organism on agar rather than in tissue culture, the first compliment fixation studies could be developed for mycoplasma. These culminated in an article in 1963 when it was first proposed that the organism responsible for causing the atypical pneumonia syndrome, known as the Eaton agent up to this time, be reclassified as *Mycoplasma pneumoniae*. Eaton and Chanock were able to confirm the *Mycoplasma* genus once the organism could be cultured using the specially prepared agar. They found than unless media contained serum or egg yolk, no organismal growth could be seen.[9,10]

Study of the organism continued to better determine the ideal treatment and effective laboratory tests to identify cases of mycoplasma pneumonia.[11,12] Although new techniques have been developed including polymerase chain reaction and other genetic studies, the cold agglutinin titers that initially sparked much of the search for the cause of mycoplasma pneumonia can still be used as a relatively reliable test if suspicious for mycoplasma. It is for this reason that it is important for modern physicians to remember the process that went into the identification of this elusive and troublesome organism.

REFERENCES

1. Meiklejohn G. The cold agglutination test in the diagnosis of primary atypical pneumonia. Proc Soc Exp Biol Med 1943;53:181,193 EOA.
2. Eaton MD. Action of aureomycin and chloromycetin on the virus of primary atypical pneumonia. Proc Soc Exp Biol Med 1950;73(1):24–9.
3. Cook MK, Chanock RM, Fox HH, et al. Role of Eaton agent in disease of lower respiratory tract. Br Med J 1960;1(5177):905–11.
4. Chanock RM, Cook MK, Fox HH, et al. Serologic evidence of infection with Eaton agent in lower respiratory illness in childhood. N Engl J Med 1960;262:648–54.
5. Evans AS, Brobst M. Bronchitis, pneumonitis and pneumonia in University of Wisconsin students. N Engl J Med 1961;265:401–9.
6. Chanock RM, Evans AS, Brobst MS. Respiratory disease in volunteers infected with Eaton agent; a preliminary report. Proc Natl Acad Sci U S A 1961;47: 401–9.
7. Chanock RM, Bloom HH, James WD, et al. Eaton agent pneumonia. JAMA 1961; 175:213–20.
8. Goodburn GM, Marmion BP, Kendall EJ. Infection with Eaton's primary atypical pneumonia agent in England. Br Med J 1963;1(5340):1266–70.
9. Chanock RM. *Mycoplasma pneumoniae*: proposed nomenclature for atypical pneumonia organism (Eaton agent). Science 1963;140:662.
10. Jansson E, Wager O, Stenstrom R, et al. Studies on Eaton PPLO pneumonia. Br Med J 1964;1:142–5.
11. Kenny GE, Grayston JT. Eaton pleuropneumonia-like organism (*Mycoplasma pneumoniae*) complement-fixing antigen: extraction with organic solvents. J Immunol 1965;95(1):19–25.
12. Alexander ER, Foy HM, Kenney GE, et al. Pneumonia due to *Mycoplasma pneumoniae*: its incidence in the membership of a co-operative medical group. N Engl J Med 1966;275(3):131–6.

Psittacosis

Andrew J. Stewardson, MBBS[a],
M. Lindsay Grayson, MBBS, MD, MSc, FRACP, FAFPHM[a,b,c,*]

KEYWORDS

- Psittacosis • *Chlamydophila psittaci*
- Atypical pneumonia • Zoonosis

Psittacosis (also known as ornithosis and parrot fever) is a systemic zoonosis caused by infection with *Chlamydophila psittaci*. A history of exposure to birds, while not always present, is a major risk factor for infection. Psittacosis is characterized by a wide range in both disease severity and in spectrum of clinical features, but it typically presents with fever, prominent headache, myalgia, and a nonproductive cough. The mainstay of diagnostic testing is serologic, although molecular techniques increasingly are utilized. Doxycycline is the treatment of choice.

MICROBIOLOGY

C psittaci are gram-negative, obligate intracellular bacteria belonging to the *Chlamydiales* order. Before the recognition of *C pneumoniae* as a species distinct from *C psittaci* in 1986,[1] the *Chlamydia* genera consisted of *C trachomatis* and *C psittaci*. Not without protest,[2] the *Chlamydiales* order was reclassified a decade ago on the basis of 16S and 23S ribosomal genetic identity (**Table 1**).[3] According to this system, the species previously named *Chlamydia psittaci* was split into four of six species of the new *Chlamydophila* genera on the basis of genetic and phenotypic distinctions: *C abortus, C psittaci, C felis, and C caviae*, which predominantly infect mammals, birds, cats, and guinea pigs, respectively. The final two *Chlamydophila* species are *C pneumoniae* and *C pecorum*.

C psittaci is divided into eight serovars according to variation in the major outer membrane protein (MOMP): serovar A to F, WC and M56. Subsequently, eight corresponding genotypes based on the sequencing of variable domains of the outer membrane protein A (ompA) gene were defined, with the later addition of genotype

[a] Department of Infectious Diseases, Austin Health, PO Box 5555, Heidelberg, Melbourne, Victoria 3084, Australia
[b] Department of Epidemiology and Preventive Medicine, Monash University, Commercial Road, Prahran, Melbourne, Victoria 3181, Australia
[c] Department of Medicine, University of Melbourne, Studley Road, Heidelberg, Melbourne, Victoria 3084, Australia
* Corresponding author. Department of Infectious Diseases, Austin Health, PO Box 5555, Heidelberg, Melbourne, Victoria 3084, Australia.
E-mail address: lindsay.grayson@austin.org.au (M.L. Grayson).

Infect Dis Clin N Am 24 (2010) 7–25
doi:10.1016/j.idc.2009.10.003

Table 1
Taxonomy of the *Chlamydiales* order

Order	Family	Genera	Species	Typical Host	Previous Taxonomy
Chlamydiales	Chlamydiaceae	*Chlamydophila*	*C abortus*	Mammals	*Chlamydia psittaci*
			C psittaci	Birds	
			C felis	Cats	
			C caviae	Guinea pigs	
			C pecorum	Mammals	*C pecorum*
			C pneumoniae	Humans	*C pneumoniae*
		Chlamydia	*C trachomatis*	People	*C trachomatis*
			C suis	Swine	
			C muridarum	Mice, hamsters	
	Parachlamydiaceae		*P acanthomaebae*		
	Waddiaceae		*W chondrophila*		
	Simkaniaceae		*S negevensis*		

Data from Bush RM, Everett KDE. Molecular evolution of the *Chlamydiaceae*. In J Syst Evol Microbiol 2001;51:203–20.

E/B (**Table 2**).[4] Each serovar/genotype is associated to a varying degree with a particular animal host.[3,4]

Illustrating the heterogeneity of this species, as well as advances in molecular diagnostic techniques, further division into 20 genotypes (with the expectation of more to come) was proposed recently on the basis of both ompA sequence analysis and multiple loci variable number of tandem repeats analysis (MLVA).[5,6]

The organism exists in two states: the extracellular, highly infectious, and metabolically inactive elementary body (350 nm diameter), and the larger intracellular, replicative, and metabolically active reticulate body (850 nm diameter).[7] After contact with a eukaryotic cell (typically a respiratory epithelial cell), the elementary body is endocytosed. Remaining inside a membrane-enclosed inclusion body and evading host immune defenses, the organism differentiates into a reticulate body that undergoes

Table 2
Serotypes and genotypes of *Chlamydophila psittaci*

Serovar	Genotype	Predominant Host Order: Examples	Human Infection Documented
A	A	Psittaformes: budgerigars, cockatiels, parakeets	Yes
B	B	Columbiforme:s pigeons, doves	Yes
C	C	Anseriformes: ducks, geese, swans	Yes
D	D	Galliformes: turkeys, pheasants, chickens	Yes[97]
E	E	Struthioniformes: ostriches, pigeons, duck	Yes[22]
F	F	Isolated from single parakeet and turkey only	Yes[97]
WC	G	Cattle	
M56	H	Rodents	
	E/B[4]	Ducks	Yes[97]

replication by means of binary fission, using ATP parasitized from the host cell.[8,9] Reticulate bodies reorganize into elementary bodies and are released from the cell. The entire developmental cycle takes over 48 hours.[10]

EPIDEMIOLOGY

Zoonotic Reservoir

Birds are the major zoonotic reservoir. Despite its name, *C psittaci* infection has been documented in 467 species from 30 bird orders, from psittaformes to ostriches to penguins.[11] Not surprisingly, given their use as pets and livestock, respectively, most human cases are associated with transmission from birds of the orders psittaformes (including budgerigars, cockatiels, cockatoos, and parakeets) and galliformes (including turkeys, pheasants, and chickens). Other orders, such as columbiformes (doves, pigeons), passiformes (canaries, finches), and anseriformes (ducks, geese, swans) are also recognized as sources of human infection. Because of the natural distribution of these bird species, in some regions such as Australia, virtually all native birds are potentially infected with *C psittaci,* thereby posing a large zoonotic reservoir.

Each bird order tends to be infected with a predominant genotype (with a varying degree of specificity between orders), with genotypes A to D associated with psittaformes, columbiformes, anseriformes, and galliformes, respectively.[12–14] Scant published data are available regarding genotype identification in clinical isolates from sporadic cases in people, but one study sequencing ompA genes in isolates from 10 patients hospitalized with psittacosis reported five genotype A isolates, three genotype B isolates, one genotype C isolate, and one novel strain.[15] Certainly these are the three most common genotypes causing human infection.

Infected birds can be asymptomatic (most common) or develop a clinical illness consisting of ruffled feathers, respiratory symptoms, conjunctivitis, or diarrhea. Factors determining morbidity, mortality, and organism excretion are incompletely understood, but bird species, maturity, stress, and concurrent illness are believed to play a role.[11] Typical scenarios for increasing bird morbidity or *C psittaci* excretion include relocation or overcrowding. The type of serovar also may be significant; for example, in psittacine birds, serovar D causes a severe, frequently fatal disease in contrast with the mild, chronic infection (with intermittent shedding) caused by serovar A.[14] Organisms can remain viable in organic material for several months.[16]

Other animals documented with *C psittaci* infection include horses,[17] cattle,[18] and koalas,[19] although transmission to people is seemingly a rare occurrence from these sources.

Transmission to Humans

Exposure to birds is the major risk factor for psittacosis. Transmission occurs either by inhalation of aerosolized organisms in dried feces or respiratory tract secretions, or by direct bird contact.[16] Consequently, those at greatest risk are individuals with leisure or occupational exposure to birds, including pet bird owners, veterinarians, pet shop employees, and poultry-processing plant employees. As a result, cases of psittacosis can range from a sporadic case in a pet bird owner to an outbreak affecting several hundred birds in a commercial flock and multiple infected workers.[20]

As an example, in one study, over 90% of fecal samples from birds (canaries, parrots, finches, budgerigars, pigeons, doves) caged in four aviaries in Turkey were polymerase chain reaction (PCR)-positive for *C psittaci* DNA.[21] In an example of commercial *C psittaci* transmission, one study followed 20 turkeys and three people in real time, monitoring with serology, culture and PCR for 15 weeks.[22] The turkeys remained positive for *C psittaci* genotype A from birth to processing at the slaughterhouse. All three people in contact with the turkeys (the farmer and the two scientists performing the study) acquired *C psittaci* genotype A with clinical features of psittacosis.

A history of direct exposure to birds, while clinically enticing, is not particularly specific. Nor is it necessary for a diagnosis of psittacosis, particularly in areas with large numbers of wild and feral bird contacts. This is illustrated by two outbreaks in Australia in townships surrounded by forested land with dense bird life.[23,24] Suggested risk factors in these cases included time spent gardening and lawn mowing.[23,24] Human-to-human transmission occurs rarely.[25] In particular, while nosocomial transmission has been suggested by some authors, stronger evidence is needed before this mode of transmission can be considered to be likely.[26,27]

From 1999 to 2006, the number of cases of psittacosis reported in the United States per year varied between 12 and 25, representing an incidence of 0.01 per 100,000 population.[28] Given the mild nature of the illness in many affected individuals, this is likely to significantly underestimate the true incidence. In studies examining the etiology of pneumonia requiring hospitalization, psittacosis accounts for less than 5% of cases.[29,30] Although psittacosis can affect any age group, the incidence peaks in middle age, between the ages of 35 and 55.[31] Children rarely present with a significant clinical illness. Furthermore, the clinical differentiation of psittacosis from illness caused by *C pneumoniae* can be difficult.

Clinical Features

As with other intracellular zoonoses such as *Coxiella burnetii* and brucella, the clinical features of psittacosis are protean; pulmonary, hepatic, central nervous system, cardiac, renal, rheumatic, and hematologic manifestations are all described, and respiratory symptoms are frequently mild or absent on presentation. Disease severity can range from subclinical infection to fulminant sepsis with multiorgan failure in previously healthy individuals,[32] which may occasionally be fatal despite appropriate treatment.[33] An illustrative case is described (**Box 1**), while the key clinical features of psittacosis are summarized and contrasted with other atypical agents of pneumonia in **Table 3**.

In reviewing the literature regarding psittacosis, interpretation of clinical reports before the introduction of MIF in the late 1980s must be tempered with the understanding that a significant proportion are likely to be due to *C pneumoniae*.

Patients hospitalized with psittacosis usually have developed symptoms over a period of 5 to 21 days after exposure, with a further week elapsing before hospital admission.[31] Symptom onset is frequently abrupt, with the most common presenting symptoms being fever, diaphoresis, headache, myalgia, and a mild cough.[31,34] If a single characteristic feature were to be identified, it would be the headache, which may be of a severity and prominence to suggest meningitis. Lumbar puncture was performed on 33% of patients with psittacosis in one large series from the 1980s.[31] Indeed, the severity of the headache warrants at least brief consideration of psittacosis and a chest radiograph in any patient with a presumed diagnosis of meningitis. Confusion also may be a presenting complaint.[23,31]

On examination, fever and an abnormal chest examination (crepitations or signs of consolidation) are the most common findings. Other signs include altered conscious state, mild neck stiffness, photophobia, hepatomegaly, splenomegaly, and pharyngitis (although pharyngitis is more characteristic of *C pneumoniae* infection). The most common symptoms and signs are summarized in **Table 4**.

Box 1
Illustrative case

A 46-year-old man presented to hospital with fever and dyspnea. He had experienced 6 days of fevers, malaise, a dry cough, anorexia and diarrhea, and had been intermittently confused for 2 days. He had bronchial breath sounds anteriorly in the right hemithorax, and chest radiograph demonstrated opacification of the right upper lobe. He had a mild neutrophila and leucopenia, and he was coagulopathic, hyponatremic, and in oliguric acute renal failure.

He was admitted to the intensive care unit with hypoxic respiratory failure and septic shock requiring mechanical ventilation and hemofiltration, and he was commenced on norepinephrine, intravenous antibiotics (ceftriaxone, ciprofloxacin, and azithromycin) and drotrecogin alfa (recombinant activated protein C). When *C psittaci* DNA was detected in his sputum by PCR, his antibiotic treatment was changed to doxycycline, initially intravenous, then oral. While the acute serum sample was negative, 2 weeks later, *Chlamydia* group antigen enzyme immunoassay (EIA) was positive, with *C psittaci* and *C pneumoniae* immunoglobulin G (IgG) titers by microimmunofluorescence (MIF) of 1:512 and 1:1024, respectively. He was discharged after 28 days.

Five weeks previously, his family had acquired a cockatiel. Three weeks after the arrival of the bird, his two children (aged 7 and 5 years) had experienced a diarrheal illness, and his wife presented to an emergency department with 5 days of fever, sweats, and a dry cough. Her chest radiograph demonstrated left middle lobe consolidation. She was treated as an outpatient with amoxycillin/clavulanic acid and made a slow recovery without further treatment. She had a positive *Chlamydia* group EIA result, and by MIF, a *C psittaci* IgG rise from a titer of <1:64 to 1:256.

The patient's parents-in-law were both admitted to hospital after the index case—his mother-in-law with pneumonia without diagnostic serologic result and his father-in-law with fever without focus (and a clear chest radiograph) but a positive *Chlamydia* group antigen and a rise in *C. psittaci* IgG from 1:128 to greater than 1:1024. They both recovered promptly with antibiotics active against *C psittaci*. The family dog was also reported to be coughing. The bird remained well but had a cloacal swab positive for *C psittaci* DNA by PCR.

This case demonstrates several key points with regards to psittacosis:

C psittaci can be excreted by a healthy-appearing bird, and excretion is increased in times of stress, such relocation. Adult patients are affected more frequently than children. The spectrum of illness ranges from mild and self-limiting (wife) to septic shock with multiorgan failure (index case).

Patients typically present with 1 week of systemic symptoms without a prominent respiratory focus. A marked neutrophilia is often not present. While still the mainstay of diagnosis, serology is limited by a lack of specificity (with significant cross-reactivity between *C psittaci* and *C pneumoniae*) and frequently by delay while waiting for a second sample.

PCR is a rapid and specific diagnostic technique.

A chest radiograph is abnormal in 80% of patients, most frequently with consolidation affecting a single lobe.[31] The presence of a normal chest radiograph, however, does not rule out the diagnosis of psittacosis. Nonspecific findings on initial blood tests include deranged liver enzymes, elevated erythrocyte sedimentation rate (ESR) and C-reactive protein (CRP), and toxic granulation or left shift of neutrophils in the absence of a marked neutrophilia. Given the lack of a neutrophilia in psittacosis, CRP, interleukin (IL)-6 and procalcitonin have been suggested as markers with which to monitor treatment response in patients where body temperature is unreliable, such as with extracorporeal lung assist or haemofiltration.[35]

In addition to headache, various more severe central nervous system manifestations are described, with meningoencephalitis being the most common.[36–39] While fever, headache, and confusion are the typical presentation, cases presenting with status epilepticus,[40] localized cerebellar ataxia,[41] and brainstem encephalitis[42] have been

Table 3
Comparison of the features of *Chlamydophila psittaci*, *Chlamydophila pneumonia*, *Mycoplasma pneumoniae*, and *Legionella pneumophila* infection

Clinical Feature	*C psittaci*	*C pneumoniae*	*M pneumoniae*	*L pneumophila*
Cough	++	+	++	+
Sputum	–	+	++	+++
Dyspnea	+	+	++	+++
Sore throat	–	++	–	–
Headache	+++	+	–	+
Confusion	+	–	–	++
Diarrhea	–	–	–	+
Chest radiograph changes	Minimal	Minimal	Disparity[a]	Often multifocal
Hyponatremia	–	–	–	++
Leukopenia	–	–	–	+
Abnormal liver function tests	+	–	+	++
Response to doxycycline	Rapid—afebrile within 48 hours	Prompt[b]	Prompt[b]	Improved but still unwell

–, rare.
+, occurs in some cases.
++, occurs in many cases.
+++, occurs frequently.
[a] Disparity between severity of chest radiograph changes and relatively minor dyspnea.
[b] Clear improvement after 48 hours, but may not be totally afebrile.

reported. Cranial nerves affected by palsies attributed to *C psittaci* include II, IV, VI and VII.[38,43,44] Transverse myelitis[45] and Guillain-Barre syndrome[46] also have been documented.

Renal complications include acute interstitial nephritis[47] and acute renal failure in severe infection and glomerulonephritis in cases of endocarditis. In contrast to the relative frequency of presenting gastrointestinal symptoms with legionellosis, severe intra-abdominal complications are rare, although hepatitis,[48] pancreatitis,[49] and acute generalized peritonism prompting exploratory laparotomy[50] have been reported.

C psittaci rarely has been reported as causing a reactive arthritis, with onset 1 week or more after the onset of symptoms of psittacosis.[51] Several different patterns of joint involvement have been described: migratory small and large joint polyarthritis, symmetric polyarthritis, and Reiter's syndrome (with asymmetric large joint arthritis, conjunctivitis and HLA B27 positivity).[51–53]

Although most patients with psittacosis are not particularly unwell, several unusual, but specific clinical presentations have been described for this disease that should alert clinicians, including fulminant psittacosis, cardiac manifestations, gestational psittacosis, and chronic follicular meningitis.

Fulminant psittacosis

Fulminant psittacosis with multiorgan failure is an infrequent but important complication of psittacosis.[33,35,37,54–60] These patients, who previously may have been healthy, develop hypoxic respiratory failure requiring mechanical ventilation accompanied by varying degrees of septic shock, impaired cognition, and renal, hepatic, and hematologic failure. Acute respiratory distress syndrome (ARDS) requiring extracorporeal lung

Table 4
Clinical features of psittacosis according to two series of 135[1] and 397[2] cases

Symptom	Frequency (%) Yung & Grayson, 1988	Frequency (%) Schmahmann, 1982	Sign	Frequency (%) Yung & Grayson, 1988	Frequency (%) Schmahmann, 1982
General					
Acute-onset	80	—			
Fever	100	79			
Sweats/diaphoresis	89	12			
Myalgia	75	28			
Rigor(s)	61	—			
Neurologic					
Headache	87	38	Altered conscious state	12	5–9
			Neck stiffness	9	5–9
			Photophobia	16	5–9
Respiratory					
Cough	78	49	Abnormal chest examination	84	—
Sputum	20	—	Pharyngitis	15	<5
Haemoptysis	8	<5			
Dyspnea	24	10			
Chest pain	17	12			
Sore throat	17	5–9			
Gastrointestinal/abdominal					
Nausea	49		Hepatomegaly	10	<5
Vomiting	38		Splenomegaly	8	<5
Diarrhea	20	5–9			
Abdominal pain	10	5–9			

Data from Yung AP, Grayson ML. Psittacosis–a review of 135 cases. Med J Aust 1988;148(5):228–33. Schmahmann JD. Psittacosis centenary—pneumotyphus reviewed. S Afr Med J 1982;62(24): 898–901.

assist has been reported.[35] Renal failure may require haemofiltration.[35,55,58,59] Hematologic complications include disseminated intravascular coagulation[61,62] and hemophagocytic syndrome.[63]

Cardiac manifestations

Cardiac manifestations of psittacosis include endocarditis, myocarditis, and pericarditis. Although often listed as a cause of culture-negative endocarditis, *C psittaci* endocarditis is rare. Published cases are summarized in **Table 5**. *C psittaci* endocarditis is characterized by negative blood cultures (using routine culture methods), the presence of cardiac vegetation, and a history of exposure to birds. Symptoms are typically present for weeks to several months before diagnosis. Endocarditis can be complicated by glomerulonephritis that may resolve with antibiotic therapy.[64–66] Cardiac

Table 5
Reported cases of *Chlamydophila psittaci* endocarditis

Age and Sex	Risk Factors	Premorbid Valvular Heart Disease	Duration of Symptoms Before Diagnosis	Extracardiac Involvement	Diagnostic Test(s)	Affected Valve(s)	Antibiotic Therapy	Cardiac Surgery	Outcome	Year Reference
62 F	Daughter with pet budgerigar	Yes	NA	NA	CF	Ao (A)	NA	No	Died	1964[65,107]
49 M	Pet budgerigar and parrot	Yes	Sudden (recent pneumonia)	Pneumonia, hepatomegaly, superficial phlebitis	CF, vegetation indirect IF	Ao (A) fingerlike	Tetracycline	No	Died	1971[65]
NA F	Multiple caged birds	Yes	3 months	Hepatomegaly, splenomegaly, myocarditis, encephalitis, proliferative glomerulonephritis	CF, valve histology and IF	Ao/Mv (A) fingerlike	Penicillin, cloxacillin	No	Died	1971[65]
57 M	Gardener; brother with budgerigar	Yes (bicuspid valve and history of rheumatic fever)	12 months	Hepatomegaly, splenomegaly	CF, valve EM	Ao (O) firm projecting vegetation	Tetracycline with rifampicin (at least 4 months)	Yes; after 4 months antibiotics with progressive heart failure	Survived	1974[66]
48 M	Fed wild pigeons	Yes	Several months	No	CF, valve histology	MV (O)	Benpenicillin with streptomcyin	Yes; elective	Survived	1975[108]
43 F	Pet budgerigar (*C psittaci* positive)	No	3 month	Splenomegaly	CF, valve histology	MV (O)	Tetracycline (10 weeks intravenous then long-term oral)	Yes; after 6 weeks of antibiotics	Survived	1977[109]

40 M	Cat	No	Months	Glomerulo-nephritis, rash, hepatitis, embolic CVA	CF	Ao (C)	Erythromycin then doxycycline 1 year	Elective (>1 year later)	Died (pneumonia 1 month postoperatively)	1979[64]
41 M[a]	Pigeon	No	Acute presentation	Brachial artery embollism	CF	Ao (C)	Chlortetracycline (1 month)	No	Survived	1980[110]
43 M	Pet pigeons	No	Pneumonia 2 months prior	Pneumonia, pulmonary embolism	CF	Ao (C)	Tetracycline 6 weeks then rifampicin 16 weeks	No	Survived	1980[111]
30 M	Pet parakeet	No – but history of intravenous drug use	9 months	No	CF and MIF on serum; EM and IF of vegetations	Ao and Mi	Erythromycin and rifampicin 6 weeks, then 4 months tetracycline	Yes—Ao and Mi replacement due to progressive heart failure	Survived	1982[112]
59M	Chicken & pheasants	No	6M	No	CF	Mi (E)	Tetracycline, Doxycyline 2 years	No	Survived	1987[113]
31F	Parakeet	No	Pneumonia 3 months prior	Popliteal aneurysm, myocarditis	Blood and throat swab culture; valve histology/IF	Mi (E, O)	Doxycycline 2-12 weeks (non-compliant)	Yes	Survived	1992[114]
79F	Pigeon exposure	No	15 days	Pneumonia	CF/MIF	Ao (E, A) "finger-like"	Erythromycin	No	Died	1993[67]

Abbrevations: A, autopsy; Ao, aortic valve; C, clinical; CF, complement fixation; E, echocardiography; F, female; IF, immunofluorescence; M, male; MIF, microimmunofluorescence; Mi, mitral valve; NA, not available; O, operative.

[a] Probable endocarditis based on changing aortic murmur and a major embolic event.

surgery frequently is required despite the early initiation of active antibiotic therapy, and the mortality in reported cases is close to 50%. On autopsy, the vegetations have been described as fingerlike projections.[65,67]

In *C psittaci*-associated myocarditis, the left ventricle is dilated, with global systolic dysfunction that recovers with treatment for *C psittaci*.[37,68–70] Electrocardiogram may demonstrate QT prolongation or T wave inversion.[70] The pathogenesis has been ascribed both to direct myocardial infection, with inclusion bodies demonstrated on biopsy,[69] and also to autoimmune-mediated damage.[71]

Gestational psittacosis

The term gestational psittacosis has been used to describe an illness consisting of multiorgan failure (coagulopathy, pulmonary and hepatic involvement in particular), intense placentitis, and fetal compromise. Many reported cases may represent what now would be regarded as infection with *C abortus*, given the association with sheep contact and the inability of contemporary diagnostic testing to distinguish reliably between the two *Chlamydophila* species.[72–75] Two cases of gestational psittacosis following exposure to psittacine birds in the United States have been reported.[76,77] These are likely to have involved *C psittaci* infection. Fetal outcome is poor, with 11 of 14 cases resulting in fetal death.[72] This compares with a single maternal death.

Chronic follicular conjunctivitis

C psittaci can be associated with unilateral chronic follicular conjunctivitis, characterized by an enlarged preauricular lymph node and punctate epithelial keratitis, in the absence of other features of psittacosis.[78] This condition has been documented in bird fanciers and laboratory staff and appears to respond to a prolonged course of up to 10 weeks of doxycycline.[78,79]

Association with lymphoma

The association between ocular adnexal mucosa-associated lymphoid tissue (MALT) lymphoma and chronic *C psittaci* infection has been the subject of significant interest over the past 5 years, largely because of two studies finding 80% of pathologic specimens positive for *C psittaci* DNA by PCR in Italy and Korea.[80,81] In addition, chlamydial elementary bodies have been demonstrated in monocytes and macrophages in ocular adnexal lymphomas,[82] and doxycycline treatment has resulted in lymphoma remission.[83] Studies from groups in other countries have not supported the association, and further investigation is required to establish the role of *C psittaci* in this condition.[84]

DIAGNOSIS

According to the Centers for Disease Control and Prevention (CDC) case definition, in the presence of an illness consistent with psittacosis, a case can be confirmed by any of the following:

- Isolation of *C psittaci* from respiratory secretions. A fourfold or greater rise in antibody titer between acute and convalescent serum samples collected 2 weeks apart (detected by complement fixation or microimmunofluorescence) to a titer of greater than or equal to 1:32
- A single IgM titer of 1:16 or greater (by microimmunofluorescence).

Culture

Culture of *C psittaci* is demanding, requires a level 3 laboratory isolation facility because of the risk of laboratory transmission and is rarely performed.

Serology

Serology remains the most widely available method for laboratory diagnosis of *C psittaci* infection, with complement fixation, microimmunofluorescence, and EIA the most commonly used techniques.

Complement fixation (CF) was the traditional method for diagnosing psittacosis before the recognition of *C pneumoniae* as a separate species 20 years ago. The presence in the serum sample of antibody active against the test antigen fixes complement, preventing the hemolysis of subsequently added erythrocytes. The antigen used is the lipopolysaccharide anchored to the outer membrane of all *Chlamydia*, including both *C psittaci* and *C pneumoniae*, and the test is thus unable to distinguish between these two species. CF is also unable to distinguish between IgM and IgG elevation.

The introduction of MIF significantly improved the sensitivity and specificity of serologic diagnosis,[85] with several psittacosis clusters being retrospectively attributed to *C pneumoniae*.[86–90] The central distinction between MIF and CF is that the former utilizes species-specific chlamydial surface antigen rather than the genus-specific lipopolysaccharide used in the latter. The surface antigen is spotted on glass slides and exposed first to test sera, then antihuman (IgG, IgM, and IgA) fluorescein-labeled immunoglobulin, and then examined for fluorescence activity. While improving on CF, cross-reactivity between species remains a significant issue with MIF, and the test is reliant on operator experience. Despite this, MIF has become the gold standard for serodiagnosis. An early study comparing CF and MIF demonstrated that after excluding patients with rheumatoid factor positivity, a single positive IgM by MIF has high specificity for *C psittaci* but poor sensitivity (19%).[85] Hence, diagnosis relies on a repeat serum sample with an increasing IgG titer in most cases.

Commercial EIA kits that utilize lipopolysaccharide (as with CF) are available, and while they do not distinguish between *C psittaci* and *C pneumoniae* infection, they have been shown to be equivalent to MIF for sensitivity for combined *C psittaci* and *C pneumoniae* infection.[91] A reasonable approach is to employ EIA as a screening test, with positive specimens undergoing MIF to give further detail regarding speciation.

The two major disadvantages of serology are the persisting issue of cross-reaction with related species, even with newer techniques[92] and the delay in confirmation while awaiting a convalescent sample in most cases.

Nucleic Acid Amplification

While not routinely available outside of reference laboratories, PCR techniques have been utilized in outbreaks for several years and can give a rapid, specific diagnosis, which is particularly important in severe infection.[93,94] Appropriate human specimens include sputum and broncho-alveolar lavage, but also blood and other tissues. PCR offers the advantages over serology of eliminating cross-reactivity with other species and facilitating detailed epidemiologic investigation.

Multiple techniques including real-time, nested, and multiplex PCR have been developed. Tests have used primers targeting the ompA and inclusion membrane protein A (incA) genes.[95,96] In addition to diagnosis, real-time PCR (RT-PCR) allows for quantitation of infectious units.[95]

With regard to epidemiologic investigations, methods recently developed to allow detailed differentiation of genotypes include real-time PCR,[97] DNA microarray assay (using 35 hybridization probes from variable domains 2 and 4 of the ompA gene),[5] and multilocus variable number tandem repeat analysis.[6]

TREATMENT

The antibiotic of choice for psittacosis is doxycycline. This is based on its intracellular activity, pharmacodynamics, and extensive clinical experience, rather than robust randomized clinical trials. Most patients will have defervesced by 48 hours of treatment with doxycycline.[31] In fulminant cases, where oral administration is not possible, or where absorption is doubtful, intravenous doxycycline can be used. Intravenous tetracycline is an alternative if an intravenous formulation of doxycycline is unavailable. Fourteen days are widely recommended for the duration of therapy. Minocycline is also has excellent in vitro activity, with the same minimum inhibitory concentration $(MIC)_{90}$ of 0.06 mg/L.[98] Minocycline has been used clinically with success. The new glycylcycline, tigecycline, has in vitro activity against *C pneumoniae* and *C trachomatis*, but clinical treatment data are lacking.[99]

Macrolides such as azithromycin, roxithromycin, and erythromycin demonstrate good in vitro activity (MIC_{90} of 0.125 mg/L, 0.25 mg/L, and 0.5 mg/L, respectively)[98,100] and are appropriate agents in pregnancy and childhood. In a mouse model of *C psittaci* pneumonia, 7 days of treatment with either azithromycin or minocycline resulted in 100% survival.[101] High-level resistance to azithromycin occurs spontaneously at a frequency of 1×10^{-8}.[102] This resistance is mediated by a single point mutation in the 23S rRNA gene but comes at a high fitness cost, minimizing its clinical significance.

Fluoroquinolones have in vitro activity against *C psittaci*, with MIC_{90} values for ciprofloxacin, levofloxacin, and both moxifloxacin and gatifloxacin of 2 mg/L, 0.5 mg/L and 0.125 mg/L, respectively.[98,100,103] In a mouse model of *C psittaci* pneumonia, gatifloxacin (5 mg/kg) also had a significantly superior 21-day survival rate of 100% (comparable to clarithromycin and minocycline) compared with the same dosage of levofloxacin (20%) and ciprofloxacin (0%).[103] Norfloxacin has poor activity.[104] Despite these in vitro data, there are few clinical studies available, such that the role of fluoroquinolones in psittacosis is not yet established, and few clinicians would recommend their use as first-line agents.

C psittaci Endocarditis

Optimal treatment for *C psittaci* endocarditis is not well defined, but in the small number of reported cases, a successful outcome frequently involves surgery in addition to antibiotic therapy. Tetracyclines (including doxycycline) are likely to be the most effective agents, and an extended course may be appropriate, particularly in the absence of valve replacement. Nevertheless, there are no clear guidelines regarding the duration of therapy.

Gestational Psittacosis

Although macrolides are a reasonable and recommended therapeutic option in pregnant women with psittacosis, successful treatment with carriage of the fetus to full term has not been documented. Both patients discussed previously with gestational psittacosis following exposure to psittacine birds were treated initially with intravenous erythromycin.[76,77] Neither responded satisfactorily to erythromycin alone, with disease progression until pregnancy was ended, by caesarian section with delivery of a healthy infant in one case and termination of pregnancy in the other. Both patients recovered after delivery in association with a change in therapy to doxycycline. Although consideration of doxycycline use during pregnancy in severe gestational psittacosis is reasonable, it is likely that the major therapeutic intervention is removal of the placenta rather than change of antibiotics from erythromycin to doxycycline, since the placenta may act as a form of sanctuary site in such cases. Because of the relative rarity of this condition, most treatment recommendations have been gleaned from clinical anecdotes.

PREVENTION

Infected birds should be treated with antibiotics under veterinary guidance. Doxycycline regimens are considered superior to chlortetracycline.[16] As *C psittaci* can persist in the environment, it is necessary to clean all potentially contaminated areas, first with removal of organic material, then disinfection. The use of protective equipment including gloves, an N95 mask (respirator), eyewear, and surgical cap while undertaking this process is recommended.[16] Appropriate health authorities should be notified of cases of psittacosis to supervise an appropriate public health response.

Many patients recovering from psittacosis ask whether they should destroy their pet birds to avoid future repeat infection; however, this is rarely necessary and generally should be discouraged, because treatment of the birds is almost always effective in either curing the disease or at least suppressing any major ongoing exposure risk. Indeed, anecdotal reports suggest that many pet shop owners routinely include some tetracycline in the drinking water of birds for sale (especially for psittacine birds such as parrots) to keep them in good health until after they are sold and are relocated into less crowded cage conditions where disease and pathogen shedding are less likely.

While no human vaccine is yet available, encouraging results have been achieved with DNA vaccines encoding *C psittaci* MOMP in poultry.[105,106] An effective veterinary vaccine would be of significant value in reducing the incidence of psittacosis in people.

REFERENCES

1. Kuo CC, Chen HH, Wang SP, et al. Identification of a new group of *Chlamydia psittaci* strains called twar. J Clin Microbiol 1986;24(6):1034–7.
2. Schachter J, Stephens RS, Timms P, et al. Radical changes to chlamydial taxonomy are not necessary just yet. Int J Syst Evol Microbiol 2001;51(1):249.
3. Everett KD, Bush RM, Andersen AA. Emended description of the order chlamydiales, proposal of *Parachlamydiaceae* fam. nov. and *Simkaniaceae* fam. nov., each containing one monotypic genus, revised taxonomy of the family *Chlamydiaceae*, including a new genus and five new species, and standards for the identification of organisms [see comment]. Int J Syst Bacteriol 1999;49(Pt 2): 415–40.
4. Geens T, Desplanques A, Van Loock M, et al. Sequencing of the *Chlamydophila psittaci* ompa gene reveals a new genotype, e/b, and the need for a rapid discriminatory genotyping method. J Clin Microbiol 2005;43(5):2456–61.
5. Sachse K, Laroucau K, Hotzel H, et al. Genotyping of *Chlamydophila psittaci* using a new DNA microarray assay based on sequence analysis of ompa genes. BMC Microbiol 2008;8:63.
6. Laroucau K, Thierry S, Vorimore F, et al. High-resolution typing of *Chlamydophila psittaci* by multilocus VNTR analysis (MLVA). Infect Genet Evol 2008;8(2): 171–81.
7. Strano AJ. Ornithosis (psittacosis). In: Connor DH, Chandler FW, editors. Pathology of infectious diseases, vol. 1. Stamford (CT): Appleton & Lang; 1997. p. 713–5.

8. Grimes JE. Zoonoses acquired from pet birds. Vet Clin North Am Small Anim Pract 1987;17(1):209–18.
9. Peeling RW, Brunham RC. *Chlamydiae* as pathogens: new species and new issues. Emerg Infect Dis 1996;2(4):307–19.
10. Vanrompay D, Ducatelle R, Haesebrouck F. *Chlamydia psittaci* infections: a review with emphasis on avian chlamydiosis. Vet Microbiol 1995;45:93–119.
11. Kaleta EF, Taday EM. Avian host range of *Chlamydophila* spp. based on isolation, antigen detection and serology. Avian Pathol 2003;32(5):435–61.
12. Andersen AA. Serotyping of *Chlamydia psittaci* isolates using serovar-specific monoclonal antibodies with the microimmunofluorescence test. J Clin Microbiol 1991;29(4):707–11.
13. Vanrompay D, Andersen AA, Ducatelle R, et al. Serotyping of European isolates of *Chlamydia psittaci* from poultry and other birds. J Clin Microbiol 1993;31(1):134–7.
14. Andersen AA. Serotyping of us isolates of *Chlamydophila psittaci* from domestic and wild birds. J Vet Diagn Invest 2005;17(5):479–82.
15. Heddema ER, van Hannen EJ, Duim B, et al. Genotyping of *Chlamydophila psittaci* in human samples. Emerg Infect Dis 2006;12(12):1989–90.
16. National Association of State and Public Health Veterinarians. Compendium of measures to control *Chlamydophila psittaci* infection among humans (psittacosis) and pet birds (avian chlamydiosis) 2008. Available at: http://www.nasphv.org/documentsCompendiaPsittacosis.html. Accessed March, 2009.
17. Theegarten D, Sachse K, Mentrup B, et al. *Chlamydophila* spp. infection in horses with recurrent airway obstruction: similarities to human chronic obstructive disease. Respir Res 2008;9:14.
18. DeGraves FJ, Gao D, Hehnen HR, et al. Quantitative detection of *Chlamydia psittaci* and *C pecorum* by high-sensitivity real-time PCR reveals high prevalence of vaginal infection in cattle. J Clin Microbiol 2003;41(4):1726–9.
19. Weigler BJ, Girjes AA, White NA, et al. Aspects of the epidemiology of *Chlamydia psittaci* infection in a population of koalas (*Phascolarctos cinereus*) in Southeastern Queensland, Australia. J Wildl Dis 1988;24(2):282–91.
20. Gaede W, Reckling KF, Dresenkamp B, et al. *Chlamydophila psittaci* infections in humans during an outbreak of psittacosis from poultry in Germany. Zoonoses Public Health 2008;55(4):184–8.
21. Sareyyupoglu B, Cantekin Z, Bas B. *Chlamydophila psittaci* DNA detection in the faeces of cage birds. Zoonoses Public Health 2007;54:237–42.
22. Verminnen K, Duquenne B, De Keukeleire D, et al. Evaluation of a *Chlamydophila psittaci* infection diagnostic platform for zoonotic risk assessment. J Clin Microbiol 2008;46(1):281–5.
23. Williams J, Tallis G, Dalton C, et al. Community outbreak of psittacosis in a rural Australian town [see comment]. Lancet 1998;351(9117):1697–9.
24. Telfer BL, Moberley SA, Hort KP, et al. Probable psittacosis outbreak linked to wild birds. Emerg Infect Dis 2005;11(3):391–7.
25. Ito I, Ishida T, Mishima M, et al. Familial cases of psittacosis: possible person-to-person transmission. Intern Med 2002;41(7):580–3.
26. Hughes C, Maharg P, Rosario P, et al. Possible nosocomial transmission of psittacosis [see comment]. Infect Control Hosp Epidemiol 1997;18(3):165–8.
27. Broholm KA, Bottiger M, Jernelius H, et al. Ornithosis as a nosocomial infection. Scand J Infect Dis 1977;9(4):263–7.
28. McNabb SJ, Jajosky RA, Hall-Baker PA, et al. Summary of notifiable diseases—United States, 2006. MMWR Morb Mortal Wkly Rep 2008;55(53):1–92.

29. Charles PG, Whitby M, Fuller AJ, et al. The etiology of community-acquired pneumonia in australia: why penicillin plus doxycycline or a macrolide is the most appropriate therapy [see comment]. Clin Infect Dis 2008;46(10):1513–21.
30. Berntsson E, Blomberg J, Lagergard T, et al. Etiology of community-acquired pneumonia in patients requiring hospitalization. Eur J Clin Microbiol 1985;4(3): 268–72.
31. Yung AP, Grayson ML. Psittacosis—a review of 135 cases. Med J Aust 1988; 148(5):228–33.
32. Heddema ER, van Hannen EJ, Duim B, et al. An outbreak of psittacosis due to *Chlamydophila psittaci* genotype a in a veterinary teaching hospital. J Med Microbiol 2006;55(11):1571–5.
33. Kovacova E, Majtan J, Botek R, et al. A fatal case of psittacosis in Slovakia, January 2006. Euro Surveill 2007;12(8):E0708021.
34. Moroney JF, Guevara R, Iverson C, et al. Detection of chlamydiosis in a shipment of pet birds, leading to recognition of an outbreak of clinically mild psittacosis in humans. Clin Infect Dis 1998;26(6):1425–9.
35. Wichert A, Lukasewitz P, Hauser MH, et al. ARDS in fulminant ornithosis and treatment with extracorporeal lung assist. Int J Artif Organs 2000;23(6):371–4.
36. Carr-Locke DL, Mair HJ. Neurological presentation of psittacosis during a small outbreak in Leicestershire. Br Med J 1976;2(6040):853–4.
37. Johnson SR, Pavord ID. Grand rounds—city hospital, Nottingham. A complicated case of community-acquired pneumonia. BMJ 1996;312(7035): 899–901.
38. Korman TM, Turnidge JD, Grayson ML. Neurological complications of chlamydial infections: case report and review. Clin Infect Dis 1997;25(4):847–51.
39. Hughes P, Chidley K, Cowie J. Neurological complications in psittacosis: a case report and literature review. Respir Med 1995;89(9):637–8.
40. Walder G, Schonherr H, Hotzel H, et al. Presence of *Chlamydophila psittaci* DNA in the central nervous system of a patient with status epilepticus. Scand J Infect Dis 2003;35(1):71–3.
41. Shee CD. Cerebellar disturbance in psittacosis. Postgrad Med J 1988;64(751): 382–3.
42. Al-Kawi MZ, Madkour MM. Brain stem encephalitis in ornithosis. J Neurol Neurosurg Psychiatr 1986;49(5):603–4.
43. Newton P, Lalvani A, Conlon CP. Psittacosis associated with bilateral 4th cranial nerve palsies. J Infect 1996;32(1):63–5.
44. Zumla A, Lipscomb G, Lewis D. Sixth cranial nerve palsy complicating psittacosis. J Neurol Neurosurg Psychiatr 1988;51(11):1462.
45. Crook T, Bannister B. Acute transverse myelitis associated with *Chlamydia psittaci* infection. J Infect 1996;32(2):151–2.
46. Grattan CE, Berman P. Chlamydial infection as a possible aetiological factor in the Guillain-Barre syndrome. Postgrad Med J 1982;58(686):776–7.
47. Branley P, Speed B. Acute interstitial nephritis due to *Chlamydia psittaci*. Aust N Z J Med 1995;25(4):365.
48. Samra Z, Pik A, Guidetti-Sharon A, et al. Hepatitis in a family infected by *Chlamydia psittaci*. J R Soc Med 1991;84(6):347–8.
49. Byrom NP, Walls J, Mair HJ. Fulminant psittacosis. Lancet 1979;1(8112):353–6.
50. Bourne D, Beck N, Summerton CB. *Chlamydia psittaci* pneumonia presenting as acute generalised peritonism. Emerg Med J 2003;20(4):386–7.
51. Lanham JG, Doyle DV. Reactive arthritis following psittacosis. Br J Rheumatol 1984;23(3):225–6.

52. Tsapas G, Klonizakis I, Casakos K, et al. Psittacosis and arthritis. Chemotherapy 1991;37(2):143–5.
53. Bhopal RS, Thomas GO. Psittacosis presenting with reiter's syndrome. Br Med J Clin Res Ed 1982;284(6329):1606.
54. Verweij PE, Meis JF, Eijk R, et al. Severe human psittacosis requiring artificial ventilation: case report and review. Clin Infect Dis 1995;20(2):440–2.
55. Pandeli V, Ernest D. A case of fulminant psittacosis. Crit Care Resusc 2006;8(1): 40–2.
56. Petrovay F, Balla E. Two fatal cases of psittacosis caused by *Chlamydophila psittaci*. J Med Microbiol 2008;57(10):1296–8.
57. Soni R, Seale JP, Young IH. Fulminant psittacosis requiring mechanical ventilation and demonstrating serological cross-reactivity between *Legionella longbeachae* and *Chlamydia psittaci*. Respirology 1999;4(2):203–5.
58. Wainwright AP, Beaumont AC, Kox WJ. Psittacosis: diagnosis and management of severe pneumonia and multi organ failure. Intensive Care Med 1987;13(6):419–21.
59. Mason AB, Jenkins P. Acute renal failure in fulminant psittacosis [see comment]. Respir Med 1994;88(3):239–40.
60. Toyokawa M, Kishimoto T, Cai Y, et al. Severe *Chlamydophila psittaci* pneumonia rapidly diagnosed by detection of antigen in sputum with an immunochromatography assay. J Infect Chemother 2004;10(4):245–9.
61. Hamilton DV. Psittacosis and disseminated intravascular coagulation. Br Med J 1975;2(5967):370.
62. Laidlaw E, Mulligan RA. Letter: psittacosis and disseminated intravascular coagulation. Br Med J 1975;2(5972):688.
63. Wong KF, Chan JK, Chan CH, et al. Psittacosis-associated hemophagocytic syndrome. Am J Med 1991;91(2):204–5.
64. Regan RJ, Dathan JR, Treharne JD. Infective endocarditis with glomerulonephritis associated with cat chlamydia (*C psittaci*) infection. Br Heart J 1979; 42(3):349–52.
65. Levison DA, Guthrie W, Ward C, et al. Infective endocarditis as part of psittacosis. Lancet 1971;2(7729):844–7.
66. Birkhead JS, Apostolov K. Endocarditis caused by a psittacosis agent. Br Heart J 1974;36(7):728–31.
67. Lamaury I, Sotto A, Le Quellec A, et al. *Chlamydia psittaci* as a cause of lethal bacterial endocarditis. Clin Infect Dis 1993;17(4):821–2.
68. Schinkel AF, Bax JJ, van der Wall EE, et al. Echocardiographic follow-up of *Chlamydia psittaci* myocarditis. Chest 2000;117(4):1203–5.
69. Walder G, Gritsch W, Wiedermann CJ, et al. Coinfection with two chlamydophila species in a case of fulminant myocarditis [see comment]. Crit Care Med 2007; 35(2):623–6.
70. Coll R, Horner I. Cardiac involvement in psittacosis. Br Med J 1967;4(5570):35–6.
71. Diaz F, Collazos J. Myopericarditis due to *Chlamydia psittaci*. The role of autoimmunity. Scand J Infect Dis 1997;29(1):93–4.
72. Jorgensen DM. Gestational psittacosis in a Montana sheep rancher. Emerg Infect Dis 1997;3(2):191–4.
73. Janssen ML, van de Wetering K, Arabin B. Sepsis due to gestational psittacosis: a multidisciplinary approach within a perinatological center—review of reported cases. Int J Fertil Womens Med 2006;51(1):17–20.
74. Walder G, Hotzel H, Brezinka C, et al. An unusual cause of sepsis during pregnancy: recognizing infection with *Chlamydophila abortus*. Obstet Gynecol 2005; 106:1215–7.

75. Hyde SR, Benirschke K. Gestational psittacosis: case report and literature review. Mod Pathol 1997;10(6):602–7.
76. Khatib R, Thirumoorthi MC, Kelly B, et al. Severe psittacosis during pregnancy and suppression of antibody response with early therapy. Scand J Infect Dis 1995;27(5):519–21.
77. Gherman RB, Leventis LL, Miller RC. *Chlamydial psittacosis* during pregnancy: a case report. Obstet Gynecol 1995;86:648–50.
78. Lietman T, Brooks D, Moncada J, et al. Chronic follicular conjunctivitis associated with *Chlamydia psittaci* or *Chlamydia pneumoniae*. Clin Infect Dis 1998; 26(6):1335–40.
79. Dean D, Shama A, Schachter J, et al. Molecular identification of an avian strain of *Chlamydia psittaci* causing severe keratoconjunctivitis in a bird fancier. Clin Infect Dis 1995;20(5):1179–85.
80. Ferreri AJ, Guidoboni M, Ponzoni M, et al. Evidence for an association between *Chlamydia psittaci* and ocular adnexal lymphomas [see comment]. J Natl Cancer Inst 2004;96(8):586–94.
81. Yoo C, Ryu MH, Huh J, et al. *Chlamydia psittaci* infection and clinicopathologic analysis of ocular adnexal lymphomas in Korea. Am J Hematol 2007;82(9): 821–3.
82. Ponzoni M, Ferreri AJ, Guidoboni M, et al. Chlamydia infection and lymphomas: association beyond ocular adnexal lymphomas highlighted by multiple detection methods. Clin Cancer Res 2008;14(18):5794–800.
83. Ferreri AJ, Ponzoni M, Guidoboni M, et al. Bacteria-eradicating therapy with doxycycline in ocular adnexal malt lymphoma: a multicenter prospective trial [see comment]. J Natl Cancer Inst 2006;98(19):1375–82.
84. Decaudin D, Dolcetti R, de Cremoux P, et al. Variable association between *Chlamydophila psittaci* infection and ocular adnexal lymphomas: methodological biases or true geographical variations? Anticancer Drugs 2008;19(8): 761–5.
85. Wong KH, Skelton SK, Daugharty H. Utility of complement fixation and microimmunofluorescence assays for detecting serologic responses in patients with clinically diagnosed psittacosis. J Clin Microbiol 1994;32(10):2417–21.
86. Grayston JT, Mordhorst C, Bruu AL, et al. Countrywide epidemics of *Chlamydia pneumoniae*, strain twar, in Scandinavia, 1981–1983. J Infect Dis 1989;159(6): 1111–4.
87. Persson K, Treharne J. Diagnosis of infection caused by *Chlamydia pneumoniae* (strain twar) in patients with Ornithosis In southern Sweden 1981–1987. Scand J Infect Dis 1989;21(6):675–9.
88. Fryden A, Kihlstrom E, Maller R, et al. A clinical and epidemiological study of Ornithosis caused by *Chlamydia psittaci* and *Chlamydia pneumoniae* (strain twar). Scand J Infect Dis 1989;21(6):681–91.
89. Pether JV, Wang SP, Grayston JT. *Chlamydia pneumoniae*, strain twar, as the cause of an outbreak in a boys' school previously called psittacosis. Epidemiol Infect 1989;103(2):395–400.
90. Wreghitt TG, Barker CE, Treharne JD, et al. A study of human respiratory tract chlamydial infections in Cambridgeshire 1986–88. Epidemiol Infect 1990; 104(3):479–88.
91. Persson K, Haidl S. Evaluation of a commercial test for antibodies to the chlamydial lipopolysaccharide (medac) for serodiagnosis of acute infections by *Chlamydia pneumoniae* (twar) and *Chlamydia psittaci*. APMIS 2000;108(2): 131–8.

92. Stralin K, Fredlund H, Olcen P. Labsystems enzyme immunoassay for *Chlamydia pneumoniae* also detects *Chlamydia psittaci* infections [comment]. J Clin Microbiol 2001;39(9):3425–6.
93. Messmer TO, Skelton SK, Moroney JF, et al. Application of a nested, multiplex PCR to psittacosis outbreaks [erratum appears in J Clin Microbiol 1998;36(6):1821]. J Clin Microbiol 1997;35(8):2043–6.
94. Madico G, Quinn TC, Boman J, et al. Touchdown enzyme time-release PCR for detection and identification of *Chlamydia trachomatis*, *C pneumoniae*, and *C psittaci* using the 16s and 16s-23s spacer rRna genes. J Clin Microbiol 2000;38(3):1085–93.
95. Branley JM, Roy B, Dwyer DE, et al. Real-time PCR detection and quantitation of *Chlamydophila psittaci* in human and avian specimens from a veterinary clinic cluster. Eur J Clin Microbiol Infect Dis 2008;27(4):269–73.
96. Menard A, Clerc M, Subtil A, et al. Development of a real-time PCR for the detection of *Chlamydia psittaci*. J Med Microbiol 2006;55(4):471–3.
97. Geens T, Dewitte A, Boon N, et al. Development of a *Chlamydophila psittaci* species-specific and genotype-specific real-time PCR. Vet Res 2005;36: 787–97.
98. Donati M, Rodriguez Fermepin M, Olmo A, et al. Comparative in vitro activity of moxifloxacin, minocycline, and azithromycin against *Chlamydia spp*. J Antimicrob Chemother 1999;43(6):825–7.
99. Roblin PM, Hammerschlag MR. In vitro activity of gar-936 against *Chlamydia pneumoniae* and *Chlamydia trachomatis*. Int J Antimicrob Agents 2000;16(1): 61–3.
100. Donati M, Pollini GM, Sparacino M, et al. Comparative in vitro activity of garenoxacin against *Chlamydia* spp. J Antimicrob Chemother 2002;50(3): 407–10.
101. Niki Y, Kimura M, Miyashita N, et al. In vitro and in vivo activities of azithromycin, a new azalide antibiotic, against *Chlamydia*. Antimicrobial Agents Chemother 1994;38(10):2296–9.
102. Binet R, Maurelli AT. Frequency of development and associated physiological cost of azithromycin resistance in *Chlamydia psittaci* 6bc and c. Trachomatis l2. Antimicrobial Agents Chemother 2007;51(12):4267–75.
103. Miyashita N, Niki Y, Kishimoto T, et al. In vitro and in vivo activities of am-1155, a new fluoroquinolone, against *Chlamydia* spp. Antimicrobial Agents Chemother 1997;41(6):1331–4.
104. Kimura M, Kishimoto T, Niki Y, et al. In vitro and in vivo antichlamydial activities of newly developed quinolone antimicrobial agents. Antimicrobial Agents Chemother 1993;37(4):801–3.
105. Vanrompay D, Cox E, Volckaert G, et al. Turkeys are protected from infection with *Chlamydia psittaci* by plasmid DNA vaccination against the major outer membrane protein. Clin Exp Immunol 1999;118(1):49–55.
106. Zhou J, Qiu C, Cao XA, et al. Construction and immunogenicity of recombinant adenovirus expressing the major outer membrane protein (momp) of *Chlamydophila psittaci* in chicks. Vaccine 2007;25(34):6367–72.
107. Grist NR, McLean C. Infections by organisms of psittacosis/lymphogranuloma venereum group in the west of Scotland. Br Med J 1964;2(5400):21–5.
108. Ward C, Sagar HJ, Cooper D, et al. Insidious endocarditis caused by *Chlamydia psittaci*. Br Med J 1975;4(5999):734–5.
109. Dick DC, McGregor CG, Mitchell KG, et al. Endocarditis as a manifestation of Chlamydia b infection (psittacosis). Br Heart J 1977;39(8):914–6.

110. Bromage D, Jeffries DJ, Philip G. Embolic phenomena in chlamydial infection. J Infect 1980;2(2):151–9.
111. Jariwalla AG, Davies BH, White J. Infective endocarditis complicating psittacosis: response to rifampicin. Br Med J 1980;280(6208):155.
112. Jones RB, Priest JB, Kuo C. Subacute chlamydial endocarditis. JAMA 1982; 247(5):655–8.
113. Walker LJ, Adgey AA. Successful treatment by doxycycline of endocarditis caused by ornithosis. Br Heart J 1987;57(1):58–60.
114. Shapiro DS, Kenney SC, Johnson M, et al. Brief report: *Chlamydia psittaci* endocarditis diagnosed by blood culture [see comment]. N Engl J Med 1992; 326(18):1192–5.

Q Fever Pneumonia

Thomas J. Marrie, MD

KEYWORDS

• Q fever • *Coxiella burnetii* • Pneumonia • Community-acquired

Q fever is a zoonosis. It had its beginnings in Brisbane, Australia, in 1936 as an outbreak of a febrile illness among abbatoir workers at the Cannon Hill Abbatoir in that city.[1] Dr E.H. Derrick, a pathologist and Director of the Laboratory of Microbiology and Pathology at the Queensland Health Department, Brisbane, was asked to investigate the outbreak. He noted that it lasted 7 to 24 days and was characterized by fever, headache, malaise, anorexia, and myalgia. Blood cultures were negative and serum samples from affected individuals had no antibodies to influenza, typhus, leptospirosis, typhoid, or paratyphoid. He named the illness Q (for query) fever.[2] Derrick sent urine and blood samples from his patients to McFarlane Burnet in Melbourne who was able to isolate an infectious agent by inoculating the material into guinea pigs.[3] To identify the agent of Rocky Mountain spotted fever, Davis collected ticks from Nine Mile Creek area in Montana, United States, and isolated an infectious agent from them. Burnet sent material from the infected guinea pigs to Cox at the National Institutes of Health in the United States and before too long he was able to show that the Nine Mile and Brisbane agents were the same.[1] Eventually, the agent was named *Coxiella burnetii* in honor of Cox and Burnet.

MICROBIOLOGY

Coxiella burnetii is a small gram-negative intracellular bacterium with a genome that is 1,995,275 base pairs long.[4] When cultured in eggs or cell cultures it exhibits antigenic variation. The wild virulent form, phase I, shifts to a frequently occurring avirulent mutant phase II. Phase II antigen is the first to be recognized by the immune system during acute Q fever, whereas high-level phase I antibodies are detected during chronic Q fever.[5] Phase II cells have a truncated lipopolysaccharide.[6] In the Nine Mile strain this shift is caused by a large chromosomal deletion. The deleted region comprises, among others, putative genes for the addition of sugars to the core oligosaccharide and for synthesis of virenose, a sugar typical of phase I lipopolysaccharide.[6] *C burnetii* targets monocytes and macrophages where it survives within the phagolysome.[7,8] Phase I bacteria escape intracellular killing by monocytes by inhibiting cathepsin fusion, the last phagosome maturation step.[9] *C burnetii* forms spores.[10] This spore stage explains the microorganism's ability to withstand harsh

Office of the Dean, Clinical Research Centre, Room C205, 5849 University Avenue, Halifax, NS B3H 4H7, Canada
E-mail address: t.marrie@dal.ca

Infect Dis Clin N Am 24 (2010) 27–41
doi:10.1016/j.idc.2009.10.004
0891-5520/10/$ – see front matter

environmental conditions.[11] It can survive for 7 to 10 months on wool at 15°C to 20°C, for more than 1 month on fresh meat in cold storage, and for more than 40 months in skim milk at room temperature.[12] Although it is destroyed by 2% formaldehyde, the organism has been isolated from infected tissues stored in formaldehyde for up to 4 to 5 months. It has also been isolated from fixed "paraffinized" tissues. Either 1% Lysol or 5% hydrogen peroxide kills *C burnetii*.

Coxiella burnetii is a Centers for Disease Control and Prevention category B bioterrorism agent.[13] These agents have the potential for large-scale dissemination but generally cause less illness and death than category A agents.[14] As a biologic warfare agent, *C burnetii* can be easily dispersed as an aerosol with a high infectivity rate and pneumonia is the major manifestation of infection. It has been calculated that a concentration of 100 cells per m^3 and an exposure time of 30 to 60 minutes can deposit more than one cell in the lung.[15]

The pathogenesis of *C burnetii* infection is fascinating. This organism not only survives in the hostile environment of the phagolysome, but it requires the acidic pH of this environment for many of it enzymes to work.[16] It induces a range of immunomodulary responses in the host, from immunosuppression in those with chronic Q fever to nonspecific stimulation after vaccination that results in regression of tumors and allows mice nonspecifically to resist infection.[16] In addition, infection with *C burnetii* induces autoantibody formation, especially to smooth muscle and to cardiac muscle.[17]

EPIDEMIOLOGY

The epidemiology of Q fever is that of its animal reservoirs and those who work with them, live or play in their environs, or use contaminated animal products. The circumstance under which exposure occurs in all of these, however, is such that one must maintain a high index of suspicion to diagnose sporadic cases of Q fever. Cattle, sheep, and goats are the most common reservoirs for *C burnetii*.[18] The organism is trophic for the placenta and the mammary glands in the females of these animals. During pregnancy, the organism reaches very high concentrations in the placenta and at the time of parturition it is aerosolized and shed into the environment. When a susceptible person inhales one or more of these organisms Q fever develops. *C burnetii* has been identified in arthropods, fish, birds, rodents, and marsupials.[19] Infected parturient cats have been the main reservoirs of *C burnetii* in Maritime Canada.[20,21] *C burnetii* has been a most successful pathogen; it is now present in at least 51 countries and the only areas known to be free of this organism are New Zealand and Antarctica.[19,22] It is not surprising that Q fever can be a travel-associated illness.[23–26]

Q fever can occur as outbreaks with an epidemic curve typical of a point source or as endemic cases. At times, the source is obvious, such as when workers on a goat farm develop a febrile illness. On other occasions, however, finding the source can be challenging as illustrated by the examples that follow.

Indirect contact with infected animals has resulted in outbreaks of Q fever, such as in Switzerland, where more than 350 persons who lived along a road over which sheep traveled from mountain pastures developed Q fever.[27] Exposure to contaminated straw, manure, or dust from farm vehicles resulted in Q fever in British residents who lived along a road traveled by these vehicles.[28] Exposure may be even more indirect, as in the case of laundry workers who developed Q fever after handling contaminated laundry from a facility that was performing Q fever research.[29] *C burnetii* can become airborne from contaminated soil during windstorms and result in infection up to 11 miles (18.3 km) distance from the point source.[30–32]

Laboratory exposure to *C burnetii* and transport of infected sheep through hospitals to research laboratories have resulted in large outbreaks of Q fever.[33–35] Rarely, Q fever has been transmitted by blood transfusion.[36] Transmission has occurred during an autopsy,[37,38] but has not been documented during clinical care of infected patients. There is one report of apparent human-to-human transmission of Q fever among members of a household.[39]

In the United States between 1948 and 1977 a total of 1168 cases were reported to the Centers for Disease Control and Prevention, a mean of 58.4 cases per year.[40] From 1978 to 1986 there was a decline in the number of reported cases to 28.5 per year. Most of the cases (67%) in this early period originated from California.[41]

From 1978 to 1999 there were 436 cases of Q fever in the United States, an average of 26 cases per year with a range of 6 to 41 cases.[41] From 2000 to 2004 there were 255 cases from 37 states, an average of 51 cases per year, range 18 to 73 cases. There was a seasonal effect, with 39% of the cases reported from April through June. Seventy-seven percent were male; the mean age was 50.5 years, the median was 51 years; and 92% were white, 6% were black, and 2% were Asian. The racial distribution of the Q fever cases was proportionally similar to that of the United States population. The age distribution of the Q fever cases differed from that of the United States population, with the Q fever cases rising with increasing age and peaking in the 50- to 59-year age group. The highest rate was in Wyoming. No cases were reported from Alabama, Alaska, Arkansas, Connecticut, and Hawaii. Q fever is not reportable in the following states: Delaware, Iowa, Vermont, and West Virginia. Hence, no data were given for these states.

McQusiton and Childs[41] noted that sheep and goats in the United States have a higher seroprevalence for *C burnetii* than cattle. McQuiston also noted an extensive wildlife reservoir for this organism in the United States.[41] Various studies have shown varying degrees of seropositivity for coyotes, gray foxes, skunks, raccoons, rabbits, deer, mice, bears, birds, and opossums.

In a study of 316 bulk milk tanks conducted throughout the United States from January 2001 through December 2003 using polymerase chain reaction (PCR) to test for the presence of *C burnetii* DNA, 94.3% of the samples were positive.[42]

An outbreak of Q fever associated with a horse-boarding ranch in Colorado in 2005 was caused by spread of infection from two herds of goats that had been acquired by the owners.[43] Twenty (53%) of 38 persons tested had serologic evidence of infection with *C burnetii*. Testing of the soil and goats using a PCR assay confirmed the presence of *C burnetii* in the soil and among the goats. One hundred and thirty-eight persons who lived within 1 mile of the ranch were also tested. Eleven (8%) had evidence of *C burnetii* infection, eight of whom had no direct contact with the ranch.

Sawyer and coworkers[44] in 1985 asked laboratories in the United States to submit to them all samples of serum that they had tested for hepatitis and for respiratory infection. Six (0.6%) of the 959 originally submitted for hepatitis testing had acute Q fever as did four (0.6%) in the respiratory cohort. They concluded that Q fever was uncommon in the United States.

Karakousis and colleagues[45] reported a case of chronic Q fever and reviewed all the published cases of chronic Q fever from the United States. They could only find seven such cases, likely a gross underestimate, from 1976 to 2004. Q fever peaked in West Germany in 1964 at 450 cases during that year.[46]

Q fever continues to be frequently diagnosed in Australia with a rate of 30 cases per million per year.[47–49] Males are predominantly involved with a male/female ratio of 5.3:1.[42] One of the unique risk factors for Q fever in Australia is kangaroo hunting.[50]

Q fever is endemic in many European countries.[46] In recent years Q fever has been seen in soldiers returning from Iraq.[51] Currently, there is a large outbreak of Q fever ongoing in the Netherlands.[52,53] It started in 2007 and to August 2008 there have been 808 cases.[52] The outbreak seems to be related to goat farming.

In many jurisdictions, Q fever is a notifiable disease. Even if reporting is not mandatory, one should report suspected or confirmed cases to the local health authorities and an investigation should be conducted to find the source of the infection.

CLINICAL PRESENTATION

Q fever as an illness is divided into two categories: acute and chronic, based on antibody titers to phase I and phase II antigen. In acute Q fever, antibodies to phase II predominate, whereas the reverse is true for chronic Q fever.[54] The major manifestations of acute and chronic Q fever are given in **Box 1**.[55,56]

One of the best descriptions of the clinical picture of Q fever is that by Huebner and colleagues in 1949.[57] In their review of 650 cases they noted five fatalities (0.8%), which is still a reasonable estimate. They also described relative bradycardia. Headache was present in about 90% of patients and retro-orbital pain was a prominent feature. They reported that photophobia occurs and that six patients relapsed following apparent recovery. They also observed relapse following treatment with streptomycin.[57] Powell and colleagues[58] in a report of 76 cases of Q fever in the 1950s noted relative bradycardia in 96% of patients, headache in 90%, diarrhea in 15, and constipation in 15. Noteworthy in this report was that 65% had hepatomegaly and 53% splenomegaly. Fever lasted on average 18 days but could persist for up to 34 days. Only three patients had pneumonia. The clinical picture that Powell and colleagues[58] describe resembles that of granulomatous hepatitis, which most often presents as fever of unknown origin.

In a study in Nova Scotia pneumonia caused by *C burnetii* (N = 21) was compared with that caused by *Mycoplasma pneumoniae* (N = 40) and *Legionella pneumophila* (N = 14).[59] The mean age did not differ among the three groups of patients, ranging from 42.3 years for those with *M pneumoniae*, to 47.1 for those with Q fever, to 61.9 years for the *L pneumophila* patients. The following symptoms were present in some or most of the patients with Q fever pneumonia: fever; chills; rigors; pleuritic chest pain; headache; nausea; vomiting; abdominal pain; diarrhea; sore throat; anorexia; myalgia; arthralgia; cough (38% had a nonproductive cough and 33%

Box 1
Major manifestations of acute and chronic Q fever

Acute Q fever

- Nonspecific febrile illness
- Pneumonia
- Hepatitis

Chronic Q fever

- Endocarditis
- Osteomyelitis
- Hepatitis
- Q fever in pregnancy

had a productive cough); and confusion. Headache was significantly more frequent among the *C burnetii* patients. Patients complain that, "this is the most severe headache that I have ever had in my life." The mean temperature at the time of admission was not different among the three groups of patients and 90% to 100% of patients were febrile at admission. About half the patients with Q fever pneumonia had crackles on auscultation and 5% had rhonchi; 29% had the physical findings of consolidation. The mean duration of fever was 2.2 days for patients with *C burnetii*, 2.45 days for those with *M pneumoniae*, and 4 days for those with Legionnaires' disease. One (4.8%) patient with Q fever pneumonia died. That patient had underlying cardiomyopathy and aspiration pneumonia complicated by *Escherichia coli* sepsis. In contrast, 5 (36%) out of 14 of the patients with Legionnaire's disease died. Except for the patient with aspiration pneumonia and sepsis, complications were uncommon among the patients with Q fever pneumonia. One patient each had deep vein thrombophlebitis, myocardial infarction, and urinary tract infection.

Most of the patients with Q fever pneumonia (70%) had a normal white blood cell count. Although the mean platelet count was normal, reactive thrombocytosis of up to 1 million platelets per mm^3 was frequently observed during recovery from Q fever pneumonia. About 50% of the patients with Q fever pneumonia had elevated liver enzymes but so did the patients with *Mycoplasma* and *Legionella*. The mean creatinine phosphokinase level among patients with Q fever pneumonia was 912 U/L (normal 18–199). Twenty-seven percent of the Q fever patients were hypoxemic compared with 38% of those with *Mycoplasma* and 54% of the *Legionella* patients. There are reports of two patients who had Q fever pneumonia with an eosinophilic pleural effusion.[60,61]

In a study of 20 patients with Q fever pneumonia in the Negev region of Israel, the mean age of the patients was 41 years, 12 were male, and the mean duration of fever was 10.5 days.[62]

A report of laboratory-acquired Q fever is instructive in that 28 (56%) of 50 had pneumonia.[33] The opacities were oval, wedge-shaped, perihilar, and on occasion resembled a coin lesion. There is a distinct entity of round pneumonia.[63] Anton[63] indicates that the most common etiology of round pneumonia in adults is Q fever. Having said that, one must be careful not to misdiagnose septic emboli associated from right-sided endocarditis as round pneumonia.

One of the largest studies of Q fever pneumonia in recent times is from the Basque region in Spain.[64] Montes and colleagues[64] reported 1261 cases of Q fever of which 1003 (79.5%) were pneumonia. Half of the patients with pneumonia were hospitalized and 10 were admitted to ICU. Unfortunately, this report lacks clinical details. Noteworthy is that during the 21 years covered by this study only two patients developed chronic Q fever.

The radiographic manifestations of Q fever pneumonia are often not distinguishable from those of pneumonia caused by other microorganisms (**Figs. 1** and **2**). Rounded opacities are not infrequently found, however, and in endemic areas can be very suggestive of Q fever pneumonia (**Fig. 3**).[65,66] Pleural effusions when they do occur are usually small and hilar adenopathy (**Fig. 4**) may occur.[59] The mean time to resolution is 30 days. In one study of 12 patients with Q fever pneumonia who had CT of the chest performed, air space involvement was seen in all patients.[67] It was lobar in three, segmental in three, patchy in three, or a combination of these patterns in three. Most (58%) had more than one lobe involved. Pleural effusions were seen in three patients and mild lymph node enlargement was noted in four patients. They also noted that chest radiography was less accurate than CT in the detection of segmental and patchy areas of consolidations.[67]

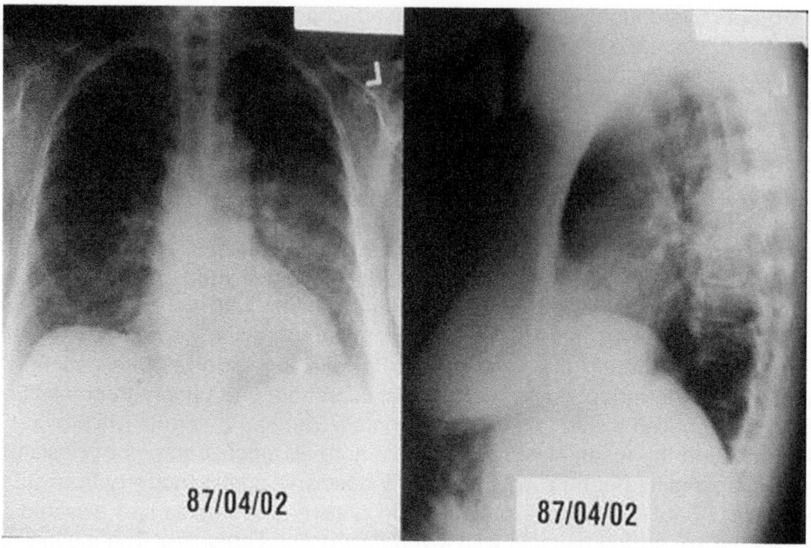

Fig. 1. Posteroanterior and lateral chest radiographs of a female patient with Q fever pneumonia. This opacity is indistinguishable from pneumonia of any cause.

There are many extrapulmonary manifestations that can occur in patients with Q fever pneumonia. One of the more troublesome ones in terms of misdiagnosis is pulmonary renal syndrome (renal failure and pulmonary infiltrates). Fortunately, anti-glomerular basement membrane antibodies and anticytoplasmic antibodies are negative in patients with Q fever.[68] Korman and colleagues[69] reported one case of acute glomerulonephritis complicating acute Q fever and two other cases from their review of the literature. There is no report of the chest radiograph on admission (for the index case) but an opacity compatible with pneumonia was present on a CT scan of the chest done later. Hematuria, usually microscopic, is common among patients with Q fever pneumonia.[70] Other extrapulmonary manifestations of acute Q fever include

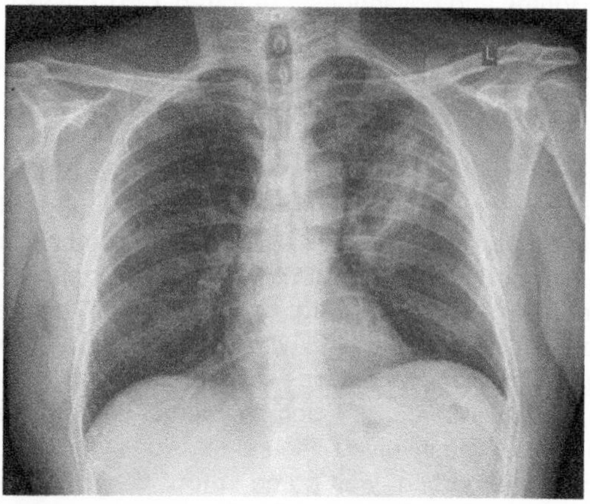

Fig. 2. Chest radiographs of a patient with Q fever pneumonia. Note the streaky opacity in the left upper lobe. L, left. (*Courtesy of* Walter Schlech III, MD.)

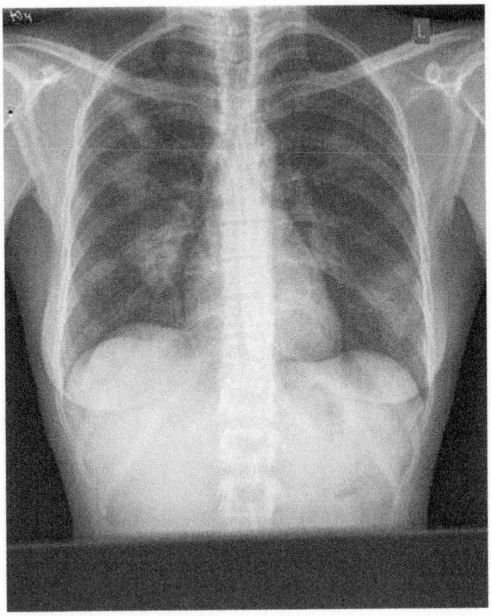

Fig. 3. Chest radiograph of a patient with Q fever pneumonia showing multiple rounded opacities in both lung fields. This appearance is suggestive of cat-related Q fever. L, left. (*Courtesy of* Walter Schlech III, MD.)

aseptic meningitis, encephalitis, Guillian-Barré syndrome, mononeuropathy, optic neuritis, pericarditis, myocarditis, hemolytic anemia, lymphadenopathy, bone marrow necrosis, hemophagocytosis, thrombocytosis, thrombocytopenia, transient hypoplastic anemia, splenic rupture, and erythema nodosum.

Q fever pneumonia can also be seen in immunocompromised hosts.[71,72] Raoult and colleagues[72] found that 5 (7.3%) of 68 of patients hospitalized with Q fever from 1987 to 1989 in Marseilles were HIV positive. They went on to estimate that in HIV-positive individuals the number of cases of Q fever was 13 times higher than that in the general population.[72]

There is a limited amount of information about the pathology of the lung in Q fever pneumonia.[73–76] Pierce and coworkers[73] found small coccobacilli within alveolar macrophages on transbronchial biopsy in a patient with Q fever. A fatal case of pneumonia in a 43-year-old man was characterized by severe intra-alveolar hemorrhagic and focal necrotizing pneumonia with associated necrotizing bronchitis. Histiocytes, lymphocytes, and plasma cells were in the alveoli. This was thought to be Q fever pneumonia on the basis of organisms seen with a modified Giemsa stain.[74] A resolving, *C burnetii* pneumonia lesion was characterized by an inflammatory pseudotumor, a lung mass composed of mixtures of macrophages, giant cells, plasma cells, and lymphocytes. The bronchiolar epithelium was focally absent, regenerated, or hyperplastic.[75] The changes that result from the inoculation of the lungs of rhesus monkeys with *C burnetii* resemble those reported from humans. The resulting consolidation was peribronchial or peribronchiolar.[76] Animal studies suggest that there are strain differences in the pulmonary manifestations of infection with *C burnetii*.[77]

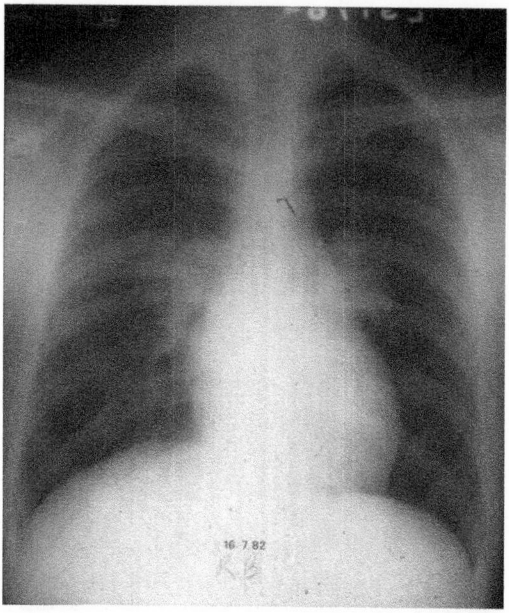

Fig. 4. Chest radiograph of a young male with Q fever. Note the extensive bilateral hilar adenopathy.

DIFFERENTIAL DIAGNOSIS

In an endemic area with the appropriate exposure history the differential diagnosis for Q fever pneumonia is very limited. In nonendemic areas the differential diagnosis includes all of the microorganisms that can cause pneumonia. Because the animal reservoir population for *C burnetii* is large the differential diagnosis often includes tularemia and plague. It is difficult to know just how commonly *C burnetii* causes pneumonia. In a study in Bristol, England, from 1974 to 1980, 4.3% of the 210 patients with pneumonia had Q fever.[78] In a study of 27 patients with atypical pneumonia in Maritime Canada, three (11%) had Q fever pneumonia.[79] In the Netherlands during an outbreak of Q fever an unexpected number of cases of pneumonia drew attention to the outbreak.[53] In a 1-year study of pneumonia, with detailed work-up for etiology including urinary antigen test for *Streptococcus pneumoniae*, 2 (0.7%) of 267 had Q fever.[80]

The major manifestations of Q fever are influenced by geography. The major manifestation of Q fever in Maritime Canada is pneumonia; however, in Taiwan 80% of patients with Q fever have hepatitis and 19% have pneumonia.[81] In Alberta, Canada (author's unpublished observations, 1999–2009), granulomatous hepatitis presenting as fever of unknown origin predominates. In southern France among 1070 patients with acute Q fever, hepatitis also predominated at 39.6%; pulmonary involvement was 16.6%, both hepatic and pulmonary was 19.5%, and isolated fever was only 14%.[82] In Thailand Q fever accounted for 1% of undifferentiated febrile illness.[83] In contrast, in the southern Spain, Q fever accounted for 10% of 233 cases of fever of intermediate duration.[84]

DIAGNOSIS

Clinical

As always a careful history is often the most important clue that the pneumonia might be caused by *C burnetii*. A history of exposure to animals whether it is as a result of occupation or avocation is important. Petting zoos have been a source of Q fever for children and adults equally.[85] One must also remember indirect exposure, such as living up to 18 km from an animal source and unusual sources, such as working in a cosmetics factory that processes ovine products.[86]

Laboratory

Because the illness is often nonspecific in clinical presentation, laboratory testing is necessary to confirm the diagnosis. Because most laboratories do not have the capability to isolate the organism, serologic tests including complement fixation and indirect immunofluorescence antibody tests are the most common means of diagnosis. A fourfold rise in antibody titer between acute and convalescent serum samples is considered diagnostic. The acute phase sample should be drawn as soon as possible in the illness and the convalescent sample 2 to 4 weeks later. When the sample is drawn early there are no detectable antibodies to *C burnetii* (phase I and phase II titers <1:8). Two weeks later phase II antibody titers of 1:128 or higher are common, whereas phase I titers are still less than 1:8 or low level positivity of 1:8 to 1:16. The immunofluorescence test is most reliable. The source and purity of the antigen, however, can affect the results. In acute Q fever, the phase II antibody response is always higher than that to phase I, whereas in chronic Q fever, the phase I antibody titer is very high often reaching levels greater than 1:16,384.

PCR has successfully been used to detect *C burnetii* DNA in cell cultures and clinical samples.[55] Several genes have been used to generate specific primers including 16S rRNA, 23S rDNA, superoxide dismutase, plasmid based sequences, and the IS1111 multicopy insertion sequence.[87]

Isolation of *C burnetii* must be done only in a biosafety level 3 containment facilities because of its extreme infectivity. The adaptation of a shell vial culture system using a human embryonic lung fibroblast (HEL cells) has improved the isolation of *C burnetii*.[88]

Serologic tests should always be interpreted with attention to the clinical picture. A pseudoepidemic of Q fever at an animal research facility was caused by a lapse in quality control of the serologic testing.[89] Seventy-five percent of those tested were seropositive; however, when the results were corrected the true seroprevalence was 25%. There was only one case of acute Q fever.

THERAPY

Empiric

Most of the time the diagnosis of Q fever pneumonia is not known at the time of presentation and empiric therapy is according to the guidelines for community-acquired pneumonia.[90] Although antimicrobial susceptibility testing of *C burnetti* because of its intracellular nature is difficult, it is apparent that there is heterogeneity in susceptibility to macrolides. Hence, if this therapy is used, the patient may or may not respond.[91,92] *C burnetii* is resistant to β-lactams and aminoglycosides and susceptible to rifampin, co-trimoxazole, tetracyclines, and quinolones. Quinolone resistance has been reported.[88]

Specific

The treatment of choice for Q fever pneumonia is doxycycline, 100 mg twice a day for 10 days. This is based on long-standing clinical practice and apparent success from observational studies and from limited clinical trial evidence.

Sobradillo and colleagues[93] from Basque Country, Spain, performed a prospective, randomized double-blind study of doxycycline and erythromycin in the treatment of pneumonia presumed to be caused by Q fever. Forty-eight patients were proved by serologic studies to have Q fever; 23 received 100 mg doxycycline twice daily, and 25 received erythromycin (500 mg every 6 hours) for 10 days. Fever resolution was faster in the doxycycline-treated group (3 $\pm$ 1.6 days versus 4.3 $\pm$ 2 days for erythromycin-treated patients; $P = .05$). The erythromycin-treated group had more gastrointestinal adverse effects (11 versus 2 for the doxycycline-treated patients; $P<.01$). By day 40, the chest radiograph was normal in 47 of the 48 patients. The authors concluded that doxycycline was more effective than erythromycin, but they recognized the self-limiting and benign nature of most cases of pneumonia caused by Q fever.

Macrolides (azithromycin, clarithromycin, and erythromycin) have all been used to treat Q fever pneumonia with success,[94–97] although in one study 15% of those treated with clarithromycin were febrile at 5 days.[95]

When one compares this information and also the in vitro data, one can conclude that β-lactams are ineffective[96]; for those who cannot tolerate doxycycline, a macrolide or quinolone may be effective.

Q fever pneumonia during pregnancy should be treated with co-trimoxazole for the duration of the pregnancy. In one retrospective study this approach reduced obstetric complications from 81% to 44%. There were no intrauterine fetal deaths in the co-trimoxazole–treated group.[98] Those patients with a "chronic Q fever serologic profile" should be treated with doxycycline and hydroxychloroquine for 1 year following delivery.[98]

There is one report of recurrent Jarisch-Herxheimer reaction complicating the treatment of Q fever pneumonia.[99]

COMPLICATIONS AND PROGNOSIS

Complications are uncommon during Q fever pneumonia and prognosis is excellent. Patients with cardiac valvular lesions who develop Q fever are at risk, however, for developing Q fever endocarditis months or years later. These patients should be followed with serologic testing every 3 months and if the serologic profile of chronic Q fever develops, they should be treated with doxycycline and hydroxychloroquine as for Q fever endocarditis. Alternatively, pre-emptive treatment with doxycycline and hydroxychloroquine can be given to these patients for 1 year.[100]

REFERENCES

1. McDade JE. Historical aspects of Q fever. In: Marrie TJ, editor, Q fever: the disease, vol. 1. Boca Raton (FL): CRC Press; 1990. p. 5–21.
2. Derrick EH. Q fever, new fever entity: clinical features, diagnosis and laboratory investigation. Med J Aust 1937;2:281–99.
3. Burnet FM, Freeman M. Experimental studies on the virus of Q fever. Med J Aust 1937;2:299–305.
4. Seshadri R, Paulsen IT, Eisen JA, et al. Complete genome sequence of the Q-fever pathogen *Coxiella burnetii*. Proc Natl Acad Sci U S A 2003;100: 5455–60.
5. Raoult D, Marrie TJ, Mege JL. Natural history and pathophysiology of Q fever. Lancet 2005;5:219–26.
6. Hoover TA, Culp DW, Vodkin MH, et al. Chromosomal DNA deletions explain phenotypic characteristics of two antigenic variants, phase II and RSA 514 (crazy), of the *Coxiella burnetii* nine mile strain. Infect Immun 2002;70:6726–33.
7. Maurin M, Raoult D. Q fever. Clin Microbiol Rev 1999;12:518–53.

8. Hackstadt T, Williams JC. Biochemical stratagem for obligate parasitism of eukaryotic cells by *Coxiella burnetii*. Proc Natl Acad Sci U S A 1981;78(5): 3240–4.
9. Ghigo E, Capo C, Tung CH, et al. *Coxiella burnetii* survival in THP-1 monocytes involves the impairment of phagosome maturation: IFN-g mediates its restoration and bacterial killing. J Immunol 2002;169:4488–95.
10. McCaul TF, Williams JC. Development cycle of *Coxiella burnetii*: structure and morphogenesis of vegetative and sporogenic differentiations. J Bacteriol. 1981;147:1063–76.
11. Sawyer LA, Fishbein DB, McDade JE. Q fever: current concepts. Rev Infect Dis 1987;9:935–46.
12. Christie AB, editor. Q fever. In: Infectious diseases, epidemiology and clinical practice. Edinburgh (UK): Churchill Livingstone; 1974. p. 876–91.
13. Karwa M, Currie B, Kvetan V. Bioterrorism: preparing for the impossible or the improbable. Crit Care Med 2005;33(1):S75–95.
14. Borchardt SM, Ritger KA, Dworkin MS. Categorization, prioritization and surveillance of potential bioterrorism agents. Infect Dis Clin North Am 2006; 20:213–25.
15. Azad AF, Radulovic S. Pathogenic rickettsiae as bioterrorism agents. Ann N Y Acad Sci 2003;990:734–8.
16. Waag DM. *Coxiella burnetii*: host and bacterial responses to infection. Vaccine 2007;25:7288–95.
17. Camacho MT, Outschoorn I, Tellez A, et al. Autoantibody profiles in the sera of patients with Q fever: characterization of antigens by immunofluorescence, immunoblot and sequence analysis. J Autoimmune Dis 2005;2:10.
18. Baca OG, Paretsky D. Q fever and *Coxiella burnetii*: a model for host-parasite interaction. Microbiol Rev 1983;47:127–49.
19. Babudieri B. Q fever: a zoonosis. Adv Vet Sci 1959;5:81–181.
20. Langley JM, Marrie TJ, Covert A, et al. Poker players' pneumonia: an urban outbreak following exposure to a parturient cat. N Engl J Med. 1988;319:354–6.
21. Marrie TJ, Durant H, Williams JC, et al. Exposure to parturient cats is a risk factor for acquisition of Q fever in Maritime Canada. J Infect Dis. 1988;158:101–8.
22. Hilbink F, Penrose M, Kovacova E, et al. Q fever is absent from New Zealand. Int J Epidemiol 1993;22:945–9.
23. Kobbe R, Kramme S, Gocht A, et al. Travel-associated *Coxiella burnetii* infections: three cases of Q fever with different clinical manifestations. Travel Med Infect Dis 2007;5:374–9.
24. Lumio J, Penttinen K, Pettersson T. Q fever in Finland: clinical, immunological and epidemiological findings. Scand J Infect Dis 1981;13:17–21.
25. Cohen NJ, Papernik M, Singleton J, et al. Q fever in an American tourist returned from Australia. Travel Med Infect Dis 2007;5:194–5.
26. Ta TH, Jiménez B, Navarro M, et al. Q fever in returned febrile travellers. J Travel Med 2008;15:126–9.
27. Dupuis G, Petite J, Peter O, et al. An important outbreak of human Q fever in a Swiss Alpine Valley. Int J Epidemiol 1987;16:282–6.
28. Salmon MM, Howells B, Glencross EJF, et al. Q fever in an urban area. Lancet. 1982;1:1002–4.
29. Oliphant JW, Gordon DA, Meis A, et al. Q fever in laundry workers presumably transmitted from contaminated clothing. Am J Hyg 1949;49:76–82.
30. Tissot-Dupont H, Torres S, Nezri M, et al. Hyperendemic focus of Q fever related to sheep and wind. Am J Epidemiol 1999;150:67–74.

31. Tissot-Dupont H, Amadei MA, Nezri M, et al. Wind in November, Q fever in December. Emerg Infect Dis 2004;10:1264–9.
32. Hawker JI, Ayres JG, Blair MR, et al. A large outbreak of Q fever in the West Midlands: windborne spread into a metropolitan area. Commun Dis Public Health 1998;1:180–7.
33. Johnson JE II, Kadull PJ. Laboratory acquired Q fever: a report of fifty cases. Am J Med 1966;41:391–403.
34. Hall CJ, Richmond SJ, Caul EO, et al. Laboratory outbreak of Q fever acquired from sheep. Lancet 1982;1:1004–6.
35. Meiklejohn G, Reimer LG, Graves PS, et al. Cryptic epidemic of Q fever in a medical school. J Infect Dis 1981;144:107–14.
36. Comment on Q fever transmitted by blood transfusion—United States [editorial]. Can Dis Wkly Rep 1977;3:210.
37. Harman JB. Q fever in Great Britain: clinical account of eight cases. Lancet 1949;2:1028–30.
38. Gerth HJ, Leidig U, Reimenschneider TH. Q-fieber-epidemie in einem Institut fur Humanpathologie. Dtsch Med Wochenschr 1982;107:1391–5 [in German].
39. Deutch DL, Peterson ET. Q fever: transmission from one human being to others. JAMA 1950;143:348–50.
40. McQusiton JH, Holman RC, McCall CL, et al. National surveillance and the epidemiology of Q fever in the United States, 1978–2004. Am J Trop Med Hyg 2006;75:36–40.
41. McQusiton JH, Childs JE. Q fever in humans and animals in the United States. Vector Borne Zoonotic Dis 2002;2:179–91.
42. Kim SG, Kim EH, Lafferty CJ, et al. *Coxiella burnetii* in bulk tank milk samples, United States. Emerg Infect Dis 2005;11:619–21.
43. Bamberg WM, Pape WJ, Beebe JL, et al. Outbreak of Q fever associated with a horse-boarding ranch, Colorado, 2005. Vector Borne Zoonotic Dis 2007;7:49–55.
44. Sawyer LA, Fishbein DB, McDade JE. Q fever in patients with hepatitis and pneumonia: results of laboratory-based surveillance in the United States. J Infect Dis 1988;158:497–8.
45. Karakousis PC, Trucksis M, Dumler JS. Chronic Q fever in the United States. J Clin Microbiol 2006;44:2238–87.
46. Hellenbrand W, Breuer T, Petersen L. Changing epidemiology of Q fever in Germany 1947–1999. Emerg Infect Dis 2001;7:789–96.
47. Marrie TJ. Epidemiology of Q fever. In: Marrie TJ, editor, Q fever: the disease, vol. 1. Boca Raton (FL): CRC Press; 1990. p. 49–70.
48. Communicable diseases Australia. Number of notifications of Q fever Australia, 1991–2006.
49. National Notifiable Diseases Surveillance System. Notification of diseases by state and territory and year 2005. Available at: http://www9.healtht.gov.au/cda/Source/Rpt_2_cfm. Accessed August 16, 2008.
50. Garner MG, Longbottom AM, Cannon RM, et al. A review of Q fever in Australia 1991–1994. Aust N Z J Public Health 1997;21:722–30.
51. Anderson AD, Smook B, Shuping E, et al. Q fever and the US military. Emerg Infect Dis 2005;11:1320–2.
52. Delsing CE, Kullberg BJ. Q fever in the Netherlands: a concise overview and implications of the largest ongoing outbreak. Neth J Med 2008;66:365–7.
53. Karagiannis I, Schimmer B, van Lier A, et al. Outbreak investigation of Q fever outbreak in a rural setting in the Netherlands. Europ Soc Clin Microbiol Infect

Dis 18th European Congress of Clinical Microbiol Infect Dis Barcelona, Spain 19–22 2008;Abstract P. 1836.
54. Fournier PE, Marrie TJ, Raoult D. Diagnosis of Q fever. J Clin Microbiol 1998;36: 1823–34.
55. Tissot-Dupont H, Raoult D, Brouqui P, et al. Epidemiologic features and clinical presentation of acute Q fever in hospitalized patients: 323 French cases. Am J Med 1992;93:427–34.
56. Haldane EV, Marrie TJ, Faulkner RS, et al. Endocarditis due to Q fever in Nova Scotia: experience with five patients in 1981–1982. J Infect Dis. 1983;148: 978–85.
57. Huebner RJ, Jellison WL. Beck MD. Q fever: a review of current knowledge. Ann Intern Med 1949;30:495–509.
58. Powell O. Q fever: clinical features in 72 cases. Australas Ann Med 1960;9: 214–23.
59. Marrie TJ. *Coxiella burnetii* (Q fever) pneumonia. Clin Infect Dis 1995; 21(Suppl 3):S253–64.
60. Murphy PP, Richardson SG. Q fever pneumonia presenting as an eosinophilic pleural effusion. Thorax 1989;44:228–9.
61. Caughey JE. Pleuropericardial lesion in Q fever. Br Med J 1977;i:1477.
62. Lieberman D, Lieberman D, Boldur I, et al. Q-fever pneumonia in the Negev Region of Israel: a review of 20 patients hospitalized over a period of one year. J Infect 1995;30:135–40.
63. Anton E. A frequent error in the etiology of round pneumonia [letter]. Chest 2004; 125:1592–3.
64. Montes M, Cilla G, Vicente D, et al. Gipuzkoa, Basque Country, Spain, (1984–2004): a hyperendemic area of Q fever. Ann N Y Acad Sci 2006; 1078:129–32.
65. Gordon JD, MacKeen AD, Marrie TJ, et al. The radiographic features of epidemic and sporadic Q fever pneumonia. J Can Assoc Radiol 1984;35:293–6.
66. Millar JK. The chest film findings in Q fever: a series of 35 cases. Clin Radiol 1978;329:371–5.
67. Voloudaki AE, Kofteridis DP, Tritou IN, et al. Q fever pneumonia: CT findings. Radiology 2000;215(3):880–3.
68. Lefebvre M, Grossi O, Agard C, et al. Systemic immune presentations of *Coxiella burnetii* infection (Q fever). Semin Arthritis Rheum 2008. [Epub ahead of print].
69. Korman TM, Spelman DW, Perry GJ, et al. Acute glomerulonephritis associated with Q fever: case report and review of renal complications. J Infect Dis 1998;26: 359–64.
70. Kosatsky T. Household outbreak of Q-fever pneumonia related to a parturient cat. Lancet 1984;ii:1447–9.
71. Larsen CP, Bell JM, Ketel BL, et al. Infection in renal transplantation: a case of acute Q fever. Am J Kidney Dis 2006;48:321–6.
72. Raoult D, Levy PY, Dupont HT. Q fever and HIV infection. AIDS. 1993;7(1): 81–6.
73. Pierce TH, Yucht SC, Gorin AB, et al. Q fever pneumonitis: diagnosis by transbronchoscopic lung biopsy. West J Med. 1979;130:453–5.
74. Perin TL. Histopathologic observations in a fatal case of Q fever. Arch Pathol 1949;47:361–5.
75. Urso FP. The pathologic findings in rickettsial pneumonia. Am J Clin Pathol 1975;64:335–42.

76. Janigan DT, Marrie TJ. An inflammatory pseudotumor of the lung in Q fever pneumonia. N Engl J Med 1983;30:86–8.
77. Stein A, Louveau C, Lepidi H, et al. Q fever pneumonia: virulence of *Coxiella burnetii* pathovars in a murine model of aerosol infection. Infect Immun 2005;73: 2469–73.
78. White RJ, Blainey AD, Harrison KJ, et al. Causes of pneumonia presenting to a district general hospital. Thorax 1981;35:566–70.
79. Marrie TJ, Haldane EV, Noble MA, et al. Causes of atypical pneumonia: results of a 1-year prospective study. Can Med Assoc J 1981;118(125):1118–23.
80. Lim WS, Macfarlane JT, Boswell TCJ, et al. Study of community-acquired pneumonia etiology (SCAPA) in adults admitted to hospital: implications for management guidelines. Thorax 2001;56:296–301.
81. Lai CH, Huang CK, Chin C, et al. Acute Q fever: an emerging and endemic disease in southern Taiwan. Scand J Infect Dis 2008;40:105–10.
82. Raoult D, Tissot-Dupont H, Foucault C, et al. Q fever 1985–1998: clinical and epidemiologic features of 1,383 infections. Medicine 2000;79:109–23.
83. Hoontrakul S, Intaranongpai W, Silpasakorn S, et al. Causes of acute, undifferentiated, febrile illness in rural Thailand: results of a prospective observational study. Ann Trop Med Parasitol 2006;100:363–70.
84. Parra Ruiz J, Peña Monje A, Tomás Jiménez C, et al. Clinical spectrum of fever of intermediate duration in the south of Spain. Eur J Clin Microbiol Infect Dis 2008; 27:993–5.
85. Porten K, Rissland J, Tigges A, et al. A super-spreading ewe infects hundreds at a farmers' market in Germany. BMC Infect Dis 2006;6:147.
86. Wade AJ, Cheng AC, Athan E, et al. Q fever outbreak at a cosmetics supply factory. Clin Infect Dis 2006;42:e50–2.
87. Stein A, Raoult D. A simple method for amplification of DNA from paraffin-embedded tissues. Nucleic Acids Res 1992;20:5237–8.
88. Raoult D, Torres H, Drancourt M. Shell-vial assay: evaluation of a new technique for determining antibiotic susceptibility, tested in 13 isolates of *Coxiella burnetii*. Antimicrob Agents Chemother 1991;35:2070–7.
89. Conti LA, Belcuore TR, Nicholson WL, et al. Pseudoepidemic of Q fever at an animal research facility. Vector Borne Zoonotic Dis 2004;4:343–50.
90. Mandell LA, Wunderink RG, Anzueto A, et al. Infectious diseases society of America/American thoracic society consensus guidelines on the management of community-acquired pneumonia in adults. Clin Infect Dis 2007;44:S27–72.
91. Gikas A, Spyridaki I, Scoulica E, et al. In vitro susceptibility of *Coxiella burnetii* to linezolid in comparison with its susceptibilities to quinolones, doxycycline and clarithromycin. Antimicrob Agents Chemother 2001;45:3276–8.
92. Yeaman MR, Mitscher LA, Baca OG. In vitro susceptibility of *Coxiella burnetii* to antibiotics, including several quinolones. Antimicrobial Agents Chemother 1987; 31:1079–84.
93. Sobradillo V, Zalacain R, Capebastegui A, et al. Antibiotic treatment in pneumonia due to Q fever. Thorax 1992;47:276–8.
94. Kuzman I, Schonwald S, Culig J, et al. The efficacy of azithromycin in the treatment of Q fever: a retrospective study. In: Proceedings of the IV International Conference on the Macrolides, Azalides, Streptogramins and Ketolides. Barcelona (Spain); 1998. p. 47.
95. Kofterids D, Gikas A, Spiradakis G, et al. Clinical response to Q fever infection to macrolides. In: Proceedings of the IV International Conference on the Macrolides, Azalides, Streptogramins, and Ketolides. Barcelona (Spain); 1998. p. 47.

96. Pérez-del-Molino A, Aguado JM, Riancho JA, et al. Erythromycin and the treatment of *Coxiella burnetii* pneumonia. J Antimicrob Chemother 1991;28:455–9.
97. Morovic M. Short report. Q fever pneumonia: are clarithromycin and moxifloxacin alternative treatments Orally? Am J Trop Med Hyg 2005;73:947–8.
98. Carcopino X, Raoult D, Bretelle F, et al. Managing Q fever during pregnancy: the benefits of long-term co-trimoxazole therapy. Clin Infect Dis 2007;45:548–55.
99. Aloizos S, Gourgiotis S, Oikonomou K, et al. Recurrent Jarish-Herxheimer reaction in a patient with Q fever pneumonia: a case report. Cases J 2008;1:360.
100. Fenollar F, Fournier PE, Carrieri MP, et al. Risk factors and prevention of Q fever endocarditis. Clin Infect Dis 2001;33:312–6.

Tularemia Pneumonia

Lora D. Thomas, MD, MPH[a,*], William Schaffner, MD[b]

KEYWORDS

• *Francisella tularensis* • Tularemia • Zoonosis • Bioterrorism

Tularemia is a zoonotic infection seen primarily in the Northern Hemisphere. It is caused by the bacteria *Francisella tularensis*, and it most commonly is acquired from arthropod bites or handling of animal carcasses such as rabbits and hares. The disease caused by *F tularensis* has been called many names including rabbit fever, deer-fly fever, and Ohara fever.[1–4] Although the ulceroglandular form of the disease is the more common manifestation of infection, *F tularensis* is known to cause pneumonia, particularly in North America.[2,5–10] This is why it is important to obtain a thorough social and exposure history when evaluating a patient with an atypical pneumonia.

HISTORICAL BACKGROUND

In the 19th century, a Japanese physician named Homma Soken described a febrile illness associated with adenopathy that presented in individuals who had eaten hare meat.[11] Several decades later, in 1911, a new pathogen was isolated from rodents suffering from a plague-like illness in Tulare County, California. This organism was named *Bacterium tularense* after the county in which it was discovered.[12] The first documented human case of infection with *B tularense* was in 1914, when a meat cutter developed conjunctivitis and lymphadenopathy. Edward Francis, then an appointed officer of the United States Public Health Service, went on to describe the clinical and epidemiologic features of the disease in 1928 after reviewing over 800 cases of infection. He eventually developed the term tularemia and was able to confirm that it was the etiology of Yato-byo or wild hare disease that had been described in Japan by both Soken and another Japanese physician named Hachiro Ohara.[13] Over the years, the pathogen underwent numerous taxonomic reclassifications, until it was finally named *Francisella tularensis* in 1947 after Francis himself.[1]

MICROBIOLOGY

F tularensis is a small gram-negative coccobacillus, with four identified subspecies. *F tularensis* subspecies *tularensis* (type A) is seen almost exclusively in North America

[a] Division of Infectious Diseases, Department of Medicine, Vanderbilt University Medical Center, A2200 MCN, 1161 21st Avenue South, Nashville, TN 37232, USA
[b] Department of Preventive Medicine, Vanderbilt University School of Medicine, 1500 21st Avenue, Nashville, TN 37212, USA
* Corresponding author.
E-mail address: lora.thomas@vanderbilt.edu (L.D. Thomas).

Infect Dis Clin N Am 24 (2010) 43–55
doi:10.1016/j.idc.2009.10.012
0891-5520/10/$ – see front matter. Published by Elsevier Inc.

and is considered the most virulent strain of *F tularensis* in both animal models and people.[1] Staples and colleagues evaluated strains of *F tularensis* type A isolated in the United States with molecular subtyping analysis and discovered two subpopulations (type A1 [east] and type A2 [west]). These two subpopulations of type A differ in their geographic distribution and disease outcomes. Type A2 isolates were identified from states west of the 100th meridian line and affected younger and more immunocompetent individuals compared with hosts afflicted with type A1 strains, which predominantly were encountered east of the 100th meridian line.[14] More recently, two genotypes of A1 isolates have been discovered: type A1a and A1b. Both of these genotypes are found primarily in the eastern United States, but data suggest that A1b causes more invasive and lethal disease than A1a or A2.[15]

F tularensis subspecies holarctica (type B) is the predominant strain in Europe and Japan, but is also present in North America. *F tularensis* type B can be differentiated from subspecies type A by its inability to ferment glycerol, and clinically it is less virulent. *F tularensis* subspecies *mediaasiatica* is found primarily in central Asia and Russia.[1] The fourth subspecies of *F tularensis* is *novicida*, causing only a handful of reported human cases in Thailand, Australia, and the United States.[16,17]

In the laboratory, *F tularensis* is a fastidious organism, requiring specific culture media to grow. It grows best when the agar is enriched with cysteine or cystine, and incubation is performed at higher temperatures (95° F to 99° F). Colonies will appear after 2 to 5 days and are greenish–white and smooth in appearance. If an enriched whole blood medium is used, alpha hemolysis may be present. Ironically, in the natural environment, *F tularensis* is a hardy bacterium in that it can survive in environmental sources, such as animal carcasses, water, and wet soil, for several weeks.[1,18]

PATHOGENESIS

F tularensis, particularly subspecies type A, is a highly virulent intracellular pathogen, requiring only 10 to 50 organisms to cause human disease. Acquisition of *F tularensis* occurs predominantly in four forms: bite from an infected arthropod, handling of an infected animal carcass, oral consumption of contaminated food or water, and inhalation of infectious droplets. The incubation period is roughly 3 to 6 days, and the mode of inoculation largely determines how the disease manifests itself. After inoculation, *F tularensis* proliferates locally and invades regional lymph nodes. It likely is disseminated by lymphohematogenous spread to multiple organs in the body, including the liver, spleen, lungs, kidneys, intestine, and central nervous system.[1,4,18] Biopsies of involved lymph nodes can show acute inflammation, necrosis, microabscesses, and even granulomatous changes. When pneumonic tularemia is present, lung biopsies may show necrotizing pneumonia with abundant fibrin, cellular debris, and neutrophilic infiltration of the alveola.[19]

Several cases of laboratory-acquired tularemia have been described, highlighting the risk involved in studying this pathogen.[9] The pathogenesis of *F tularensis* is still not understood well, but its ability to survive and replicate in macrophages appears to be its most prominent virulence feature.[20] Like other gram-negative organisms, *F tularensis* contains a lipopolysaccharide (LPS), but it behaves as an atypical endotoxin, in that it elicits a weak cytokine response compared with other gram-negative bacteria. Another possible source of virulence of *F tularensis* is its capsule. Predominantly composed of lipids, the capsule is believed to protect *F tularensis* from lysis in the serum.[21]

EPIDEMIOLOGY

Incidence

Tularemia has a worldwide distribution in the Northern Hemisphere, but its exact incidence is unknown. It was frequent in the United States before World War II, when a peak of 2291 cases occurred in 1939. Since 1958, the number of tularemia cases in the United States has declined steadily and since 1967, only 100 to 200 cases per year have been reported. The reasons for this decline are not fully known, but several theories have been postulated, including better awareness regarding arthropod bite prevention, less hunting and trapping, and a reduction in size of rural populations. Those infected are overwhelmingly male (greater than 70%), and while most of those infected are adults, the highest incidence of disease in the years between 1990 and 2000 was in children ages 1 to 14, and in adults over 75 years of age.[22] Tularemia occurs most commonly between the months of May and September.[15]

Risk Factors

When evaluating a patient with community-acquired pneumonia, it is important for the clinician to ask detailed questions regarding the patient's personal, social, and occupational history. *F tularensis* infects multiple terrestrial and aquatic mammals, so suspicion should be raised if a patient relates a history of exposure to a potentially infected animal. Mammals most famous for transmitting tularemia include lagomorphs, or rabbits and hares. In the United States, most lagomorphs that have transmitted tularemia to people had been infected with the type A strain. Domesticated cats, thought to be an incidental host of tularemia, are increasingly being recognized as a source of infection to people, and they also transmit type A strains. In fact, a recent study found that more than 80% of human cases of tularemia type A acquired from animal contact occur after exposure to domesticated cats or lagomorphs.[15] Other rodents, such as voles, squirrels, muskrats, mice, and beavers can harbor *F tularensis*, but type B strains are more frequent in these animals. Skinning or eating infected animals is the primary mode of transmission, although scratches and bites explain most of the cases acquired from domesticated cats.[23]

Blood-feeding arthropods serve as another vector of transmission. Multiple tick species including the dog tick, wood tick, and Lone Star tick have been found to harbor *F tularensis*, and most tick-acquired tularemia involves type A strains. Deer flies and mosquitoes are also possible vectors, although mosquito-transmitted tularemia is seen predominantly in Europe and Russia.[18]

Data in patients with pneumonic tularemia suggest that these patients are less likely to remember or identify a vector exposure in their history compared with patients without pneumonia.[6] Because tularemia pneumonia is occasionally acquired through infected aerosolized droplets, this potentially can occur without any evidence of animal or arthropod exposure. It is believed that *F tularensis* can become aerosolized through lawn mowing or brush cutting, which can explain why landscapers and farmers are at increased risk of developing pneumonic tularemia.[7] Pneumonia related to tularemia has been described in two adolescents who had run over a rabbit with a lawnmower, thus coining the phrase "lawnmower tularemia".[24]

Geographic Distribution

In the United States, human cases of tularemia have been diagnosed in every state but Hawaii. Most cases are concentrated in the south–central United States, with the majority occurring in Arkansas, Oklahoma, Texas, Missouri, and Louisiana.

Substantial numbers of cases are also reported in the mountain states such as Montana, Utah, and Colorado.[22] Infections with *F tularensis* types A and B occur throughout the United States. In Europe and Russia, *F tularensis* type B is the primary strain, and outbreaks have been reported within the past decade in Spain, Scandinavia, Turkey, and Kosovo.[25–27] Type B tularemia also occurs in Japan.[28]

Outbreaks of Pulmonary Tularemia: Martha's Vineyard

In the summer of 1978, seven individuals who had been staying at a cottage in Martha's Vineyard developed an acute febrile illness within 2 weeks of their cottage residence. None of the affected individuals had any skin or oropharyngeal lesions, but five developed pneumonia, and all seven were diagnosed with tularemia by serology. Specimens of water, soil, and dust debris taken from around the cottage tested negative for *F tularensis*, but the group's two pet dogs, which reportedly captured rabbits near the house, had serologic evidence of recent infection. An island-wide investigation revealed that eight other people in Martha's Vineyard had evidence of tularemia infection, seven of whom had pleuropulmonary disease. Two of those individuals were gardeners, and one was a sheepshearer.[29]

In 2000, a second outbreak of primary pneumonic tularemia was reported from Martha's Vineyard. Fifteen cases of tularemia were identified, 11 of which had pulmonary disease. One of the patients died, who ultimately grew *F tularensis* type A from his blood and lung tissue. A case–control study identified recent lawn mowing or brush cutting as significant risk factors for acquiring tularemia. Multiple cultures were performed of lawnmower filters, cut grass, soil, and water, all of which were negative for *F tularensis*. It was hypothesized that animal excrement infected with *F tularensis* underwent mechanical aerosolization during lawn mowing, which ultimately was inhaled by the affected individuals.[30] Between 2000 and 2006, 59 cases of tularemia were reported from Martha's Vineyard, 64% of which had a primary pneumonic presentation. These cases typically involved young male landscapers who would present with high fevers (up to 104°F), but few localizing signs of infection. A nonproductive cough usually developed 2 to 4 days into the illness. Seroprevalence studies in insects and animals on the island have documented that dog ticks, skunks, and raccoons are the primary reservoirs of this disease.[7] Why tularemia commonly presents as pneumonic disease on this island has yet to be elucidated.

CLINICAL MANIFESTATIONS

Different clinical syndromes have been described with tularemia, manifestations that are determined by the infecting strain of *F tularensis* and mode of acquisition. Ulceroglandular tularemia is the most common form (up to 80% of cases) and often originates as an infected skin lesion that eventually leads to localized lymphadenopathy.[2] The original skin lesion erupts after a tick bite or animal contact, and the lesion eventually ulcerates with raised edges. Glandular tularemia is similar to ulceroglandular tularemia in that localized lymphadenopathy is present, but without a skin lesion. Oculoglandular tularemia occurs when the organism is introduced through the conjunctiva, causing painful conjunctivitis and lymphadenopathy in the preauricular, submandibular, and cervical regions. Oropharyngeal tularemia often is acquired by consuming contaminated food or water, or it can be acquired through the respiratory route with contaminated droplets. It usually will present as a painful exudative pharyngitis or tonsillitis.[1–4]

Typhoidal tularemia refers to the systemic form of infection with *F tularensis* and may develop after any mode of acquisition. It is seen less commonly than ulceroglandular disease and accounts for up to 30% of cases.[3] Typhoidal tularemia often presents with high fevers, headache, myalgias, prostration, vomiting, and diarrhea. Some of the more severe manifestations of tularemia are seen with the typhoidal form of disease such as renal failure, rhabdomyolisis, pericarditis, meningitis, and erythema nodosum.[2,31] As would be expected, typhoidal disease is associated with higher morbidity and mortality. Because of its increased virulence, *F tularensis* type A is associated more commonly with typhoidal disease.[15]

Pneumonic tularemia can be seen with either ulceroglandular or typhoidal disease, although it is much more common with typhoidal infection. In this situation, it is thought that pneumonia is a complication of hematogenous seeding of the lungs. One Louisiana study found that 44% of typhoidal cases of tularemia presented with pleuropulmonary disease, while only 17% of ulceroglandular cases had pneumonia.[3] Because tularemia pneumonia is a more invasive form of infection, it is more likely to be caused by *F tularensis* type A, and as such, it is much more common in North America compared with other parts of the world (**Table 1**). Scofield and colleagues[6] examined factors associated with pneumonic tularemia among cases in Oklahoma and identified increased age, absence of a known vector exposure, and typhoidal illness (versus ulceroglandular disease) as characteristics associated with pneumonia. Primary pneumonic tularemia (as opposed to secondary pneumonia seen in ulceroglandular or typhoidal disease) is considered to be a separate entity acquired from inhalation of organisms. This form of tularemia pneumonia is uncommon and primarily has been described in those working in occupations that put the individual at increased risk of aerosolized exposure such as laboratory workers, landscapers, farmers, and sheapshearers.[18]

When a patient infected with *F tularensis* presents with pneumonia, it is likely that the respiratory symptoms began a few days and even weeks after initial symptoms occurred. High fevers (as high as 104°F) will occur abruptly, and headache is a prominent feature. Within time, a nonproductive cough with or without pleuritic chest pain (which occurs in about one third of cases) may occur.[5–7] Differentiating pneumonic tularemia from other community-acquired pneumonias can be difficult. That is why it is important for the clinician to have a high index of suspicion and to inquire about appropriate risk factors. Of note, the relative bradycardia that has been described with other atypical pneumonias, such as *Legionella* and psittacosis, is usually absent in pneumonic tularemia.[5]

Radiographic Studies

The radiographic features of pulmonary tularemia are highly variable, as can be seen in **Table 2**. Some reports describe multilobar patchy opacities as the primary radiographic pattern in patients with pneumonic tularemia,[8,10] while others note more unilobar consolidations.[2,6] Ovoid opacities, a feature that historically has been considered pathognomonic for tularemia pneumonia, are seen in a minority of cases. Pleural effusions and hilar adenopathy are common.

Fig. 1A is a chest radiograph of a 26-year-old man who was the owner of a junk yard. He was admitted to a hospital in Nashville, Tennessee with fever, pneumonia, and encephalopathy. As can be seen in the radiograph, he had an extensive right multilobar pneumonia. Cerebrospinal fluid analysis revealed 15 leukocytes that were predominantly neutrophils and monocytes. The patient lived in a trailer. The crawl space under the trailer was littered with dead rabbits that were placed there by the patient's dog. Shortly after his admission, a nurse combed a tick out of the patient's hair that had been attached to his scalp (**Fig. 1**B). Thus, he had two risk factors for

Table 1
Proportion of tularemia cases with pulmonary involvement based on geographic location

References	Years that Cases Occurred	Geographic Region	Total Number of Tularemia Cases	Number (%) of Pulmonary Cases	Total Mortality	Mortality in Pulmonary Cases
United States						
2	1949–79	Tennessee	88	36 (41%)	2 (2%)	2 (6%)
6	1982–87	Oklahoma	128	32 (25%)	5 (4%)	4 (13%)
7	2000–06	Massachusetts[a]	59	38 (64%)	1 (2%)	1 (3%)
Europe						
26	2000–04	Sweden	234	11 (5%)	0 (0%)	0 (0%)
25	1997	Spain	140	5 (4%)	NA	0 (0%)
27	1988–98	Turkey	205	1 (0.5%)	0 (0%)	0 (0%)
Asia						
28	1924–87	Japan	1355	0 (0%)	0 (0%)	—

Abbreviation: NA, information not available.
[a] Martha's Vineyard, Massachusetts.

Table 2
Radiographic patterns in pneumonic tularemia

References	10	6	8	2
Number of cases reviewed	29	32	50	37
Radiographic pattern				
Infiltrates	93%	94%	92%	97%
Unilobar	28%	60%	18%	61%
Multilobar/diffuse	65%	34%	74%	30%
Pleural effusion	21%	25%	30%	32%
Hilar adenopathy	45%	NA	32%	NA
Oval density	7%	NA	8%	NA

Abbreviation: NA, information not available.

tularemia: exposure to rabbits and ticks. The patient's serologic testing revealed a diagnostic rise in *F tularensis* titers.

Several aspects of pneumonic tularemia can mimic features of pulmonary tuberculosis. Analysis of pleural fluid in patients with tularemia usually reveals a lymphocyte-rich exudate with high concentrations of adenosine deaminase, characteristics that are also seen in pleuritic tuberculosis.[32] Additionally, pleural biopsies in both diseases

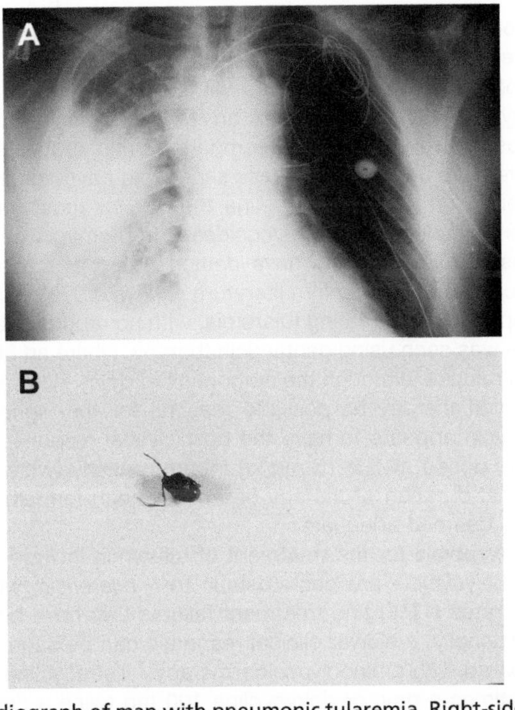

Fig. 1. (*A*) Chest radiograph of man with pneumonic tularemia. Right-sided multilobar infiltrates are seen. (*Courtesy of* Barney S. Graham, MD, PhD, National Institutes of Health, Bethesda, Maryland.) (*B*) Tick that was combed out of patient's hair after admission. (*Courtesy of* Barney S. Graham, MD, PhD, National Institutes of Health, Bethesda, Maryland.)

can reveal granulomas, and tularemia patients also can present with apical infiltrates or a military pattern on chest radiograph.[8]

DIAGNOSIS

Because the organism is difficult to grow using standard culture media (and can expose laboratory workers to the risk of infection), serologic testing is often the preferred method for diagnosing tularemia. Most commercially available serologic tests employ agglutination or enzyme-linked immunosorbent assay (ELISA) methodology. A fourfold rise in antibody levels between acute and convalescent immunoglobulin G (IgG) titers, an acute microagglutination titer of 1:128, or an acute tube agglutination titer of 1:160 is presumptive of infection.[18] The downside to using serology in the early phase of the illness is its poor sensitivity, because most individuals do not develop detectable antibody levels until the second week of illness,[33] and a lone positive antibody titer may be indicative of remote infection. Polymerase chain reaction (PCR) assays are being used increasingly in the diagnosis of tularemia and can be performed on a number of clinical specimens, including ulcer swabs, lymph node aspirations, tissue, and blood. In one study of patients with ulceroglandular tularemia, PCR performed on wound swabs showed a sensitivity of 78% and a specificity of 96%.[34] The sensitivity of these assays performed on blood is considerably lower, which may be from inhibitory compounds present in the blood.[1] There are few data regarding use of PCR techniques on respiratory specimens, outside of lung tissue.

TREATMENT

Early recognition of infection with *F tularensis* followed by prompt, appropriate treatment is crucial in reducing morbidity from tularemia. In an evaluation to identify factors associated with poor outcome in patients with tularemia, Penn and Kinasewitz[35] showed that delayed therapy led to more adverse outcomes and mortality. There have been no prospective clinical trials comparing antimicrobial agents in treating tularemia, but there have been multiple case series that have documented the effectiveness of different therapies.[36–38] First-line therapy for most forms of tularemia, including pneumonia, includes aminoglycosides. Streptomycin and gentamicin are bactericidal against *F tularensis* and have demonstrated effectiveness in both the laboratory and in clinical tularemia. In a literature review, a 97% cure rate was documented using streptomycin in treating tularemia, with no reported relapses. A slightly higher relapse rate was seen using gentamicin therapy, where an 86% cure rate was observed, and 6% relapse (although the authors cited delay in initiation of therapy or shortened duration of therapy as possible reasons for the higher relapse rate).[36] Because streptomycin appears to have the best clinical response, it is considered the drug of choice, dosed at 7.5–15 mg/kg intramuscularly twice a day for adults. Although the optimal duration of therapy has never been formally studied, 7 to 10 days of therapy are deemed adequate.[18]

Alternative antimicrobials for the treatment of tularemia include the tetracyclines. Tetracycline and doxycycline are bacterostatic to *F tularensis*, which may explain the higher relapse rates (12%) and treatment failures that have been reported with their use.[36,38] Additionally, a slower clinical response can be seen with tetracycline/doxycycline compared with aminoglycoside therapy.[7] Tetracycline 500 mg orally or intravenously four times a day, or doxycycline 100 mg twice a day can be used in adults, but the duration of therapy is longer: 14 days.

Chloramphenicol also has been used successfully in treating cases of tularemia, although its relapse rate is 21%. In general, the use of chloramphenicol has fallen out of favor because of its toxicities, including blood dyscrasias. In the case of tularemic meningitis, however, some have recommended that both chloramphenicol and streptomycin be used in combination, because of streptomycin's unreliable penetration in the cerebral spinal fluid.[18] The quinolones have excellent in vitro, bactericidal activity against *F tularensis*. Several cases, including cases of *F tularensis* pneumonia, have been described where patients were treated successfully with quinolone therapy.[37] In an outbreak of oropharyngeal tularemia in Turkey, patients receiving quinolone therapy had similar outcomes compared with patients who received aminoglycosides.[38] Most *F tularensis* strains are resistant to beta-lactam antibiotics and azithromycin.[39]

Box 1
Working Group Consensus recommendation for treatment of patients with tularemia in a contained casualty setting

Adults

First-line therapy

- Streptomycin, 1 gm intramuscularly twice daily
- Gentamicin 5 mg/kg intramuscularly or intravenously once daily

Second-line therapy

- Doxycycline 100 mg intravenously twice daily
- Chloramphenicol 15 mg/kg intravenously four times daily
- Ciprofloxacin 400 mg intravenously twice daily

Children

First-line therapy

- Streptomycin 15 mg/kg intramuscularly twice daily (not to exceed 2 g/d)
- Gentamicin 2.5 mg/kg intramuscularly or intravenously three times daily

Second-line therapy

- Doxycycline 100 mg intravenously twice daily if weight ≥45 kg; 2.2 mg/kg intravenously twice daily if weight <45 kg
- Chloramphenicol 15 mg/kg intravenously four times daily
- Ciprofloxacin 15 mg/kg intravenously twice daily

Pregnant Women

First-line therapy

- Gentamicin 5 mg/kg intramuscularly or intravenously once daily
- Streptomycin 1 g intravenously twice daily

Second-line therapy

- Doxycycline 100 mg intravenously twice daily
- Ciprofloxacin 400 mg intravenously twice daily

Duration of therapy for streptomycin, gentamicin, and ciprofloxacin is 10 days.

Duration of therapy for doxycycline, and chloramphenicol is 2 to 3 weeks.

Patients treated with intramuscular or intravenous doxycycline, ciprofloxacin, or chloramphenicol can switch to oral therapy when clinically indicated.

Data from Dennis DT, Inglesby TV, Henderson DA, et al. Tularemia as a biologic weapon: medical and public health management. JAMA 2001;285(21):2763–73.

BIOTERRORISM THREAT

Several characteristics of *F tularensis* have made it an attractive agent to potentially use as a biologic weapon. Two of the more obvious characteristics include its ability to be acquired by the respiratory route and to cause infection with a small number of organisms. Historically, both the United States and the former Soviet Union have had programs developing weapons containing *F tularensis*. The United States reportedly ceased their developments in the early 1970s, after signing the 1972 Convention on the Prohibition of Development, Production, and Stockpiling of Bacteriological and Toxin Weapons and their Destruction. The former Soviet Union continued with their biologic warfare programs well into the 1990s, developing strains of *F tularensis* that were both antibiotic- and vaccine-resistant.[40] After Sept. 11, 2001, and the events of the postal anthrax outbreak, there has been renewed concern regarding *F tularensis* being used as a biologic weapon.

The Working Group on Civilian Biodefense published a consensus statement regarding the use of *F tularensis* as a biologic weapon.[41] They explained that the most likely method that would be used to infect a large population would be through aerosol release, and if this occurred in a densely populated area, large numbers of cases involving an acute febrile illness would arise in 3 to 5 days. Pleuropneumonic disease could develop in the ensuing days and weeks, creating a substantial number of cases. Airborne exposure of *F tularensis* also can cause eye contamination, resulting in ocular tularemia, or pharyngitis with cervical adenopathy. In contrast to infections caused by other bioterrorist pathogens, it generally is believed that a slower progression of disease would be seen in the setting of a tularemia outbreak. In the early stages of the outbreak, this characteristic might distinguish this disease from that caused by *Yersinia pestis* (where a rapid progression to severe pneumonia would be seen) or *Bacillus anthracis* (symmetric mediastinal widening without presence of

Box 2
Working Group Consensus recommendations for treatment of patients with tularemia in a mass casualty setting and for postexposure prophylaxis

Adults

First-line therapy

- Doxycycline 100 mg by mouth twice daily
- Ciprofloxacin 500 mg by mouth twice daily

Children

First-line therapy

- Doxycycline 100 mg by mouth twice daily if weight ≥45 kg; 2.2 mg/kg by mouth twice daily if weight <45 kg
- Ciprofloxacin 15 mg/kg by mouth twice daily (not to exceed 1 g/d)

Pregnant Women

Fist-line therapy

- Ciprofloxacin 500 mg by mouth twice daily
- Doxycycline 100 mg by mouth twice daily

Duration of all recommended therapies is 14 days.

Data from Dennis DT, Inglesby TV, Henderson DA, et al. Tularemia as a biologic weapon: medical and public health management. JAMA 2001;285(21):2763–73.

bronchopneumonia). The Working Group Consensus made recommendations for treatment of tularemia in both contained and mass casualty settings; these are shown in **Boxes 1** and **2**.

Because of the fear of a bioterrorism attack, there has been increased interest in developing an effective vaccine. A live vaccine strain (LVS) tularemia vaccine has been in development in the United States since the 1950s. It is administered by scarification, requiring a bifurcated needle to make multiple inoculations in much the same way that the smallpox vaccine is given. In a retrospective study of civilians who worked in a military laboratory at Fort Detrick, Maryland, the incidence of typhoidal tularemia fell from 5.70 to 0.27 cases per 1000 employee years when employees who had been vaccinated with the LVS vaccine were compared with employees who had been vaccinated with a killed tularemia vaccine. Incidence of ulceroglandular disease did not change, although the individuals that received the LVS vaccine suffered milder symptoms.[42]

SUMMARY

F tularensis is a zoonotic infection that can be acquired in multiple ways, including a bite from an arthropod, the handling of animal carcasses, consumption of contaminated food and water, or inhalation of infected particles. The most virulent subspecies of *F tularensis* is type A, which is almost exclusively seen in North America. Pneumonia can occur in tularemia, as either a primary process from direct inhalation, or as a secondary manifestation of ulceroglandular or typhoidal disease. Although streptomycin and gentamicin remain the drugs of choice for most forms of tularemia, doxycycline and the quinolones also have activity against *F tularensis*. Because of its high virulence, *F tularensis* could be used as a potential bioterrorist weapon.

REFERENCES

1. Ellis J, Oyston PC, Green M, et al. Tularemia. Clin Microbiol Rev 2002;15(4):631–46.
2. Evans ME, Gregory DW, Schaffner W, et al. Tularemia: a 30-year experience with 88 cases. Medicine (Baltimore) 1985;64(4):251–69.
3. Dienst FT. Tularemia: a perusal of three hundred thirty-nine cases. J La State Med Soc 1963;115:114–27.
4. Titball RW, Sjostedt A. Francisella tularensis: an overview. ASM News 2003;69(11):558–63.
5. Gill V, Cunha BA. Tularemia pneumonia. Semin Respir Infect 1997;12(1):61–7.
6. Scofield RH, Lopez EJ, McNabb SJ. Tularemia pneumonia in Oklahoma, 1982–1987. J Okla State Med Assoc 1992;85(4):165–70.
7. Matyas BT, Nieder HS, Telford SR. Pneumonic tularemia on Martha's Vineyard: clinical epidemiologic, and ecological characteristics. Ann N Y Acad Sci 2007;1105:351–77.
8. Rubin SA. Radiographic spectrum of pleuropulmonary tularemia. AJR Am J Roentgenol 1978;131(2):277–81.
9. Overholt EL, Tigertt WD, Kadull PJ, et al. An analysis of forty-two cases of laboratory-acquired tularemia. Am J Med 1961;30:785–806.
10. Miller RP, Bates JH. Pleuropulmonary tularemia. Am Rev Respir Dis 1969;99(1):31–41.
11. Ohara S. Studies on Yato-Byo (Ohara's disease, tularemia in Japan), report I. Jpn J Exp Med 1954;24(2):69–79.

12. McCoy GW, Chapin CW. Further observations on a plague-like disease of rodents with a preliminary note on the causative agent *Bacterium tularense*. J Infect Dis 1912;10:61–72.
13. Francis E. A summary of the present knowledge of tularemia. Medicine (Baltimore) 1928;7:411–32.
14. Staples JE, Kubota KA, Chalcraft LG, et al. Epidemiologic and molecular analysis of human tularemia, United States, 1964–2004. Emerg Infect Dis 2006;12(7):1113–8.
15. Kugeler KJ, Mead PS, Janusz AM, et al. Molecular epidemiology of *Francisella tularensis* in the United States. Clin Infect Dis 2009;48(7):863–70.
16. Leelaporn A, Yongyod S, Limsrivanichakorn S, et al. *Francisella novicida* bacteremia, Thailand. Emerg Infect Dis 2008;14(12):1935–7.
17. Hollis DG, Weaver RE, Steigerwalt AG, et al. *Francisella philomiragia* comb. nov. (formerly Yersinia philomiragia) and *Francisella tularensis* biogroup *novicida* (formerly *Francisella novicida*) associated with human disease. J Clin Microbiol 1989;27(7):1601–8.
18. Penn RL. *Francisella tularensis* (Tularemia). In: Mandell GL, Bennett JE, Dolin R, editors. Mandell, Douglas, and Bennett's principles and practice of infectious diseases. Philadelphia: Elsevier Churchill Livingstone; 2005. p. 2674–86.
19. Lamps LW, Havens JM, Sjostedt A, et al. Histologic and molecular diagnosis of tularemia: a potential bioterrorism agent endemic to North America. Mod Pathol 2004;17(5):489–95.
20. Barker JR, Klose KE. Molecular and genetic basis of pathogenesis in *Francisella tularensis*. Ann N Y Acad Sci 2007;1105:138–59.
21. Sjostedt A. Intracellular survival mechanism of *Francisella tularensis*, a stealth pathogen. Microbes Infect 2006;8(2):561–7.
22. Tularemia. United States, 1990–2000. Centers for Disease Control and Prevention. MMWR Morb Mortal Wkly Rep 2002;51(9):181–4.
23. Evans ME, McGee ZA, Hunter PT, et al. Tularemia and the tomcat. JAMA 1981; 246(12):1343.
24. McCarthy VP, Murphy MD. Lawnmower tularemia. Pediatr Infect Dis J 1990;9(4): 298–300.
25. Bellido-Casado J, Perez-Castrillon JL, Bachiller-Luque P, et al. Report on five cases of tularaemic pneumonia in a tularaemia outbreak in Spain. Eur J Clin Microbiol Infect Dis 2000;19(3):218–20.
26. Eliasson H, Back E. Tularaemia in an emergent area of Sweden: an analysis of 234 cases in five years. Scand J Infect Dis 2007;39(10):880–9.
27. Helvaci S, Gedikoglu S, Akalin H, et al. Tularemia in Bursa, Turkey: 205 cases in ten years. Eur J Epidemiol 2000;16(3):271–6.
28. Ohara Y, Sato T, Fujita H, et al. Clinical manifestations of tularemia in Japan—analysis of 1355 cases observed between 1924 and 1987. Infection 1991; 19(1):14–7.
29. Teutsch SM, Martone WJ, Brink EW, et al. Pneumonic tularemia on Martha's Vineyard. N Engl J Med 1979;301(15):826–8.
30. Feldman KA, Enscore RE, Lathrop SL, et al. An outbreak of primary pneumonic tularemia on Martha's Vineyard. N Engl J Med 2001;345(22):1601–6.
31. Kaiser AB, Rieves D, Price AH, et al. Tularemia and rhabdomyolysis. JAMA 1985; 253(2):241–3.
32. Pettersson T, Nyberg P, Nordstrom D, et al. Similar pleural fluid findings in pleuropulmonary tularemia and tuberculous pleurisy. Chest 1996;109(2):572–5.
33. Koskela P, Salminen A. Humoral immunity against *Francisella tularensis* after natural infection. J Clin Microbiol 1985;22(6):973–9.

34. Eliasson H, Sjostedt A, Back E. Clinical use of diagnostic PCR for *Francisella tularensis* in patients with suspected ulceroglandular tularaemia. Scand J Infect Dis 2005;37:833–7.
35. Penn RL, Kinasewitz GT. Factors associated with a poor outcome in tularemia. Arch Intern Med 1987;147(2):265–8.
36. Enderlin G, Morales L, Jacobs RF, et al. Streptomycin and alternative agents for the treatment of tularemia: review of the literature. Clin Infect Dis 1994;19(1):42–7.
37. Limaye AP, Hooper CJ. Treatment of tularemia with fluoroquinolones: two cases and review. Clin Infect Dis 1999;29(4):922–4.
38. Meric M, Willke A, Finke EJ, et al. Evaluation of clinical, laboratory, and therapeutic features of 145 tularemia cases: the role of quinolones in oropharyngeal tularemia. APMIS 2008;116(1):66–73.
39. Ikaheimo I, Syrjala H, Karhukorpi J, et al. In vitro antibiotic susceptibility of *Francisella tularensis* isolated from humans and animals. J Antimicrob Chemother 2000;46(2):287–90.
40. Oyston PC, Sjostedt A, Titball RW. Tularemia: bioterrorism defence renews interest in *Francisella tularensis*. Nat Rev Microbiol 2004;2(12):967–78.
41. Dennis DT, Inglesby TV, Henderson DA, et al. Tularemia as a biological weapon: medical and public health management. JAMA 2001;285(21):2763–73.
42. Burke DS. Immunization against tularemia: analysis of the effectiveness of live *Francisella tularensis* vaccine in prevention of laboratory-acquired tularemia. J Infect Dis 1977;135(1):55–60.

Mycoplasma Pneumonia and Its Complications

Leon G. Smith, MD, MACP[a,b,c,*]

KEYWORDS

- Mycoplasma pneumoniae • Extrapulmonary
- Atypical pneumonia • Neurological

Mycoplasma pneumoniae is an extremely interesting, very small, free-living organism that has no cell wall and that attaches readily to mucosal surfaces, such as the respiratory tract. It took years of investigation before *M pneumoniae* was found to be the most common cause of atypical pneumonia. *M pneumonia* occurs in colleges, armed forces recruiting camps, and schools and is most common in children and young adults. Years ago, *M pneumoniae* was called "walking pneumonia," because there was a discrepancy seen on chest radiograph with relatively few symptoms. The most common symptom is bronchitis, with symptoms persisting for weeks with a nonproductive cough and no fever initially. Later, nonbloody sputum develops with fever, headache, coryza, otitis media, and malaise. There is no exudate in the red pharynx, but bullae can be seen on the ear drum in children, which is highly diagnostic of *M pneumonia*. Pulmonary infiltrates are often scattered throughout both lung fields. *M pneumoniae* is the most common cause of pneumonia in young adults and teenagers, increasing again in frequency in elderly people. Hospitalization is rarely required unless the individual is very sick or has complications. On examination, inspiratory respiratory rales are found in all lung fields. With children, the onset of wheezing with subsequent asthma can be a predominant finding.[1–13]

The white blood cell count is often normal. However, extensive pneumonia can produce a profound leukocytosis with neutrophils. Toxicity is rare until the late stages of the illness. The sputum, unlike bacteria, is filled with lymphocytes and not neutrophils, unless secondary bacterial invasion is present. Chest radiograph shows unilateral or bilateral infiltrates, and rarely lobar consolidation, and up to 25% have small pleural effusions. Pleuritic chest pain is rare, as distinct from pneumococcal pneumonia.

[a] Infectious Disease Foundation of Saint Michael's Medical Center, 111 Central Avenue, Newark, NJ 07102, USA
[b] Department of Medicine, Saint Michael's Medical Center in Newark, NJ, USA
[c] Department of Preventive Medicine, New Jersey Medical School, NJ, USA
* Corresponding author. Infectious Disease Foundation of Saint Michael's Medical Center, 111 Central Avenue, Newark, NJ 07102.
E-mail address: lgsmithmd@aol.com

Infect Dis Clin N Am 24 (2010) 57–60
doi:10.1016/j.idc.2009.10.006
id.theclinics.com

Most patients are treated empirically because of the frequency and lack of toxicity as compared with streptococcal pneumonia and that of other bacteria. In most cases, the diagnosis is made clinically or by epidemiology in the community. Although there are excellent culture techniques and even polymerase chain reaction (PCR) tests to detect this organism, it is practical to treat empirically and obtain *M pneumoniae* in nonresponders by new serological tests, such as IGM and IGG using enzyme-linked immunosorbent assays. These are the most common tests done today. Cold agglutinins are unpredictable, unreliable, and less sensitive. The more difficult tests, such as the complement fixation test, seem outdated. Paired serum samples taken 2 to 4 weeks apart to detect increase in antibody level is preferred to one determination to see a significant increase. PCR assay on sputum and mucosal cells may soon become a rapid diagnostic test for the fastidious, hard-to-grow organism.

COMPLICATIONS

This organism, by direct invasion or by immunity, can cause several complex illnesses, including skin rashes, such as erythema multiform and other rashes; pericarditis, rare but difficult to diagnose; hemolytic anemia due to cold agglutinin production;

Box 1
***M pneumoniae* pearls**

M pneumoniae can have the following malfunctions:

- Neurological complications in 6% of hospitalized patients
- Cerebellar syndrome
- Bell and cranial nerve palsies
- Aseptic meningitis
- Coma
- Optic neuritis
- Acute psychosis
- Diplopia
- Guillain-Barré syndrome
- Peripheral neuropathy

M pneumoniae

- Can be found in neural tissue by PCR
- Can produce chronic pneumonia in a normal host
- Causes pneumonia, except in carcinoma, or ruptures the esophagus as a secondary invader
- Is increasing in frequency in nursing homes
- Can be found in the solid and surface water and increases in frequency during the rainy season; can be a tourist disease or may have an incubation period of many years
- Can resemble tuberculosis on radiograph
- Can be associated with bronchiolitis obliterans organizing pneumonia
- Can cause hemophilialike illness and rhabdomyolysis and polyarthralgia
- Is associated with onset of asthma

prolonged arthralgia, and rarely, arthritis lasting many months; severe neurological diseases, including most commonly, Guillain-Barré syndrome, meningoencephalitis, peripheral neuritis, uveitis, coma, transverse myelitis, optic neuritis, radiculitis, and other more rare neurological entities. It is always wise, especially with neurological disease of unknown cause, to search for mycoplasma serologically. The response to therapy of these extrapulmonary complications is unpredictable but sometimes can be miraculous. The organism can be found in cerebrospinal fluid and in neural tissue by PCR. Most think that the extrapulmonary complications are more likely to be autoimmune response, and some recommend use of steroid therapy.

M pneumoniae infection is self-limited in most cases, as noted in military bases. However, it has been proved that tetracycline or erythromycin compounds are still very effective against the cell-wall–deprived organism. Antibiotic susceptibility is not needed as with bacterial pathogens. Today, the second generation tetracyclines and macrolides are the drugs of choice. Cell-wall antibiotics, such as penicillin, ampicillin, cephalosporin, and vancomycin are ineffective. Doxycycline, 200 mg as a first dose and 100 mg every 12 hours for 10 to 14 days, remains extremely effective and popular. Azithromycin, 500 mg followed by 250 mg/d for 4 days, is equally effective. Clarithromycin, 500 mg every 12 hours for 7 to 14 days is acceptable. The quinolones are also effective, such as levofloxacin (Levoquin) at 500 mg/d for 5 days. These are all adequate recommendations.

M pneumoniae "pearls" are shown in **Box 1**.

SUMMARY

M pneumoniae continues to be the most frequent cause of atypical pneumonia. Fortunately, the antibiotics listed are generally very effective. Major skills are needed to detect *M pneumoniae* extrapulmonary diseases, which require a special heightened awareness and sensitivity. It is not known whether early therapy prevents dreaded complications.

REFERENCES

1. Stamm B, Moschopulos M, Hungerbuehler H, et al. Neuroinvasion by *Mycoplasma pneumoniae* in acute disseminated encephalomyelitis. Emerg Infect Dis 2008;14(4):641–3.
2. Kim MS, Kilgore PE, Kang JS, et al. Transient acquired hemophilia associated with *Mycoplasma pneumoniae* pneumonia. J Korean Med Sci 2008;23:138–41.
3. Daxboeck F. *Mycoplasma pneumoniae* central nervous system infections. Curr Opin Neurol 2006;19(4):374–8.
4. Sutherland RE, Martin RJ. Asthma and atypical bacterial infection. Chest 2007; 132:1962–6.
5. Vazquez JL, Vazquez I, Gonzalez ML, et al. Pneumomediastinum and pneumothorax as presenting signs in severe *Mycoplasma pneumoniae* pneumonia. Pediatr Radiol 2007;37(12):1286(3).
6. Cunha BA. The atypical pneumonias: clinical diagnosis and importance. Clin Microbiol Infect 2006;12(Suppl 3):12–24.
7. Atkinson TP, Balish MF, Waites KB. Epidemiology, clinical manifestations, pathogenesis and laboratory detection of *Mycoplasma pneumoniae* infections. FEMS Microbiol Rev 2008;32(6):956–73.
8. Sanchez-Vargas FM, Gomez-Duarte OG. *Mycoplasma pneumoniae* – an emerging extra-pulmonary pathogen. Clin Microbiol Infect 2008;14:105–15.

9. Nisar N, Guleria R, Kumar S, et al. *Mycoplasma pneumoniae* and its role in asthma. Postgrad Med J 2007;83:100–4.
10. Teig N, Anders A, Schmidt C, et al. *Chlamydophila pneumoniae* and *Mycoplasma pneumoniae* in respiratory specimens of children with chronic lung diseases. Thorax 2005;60:962–6.
11. Shankar EM, Kumarasamy N, Vignesh R, et al. Epidemiological studies on pulmonary pathogens in HIV-positive and -negative subjects with or without community-acquired pneumonia with special emphasis on *Mycoplasma pneumoniae*. Jpn J Infect Dis 2007;60:337–41.
12. Hammerschlag MR. *Mycoplasma pneumoniae* infections. Curr Opin Infect Dis 2001;14:181–6.
13. Clyde WA Jr. Clinical overview of typical *Mycoplasma pneumoniae* infections. Clin Infect Dis 1993;17(Suppl 1):S32–6.

Chlamydophila pneumoniae

Almudena Burillo, MD, PhD[a], Emilio Bouza, MD, PhD[b,c,d,*]

KEYWORDS

• Pneumonia • *Chlamydophila pneumoniae*
• Diagnosis • Treatment

The bacterial family Chlamydiaceae includes the human pathogens *Chlamydia trachomatis*, *Chlamydophila psittaci*, and *Chlamydophila pneumoniae*.[1] The most recently identified *C pneumoniae* shares with *C trachomatis* and *C psittaci* the unique chlamydial developmental cycle but differs from those two species in several important characteristics. Unlike *C trachomatis*, *C pneumoniae* is not sexually transmitted but is spread by aerosolized respiratory secretions. Meanwhile, unlike *C psittaci*, *C pneumoniae* is not a zoonosic pathogen. *C pneumoniae* isolates show relatively limited genotypic or phenotypic variation, and presently only a single serovar or strain of *C pneumoniae* is recognized.

C pneumoniae is a common cause of acute respiratory infection, including community-acquired pneumonia (CAP), pharyngitis, bronchitis, sinusitis, and exacerbations of chronic bronchitis.[2,3] Moreover, in the past 20 years, a heterogeneous spectrum of extrapulmonary diseases has been linked to *C pneumoniae*, including atherosclerotic cardiovascular disease.[4–8] The organism has been identified in atherosclerotic lesions of patients by culture, immunohistochemistry, polymerase chain reaction (PCR), and electron microscopy. Nevertheless, the organism's role in atherosclerosis has been questioned by discrepancies among the results of animal studies. Large-scale treatment studies have not been able to detect a modified risk or rate of cardiovascular events in treated patients. Further diseases linked to *C pneumoniae* are multiple sclerosis,[9–14] asthma,[15,16] age-related macular degeneration,[17] Alzheimer disease,[10] chronic fatigue syndrome,[18] and chronic skin wounds.[19] However, a causal relationship between these diseases and *C pneumoniae* infection has not been confirmed.[20]

[a] Clinical Microbiology Department, Hospital Universitario de Móstoles, C/Río Júcar, s/n, 28935 Móstoles, Madrid, Spain
[b] Microbiology Department, Universidad Complutense, Madrid, Spain
[c] Clinical Microbiology and Infectious Diseases Department, Hospital General Universitario Gregorio Marañón, C/Dr Esquerdo, 46, 28007 Madrid, Spain
[d] CIBER de Enfermedades Respiratorias (CIBERES), Spain
* Corresponding author. Department of Clinical Microbiology and Infectious Diseases, Hospital General Universitario Gregorio Marañón, C/Dr Esquerdo, 46, 28007 Madrid, Spain.
E-mail address: ebouza@microb.net (E. Bouza).

Infect Dis Clin N Am 24 (2010) 61–71
doi:10.1016/j.idc.2009.10.002
0891-5520/10/$ – see front matter

MICROBIOLOGY

Chlamydiae are differentiated from all other bacteria by their unique developmental cycle, which is related to the laboratory diagnosis of the infections they cause, clinical course, and antibiotic therapy. Chlamydiae have cell walls with inner and outer membranes. They replicate by binary fission; contain DNA, RNA, and ribosomes; and synthesize some proteins. They cannot synthesize adenosine triphosphate or guanosine triphosphate and must rely on the host cell for adenosine triphosphate. The cell wall contains a common lipopolysaccharide that differs from the lipopolysaccharide of other bacteria in that it is less endotoxic. Surface-associated chlamydial macromolecules, including MOMP (major outer membrane protein), OmcB (OMP 2) and lipopolysaccharide, may induce a strong antibody response in infected individuals. OmcB binds heparin and this may be related to mammalian host cell adhesion and entry.[21]

The metabolically inactive infectious form of the organism is a small, dense elementary body. Elementary bodies each have a rigid cell wall, a result of disulfide cross-linking of envelope proteins, enabling survival outside the host cell for a limited time. After host cell infection by receptor-mediated endocytosis, the elementary body differentiates into reticulate bodies. These reticulate bodies are the larger, metabolically active noninfectious form of the organism. Inside the host cell, the reticulate bodies divide by binary fission, forming microcolonies referred to as intracytoplasmic inclusions. During this process, chlamydial antigens are released onto the host cell surface, inducing a host immune response. After 48 to 72 hours, the reticulate bodies reorganize themselves and condense to form new elementary bodies. After host cell lysis, the elementary bodies are released and initiate a new infectious cycle.[1]

The first *C pneumoniae* isolates were obtained from conjunctival cultures of children during trachoma vaccine studies in the 1960s. The organism is not, however, associated with eye infection and its role as a human pathogen was not fully defined until 1983, when the first respiratory isolate was obtained.[22] Since then, *C pneumoniae* has been identified as an significant cause of community-acquired respiratory infections, responsible for an estimated 10% of CAP cases and 5% of bronchitis cases.

The first *C pneumoniae* isolates were obtained in yolk-sac cultures, the only method available for the isolation of Chlamydiae, and these isolates were thought to represent strains of *C psittaci* based on inclusion morphology. After the introduction of new cell culture methods, it was observed that the organism has a characteristic pear-shaped elementary body surrounded by a periplasmic space, which is morphologically distinct from the round elementary bodies of *C trachomatis* and *C psittaci*. DNA homology studies have revealed that *C pneumoniae* isolates have less than 5% DNA homology with *C trachomatis* and less than 10% with *C psittaci*, although they are highly related (>95%) among themselves. Since only one strain or serovar of *C pneumoniae* has been identified, the strain name TWAR (after the designation of two of the initial isolates, TW-183 and AR-39) is today synonymous with *C pneumoniae*.

Mounting evidence indicates that such factors as gamma interferon, antibiotics, and nutrient deprivation may drive Chlamydiae into a state of persistence.[23] However, the clinical significance of chlamydial persistence is still a matter of debate since there are no diagnostic tools to detect persistence in the human host.

EPIDEMIOLOGY

This organism is widely spread in both industrialized and developing countries. Serological evidence of previous infection can be found in some 50% of young adults and

75% of elderly persons. Primary infection occurs mainly in school-aged children, while reinfection is observed in adults.

The pathogen is estimated to cause 3% to 10% of cases of CAP among adults.[24,25] The estimated number of cases of *C pneumoniae* pneumonia in the United States is 100 cases per 100,000 inhabitants.[26] In a recent study on the epidemiology of severe CAP caused by *Legionella longbeachae*, *Mycoplasma pneumoniae*, and *C pneumoniae* in Thailand, the incidence of *C pneumoniae* CAP was 3 to 23 cases per 100,000 inhabitants. Rates were highest among patients aged under 1 year (18–166 cases per 100,000 inhabitants) and those aged 70 years or older (23–201 cases per 100,000 inhabitants). This pathogen was associated with 15% of all cases of pneumonia.[27]

In a study that included 4337 patients and addressed the incidence of CAP due to atypical pathogens in the different world regions, some 7% were attributed to *C pneumoniae* (North America 8%, Europe 7%, Latin America 6%, and Asia/Africa 5%).[28]

Rates of *C pneumoniae* infection do not vary significantly by season.[26] Epidemiological studies suggest a 4-year cycle in the incidence of *C pneumoniae* pneumonia. The exact mode of transmission is unknown and spread via droplets has been proposed. Outbreaks of respiratory infection have been reported in nursing homes, in schools, and among military recruits and families.

CLINICAL MANIFESTATIONS

C pneumoniae is a significant cause of both lower and upper respiratory tract infections. Pneumonia and bronchitis are the most common, while upper respiratory infections, including sinusitis, pharyngitis, and laryngitis, may also occur, either in isolation or in conjunction with a lower respiratory infection. Clinical presentations vary widely from mild disease to severe CAP.

The 21-day incubation period of infection due to *C pneumoniae* is longer than that of many other respiratory pathogens. Most patients with *C pneumoniae* infection are asymptomatic, and the course of respiratory illness is relatively mild. The clinical symptoms of *C pneumoniae* infection are nonspecific and do not differ significantly from those caused by other atypical organisms, such as *Mycoplasma pneumoniae* and respiratory viruses.[29] Upper respiratory signs and symptoms, such as rhinitis, sore throat, or hoarseness, may be reported initially.[30] The most important clinical finding to differentiate *M pneumoniae* from *C pneumoniae* is the presence or absence of laryngitis. Although not all patients with *C pneumoniae* CAP suffer laryngitis, most do. Fever may be accompanied by myalgia and chills. These signs and symptoms may then subside over days to weeks, followed by the onset of cough, which is a predominant feature of *C pneumoniae* respiratory infections, resulting in a biphasic pattern of illness symptoms with a protracted course.[31,32] This symptom pattern may delay the first consultation and makes determination of the real onset of illness difficult. Other investigators, however, have not found this pathogen to cause persistent cough.[33] Patients with *C pneumoniae* suffer from headache more frequently than patients with *Streptococcus pneumoniae* pneumonia.[34]

After gradual onset, symptoms due to *C pneumoniae* respiratory infection may continue over extended periods, with persistence of cough and malaise for several weeks or months despite appropriate antibiotic therapy.

An infection with this organism may precede asthma onset, exacerbate asthma, or make asthma control more difficult. Its ability to elicit a TH2 response and promote airway inflammation may be the common feature of its atopic inflammatory response.[35]

C pneumoniae may present as severe CAP in patients with severely compromised respiratory function.[36] It has also been associated with acute respiratory exacerbations in patients with cystic fibrosis and with acute chest syndrome in children with sickle cell disease.[37,38] Severe or life-threatening *C pneumoniae* infections have been described in patients with acute leukemia and treatment-induced neutropenia.[39]

Few investigations have specifically examined prevalence rates of atypical pathogens causing CAP requiring intensive care unit management. In most studies, *C pneumoniae* is not considered despite having been reported to cause 10% of CAP treated in the intensive care unit.[40]

A single, subsegmental, patchy infiltrate is the classic radiographic appearance of atypical pneumonias and this is commonly seen in *C pneumoniae* infection.[25] However, this pattern is also common in cases of pneumonia caused by typical bacterial pathogens, including *S pneumoniae*.[34] Infiltrates are sometimes described as funnel-shaped and, if present, may be a clue to diagnosis.[41] Other radiographic features, such as lobar or sublobar consolidation, interstitial infiltrates, bilateral involvement, pleural effusion, and hilar adenopathy, may be present in *C pneumoniae* infection, although less frequently.[42,43] Hence, the pattern of infiltrates observed in a chest radiograph is not a reliable indicator of the probable etiologic agent in cases of CAP. As with other atypical pathogens, the white blood cell count is usually not elevated[42] and other laboratory findings are nonspecific to *C pneumoniae* infection.

DIAGNOSIS

Because of the diversity and varying quality of the different tests and interpretative criteria, the main concern in making a diagnosis is the diagnostic accuracy of testing.[44]

The current concept is that asymptomatic carriage of these pathogens is rare, so isolation is equivalent to a diagnosis of infection.[45,46]

The reference standard for identifying infections caused by *C pneumoniae* is culture. Since the pathogen is an obligate intracellular organism, specimen collection should aim to include the host cells that harbor the organisms. Culture must be performed in vitro using laboratory-propagated cell lines. Samples are obtained using nasopharyngeal swabs. Specimens need to be kept at 4°C to 8°C in specialized transport media such that overall culture sensitivity is relatively low (50%–70%).

Most commonly used serological assay formats include the complement fixation test, the microimmunofluorescence (MIF) test, and enzyme immunoassay to detect immunoglobulin M (IgM), immunoglobulin A (IgA), immunoglobulin G (IgG), or antibody classes showing family, species, or serotype specificity. Complement fixation serology is not helpful because it is insensitive and detects all *Chlamydia* spp, not just *C pneumoniae*. The MIF test, which was developed by Wang and Grayston in the early 1970s, is still considered the method of choice for serodiagnosis of acute *C pneumoniae* infection, according to Centers for Disease Control and Prevention recommendations.[47] This method can detect a species response and shows a sensitivity of 50% to 90% using paired sera. The assay uses purified formalinized elementary bodies of representative strains or serovars of *C trachomatis*, *C psittaci*, and *C pneumoniae* dotted in a specific pattern on glass slides. A detailed description of the method can be found elsewhere.[48]

The criteria used to identify acute *C pneumoniae* infection generally include paired sera in which at least a fourfold rise in titer is detected, and single serum samples with IgM levels greater than or equal to 1:16 and/or IgG greater than or equal to 1:512. Because IgM antibodies appear approximately 2 to 3 weeks after illness onset, levels may not be detectable in specimens obtained early in the course of illness.[46] In addition, *C pneumoniae* infection does not consistently induce protective immunity and reinfection is common, substantially more so than primary infection in older persons. In cases of reinfection, IgM antibodies may not appear. Thus, failure to detect anti–*C pneumoniae* IgM in a serum specimen obtained in the context of acute respiratory illness does not exclude *C pneumoniae* as a possible cause. Besides, patients with previous infection may have IgG levels approaching the cutoff titer for several years. Preexisting antibodies are indicated by IgG titers greater than 16 and less than 512 and this is suggestive of past infection. The usefulness of IgA as a diagnostic marker in acute or chronic *C pneumoniae* infections has not been demonstrated.

The MIF assay format is technically demanding, time consuming, and less useful for higher volume testing. In addition, subjective reading may contribute to intra- and interlaboratory variation in MIF assay results.[49] Hence, a well-trained and experienced laboratory staff is needed. A few standardized kits based on the MIF assay have been developed and marketed.[1] Initial studies suggest that their performance characteristics correspond well with the classic MIF method, yet none has been cleared by the Food and Drug Administration for use in the United States for the diagnosis of *C pneumoniae* infection.

The results of DNA amplification studies using PCR or PCR–enzyme immunoassay techniques for *C pneumoniae* have been promising. The lack of a true gold standard makes it difficult to assess this method, Following a report on the need to standardize these assays,[47] specific guidelines were introduced and it is now recommended that the performance of newly developed PCR protocols should be compared with at least one of four assays that target the *PSTI* fragment,[50] the ompA gene,[51] or the 16S rRNA gene.[52,53] Notwithstanding, all these assays must be considered research tools, because no commercial Food and Drug Administration–cleared assays are currently available.[54] Oosterheert and colleagues[55] showed that the rapid detection of viral and atypical bacterial pathogens by real-time PCR for patients with lower respiratory tract infection increases the diagnostic yield considerably, but this measure was not found to reduce antibiotic use or costs. This study included no infections by *C pneumoniae*.

In a recent study, two methods were evaluated for the diagnosis of *C pneumoniae* infection during an outbreak in a military community. One used *C pneumoniae* PCR, as described by Tong and Sillis.[51] The other used *C pneumoniae* IgM antibody and IgG seroconversion assays.[46] The sensitivity of PCR was lower (68%) than that of MIF IgM (79%), though specificity and positive predictive values were higher (93% and 81% vs 86% and 67%, respectively). This may be attributable to PCR becoming negative after days to months because of clearance of the organism following antibiotic treatment,[56] thus appearing as a false negative. This study reveals the importance of sample timing when comparing PCR and serological techniques.

According to the Infectious Diseases Society of America/American Thoracic Society consensus guidelines on the management of CAP in adults, routine diagnostic tests to identify an etiologic diagnosis are optional for outpatients with CAP (moderate recommendation; level III evidence).[57] This guideline stresses that management of patients according to the results of a single acute-phase serologic test is unreliable because initial antibiotic therapy will be completed before the earliest time a convalescent-phase specimen may be confirmed.

TREATMENT

The agents erythromycin, tetracycline, and doxycycline show in vitro activity against *C pneumoniae* and are used as first-line therapy for acute respiratory infections caused by this organism. Its in vitro resistance to penicillin, ampicillin, or sulfa drugs means these drugs are not recommended for the treatment of a suspected *C pneumoniae* infection. Given that symptoms of *C pneumoniae* infection often reappear after a short or conventional course of antibiotics, and persistent infection after treatment has been culture-proven, intensive long-term treatment is recommended.

Mainstay treatment regimens for adults are tetracycline 500 mg four times daily for 14 days; doxycycline 100 mg twice daily for 14 days; or erythromycin 500 mg four times daily for 14 days, or 250 mg four times daily for 21 days if the former dose is not tolerated. Tetracyclines should not be given to children under 8 years old. Erythromycin (30–50 mg/kg/d divided every 6 hours) is the drug of choice in these patients.

A second course of antibiotics may be beneficial when such symptoms as cough or malaise persist after treatment. Tetracycline or doxycycline is recommended for the second course. Although *C pneumoniae* infections may be long-lasting, they rarely give rise to serious sequelae and most patients make a complete recovery.

Many respiratory infection studies have been based on identifying persons infected with *C pneumoniae* through blood samples obtained in the acute and convalescent stages. However, despite accurately identifying infected persons, these studies provide little information on whether antibiotic treatment serves to eliminate the bacterium. The first time *C pneumoniae* was described as a causal agent of human respiratory infections, patients were identified by nasopharyngeal culture and serology, but cultures were not repeated posttreatment to document eradication. In this study, 1 g of erythromycin per day taken orally for 5 to 10 days was unable to resolve symptoms such that Grayston and colleagues[22] later recommended either 2 g of tetracycline per day for 7 to 10 days or 1 g per day for 21 days.

In a study by Lipsky and colleagues,[58] a clinical response to ofloxacin (400 mg given twice daily for 10 days) was reported in patients with pneumonia and bronchitis caused by *C pneumoniae*. Infection was defined according to acute- and convalescent-stage sera. Although older quinolones, such as ofloxacin, are not highly active against *C pneumoniae*, the newer quinolone agents, such as levofloxacin, gatifloxacin, gemifloxacin, and moxifloxacin, show good in vitro action. Gatifloxacin is no longer marketed in the United States.

More recent results include those of several clinical trials in which nasopharyngeal cultures were one of the methods used to measure the microbiologic efficacy of antimicrobial therapy against *C pneumoniae* infection. The first of these was a randomized controlled trial of clarithromycin (15 mg/kg per day for 10 days) versus erythromycin suspension (40 mg/kg per day for 10 days) used to treat 3- to 12-year-olds in whom CAP had been radiographically proven.[59] Of the 260 children enrolled, 74 (28%) showed PCR or throat swab evidence of infection with *C pneumoniae*. Among 33 patients in whom *C pneumoniae* had been isolated from nasopharyngeal cultures obtained before antibiotic treatment, bacteriologic eradication was documented in 79% (15 of 19) of those treated with clarithromycin compared to 86% (12 of 14) of those receiving erythromycin. The minimum inhibitory concentrations of erythromycin and clarithromycin for isolates obtained from children testing positive both before and after therapy remained unchanged during treatment.[60] Notwithstanding, all the children with persistent infection improved clinically, and chest radiographs indicated complete resolution of the infection.

In a similar study, in 36 of 456 (8%) children aged 6 months to 16 years treated with azithromycin for CAP, *C pneumoniae* was isolated from pretreatment nasopharyngeal cultures and was eradicated in 19 of the 23 (83%) children evaluable after treatment.[61]

In an open study of azithromycin (1.5-g oral dose given over 5 days) used to treat CAP in adults,[62] *C pneumoniae* infection was culture identified in 10 of 48 (21%)

patients at the study outset. After treatment, 7 of the 10 culture-positive patients were culture-negative. The isolate obtained at this time in 1 persistently infected patient showed a MIC four times higher (0.25 μg/mL vs 0.062 μg/mL) than the initial isolate, though still within the range considered to indicate antibiotic susceptibility. All patients improved clinically. Persistence of *C pneumoniae* in nasopharyngeal specimens following treatment has also been observed in a small subset of patients receiving moxifloxacin to treat CAP.[63]

It has been well established that *C pneumoniae* may persist after antimicrobial therapy with agents to which it is susceptible in vitro. The above-mentioned studies confirm its persistence after azithromycin, clarithromycin, erythromycin, or moxifloxacin treatment although clinical symptoms improved. In several patients with nasopharyngeal culture-positive *C pneumoniae* acute respiratory illness, Hammerschlag and colleagues[64] also reported the persistence of positive cultures and symptoms following 2 weeks of erythromycin or 30 days of tetracycline or doxycycline treatment. These findings reveal the lack of a clear link between in vitro susceptibility and nasopharyngeal eradication, and between eradication and a clinical response.

The above reports do, however, suggest that azithromycin and clarithromycin are as effective or more effective than doxycycline or erythromycin therapy for a *C pneumoniae* respiratory infection. These drugs attain high intracellular and tissue levels and have been demonstrated effective against *C pneumoniae* in vitro. Also, given they are better tolerated than erythromycin with fewer gastrointestinal side effects, they may be preferable in certain situations. Recommended doses for respiratory infections in adults are 500 mg on day 1 then 250 mg a day on days 2 through 5 for azithromycin and 500 mg twice a day for 10 to 14 days for clarithromycin. Recommended pediatric doses are 5 to 12 mg/kg once daily of azithromycin and 7.5 mg/kg/d divided twice a day of clarithromycin. In adults, newer quinolone agents are being increasingly used for empiric treatment of respiratory infections potentially due to *C pneumoniae*.

Despite this, a recent meta-analysis of trials conducted in hospitalized patients with CAP revealed no survival or clinical benefits of empirical atypical-coverage drugs (macrolides or fluoroquinolones vs beta-lactam agents).[65] The trials examined in this meta-analysis did not provide compelling evidence of a need to treat CAP caused by atypical pathogens, with the exception of legionnaires disease. However, in a recent retrospective study of 27,330 Medicare hospitalized patients with CAP, initial treatment with a second- or third-generation cephalosporin plus a macrolide or initial treatment with a fluoroquinolone were associated with reduced 30-day mortality, compared to third-generation cephalosporin monotherapy.[66] The investigators of this study, however, admitted the limitations of nonexperimental cohort studies designed to identify correlations between factors, such as antibiotic selection and patient outcomes.

Despite the shortcomings of these studies, the routine use of agents to treat respiratory infections caused by atypical pathogens is standard practice in the United States, Canada, and several other countries. This means that conducting controlled trials to address these issues is ethically difficult and practically impossible.[45] Further limitations include diagnostic difficulties in testing for *C pneumoniae* and the need for a prompt start of therapy in patients requiring hospitalization. Thus, studies designed to assess the use of specific agents, except for those studies that use retrospective methods, are difficult to conduct because of ethical and logistical barriers.

Despite these barriers, an assessment of emergency physician (EP) understanding of Centers for Medicare and Medicaid Services (CMS) core measures for non–intensive care unit patients with CAP treatment guidelines has been recently published. This report determined self-reported effects on antibiotic prescribing patterns in non–intensive care unit CAP patients.[67] A 121 emergency physician responders (81%) were aware of CMS CAP guidelines. Nearly all physicians (96%; 95% CI 93%–99%) reported an institutional commitment to meet these core measures, and 84% (95% CI 78%–90%) claimed they had a department-based CAP protocol. Over half the responders (55%; 95% CI 47%–70%) reported prescribing antibiotics to patients they did not believe had pneumonia to comply with the CMS guidelines. Only 40% (95% CI 32%–48%) of emergency physicians thought that CAP awareness and the expedient care resulting from these guidelines improved overall pneumonia-related patient care. The limitation of this study is that it lacks outcome-based data.

SUMMARY

C pneumoniae commonly causes acute respiratory infections, including pneumonia and bronchitis, spread by aerosolized respiratory secretions. Clinical presentations vary widely from mild disease to the less frequent severe CAP. Patients initially complain of such symptoms as rhinitis, sore throat, or hoarseness, which may subside and give way to cough days or weeks later. *C pneumoniae* infection is not usually serious and its diagnosis, though culture-based, is delayed in relation to the onset of symptoms, antibiotic treatment, and resolution. To date, no rapid, standardized accurate diagnostic methods exist. The benefits of the use of antimicrobials have not been clearly established, although it is recommended in North American guidelines for the treatment of patients with *C pneumoniae* CAP. The role played by this pathogen in other diseases has yet to be determined.

REFERENCES

1. Essig A. *Chlamydia* and *Chlamydophila*. In: Murray PR, Baron EJ, Jorgensen JH, et al, editors. Manual of clinical microbiology. 9th edition. Washington, DC: ASM; 2007. p. 1021.
2. Grayston JT, Aldous MB, Easton A, et al. Evidence that *Chlamydia pneumoniae* causes pneumonia and bronchitis. J Infect Dis 1993;168:1231.
3. Sopena N, Pedro-Botet ML, Sabria M, et al. Comparative study of community-acquired pneumonia caused by *Streptococcus pneumoniae*, *Legionella pneumophila* or *Chlamydia pneumoniae*. Scand J Infect Dis 2004;36:330.
4. Andraws R, Berger JS, Brown DL. Effects of antibiotic therapy on outcomes of patients with coronary artery disease: a meta-analysis of randomized controlled trials. JAMA 2005;293:2641.
5. de Barbeyrac B, Bebear C. [Chlamydial pathogenesis: diagnostic and therapeutic consequences]. Arch Pediatr 2005;12:S26 [in French].
6. Kuppuswamy VC, Gupta S. Antibiotic therapy for coronary heart disease: the myth and the reality. Timely Top Med Cardiovasc Dis 2006;10:E2.
7. Saikku P, Leinonen M, Mattila K, et al. Serological evidence of an association of a novel *Chlamydia*, TWAR, with chronic coronary heart disease and acute myocardial infarction. Lancet 1988;2:983.
8. West SK, Kohlhepp SJ, Jin R, et al. Detection of circulating *Chlamydophila pneumoniae* in patients with coronary artery disease and healthy control subjects. Clin Infect Dis 2009;48:560.
9. Greenlee JE, Rose JW. Controversies in neurological infectious diseases. Semin Neurol 2000;20:375.
10. Horvath Z, Vecsei L. [The significance of *Chlamydia pneumoniae* in selected neurologic disorders]. Ideggyogy Sz 2006;59:4 [in Hungarian].

11. Moses H Jr, Sriram S. An infectious basis for multiple sclerosis: perspectives on the role of *Chlamydia pneumoniae* and other agents. BioDrugs 2001;15:199.
12. Sriram S, Ljunggren-Rose A, Yao SY, et al. Detection of chlamydial bodies and antigens in the central nervous system of patients with multiple sclerosis. J Infect Dis 2005;192:1219.
13. Swanborg RH, Whittum-Hudson JA, Hudson AP. Human herpesvirus 6 and *Chlamydia pneumoniae* as etiologic agents in multiple sclerosis—a critical review. Microbes Infect 2002;4:1327.
14. Swanborg RH, Whittum-Hudson JA, Hudson AP. Infectious agents and multiple sclerosis—Are *Chlamydia pneumoniae* and human herpes virus 6 involved? J Neuroimmunol 2003;136:1.
15. Johnston SL, Blasi F, Black PN, et al. The effect of telithromycin in acute exacerbations of asthma. N Engl J Med 2006;354:1589.
16. Little FF. Treating acute asthma with antibiotics—not quite yet. N Engl J Med 2006;354:1632.
17. Baird PN, Robman LD, Richardson AJ, et al. Gene-environment interaction in progression of AMD: the CFH gene, smoking and exposure to chronic infection. Hum Mol Genet 2008;17:1299.
18. Chia JK, Chia LY. Chronic *Chlamydia pneumoniae* infection: a treatable cause of chronic fatigue syndrome. Clin Infect Dis 1999;29:452.
19. King LE Jr, Stratton CW, Mitchell WM. *Chlamydia pneumoniae* and chronic skin wounds: a focused review. J Investig Dermatol Symp Proc 2001;6:233.
20. Blasi F, Tarsia P, Aliberti S. *Chlamydophila pneumoniae*. Clin Microbiol Infect 2009;15:29.
21. Stephens RS, Kalman S, Lammel C, et al. Genome sequence of an obligate intracellular pathogen of humans: *Chlamydia trachomatis*. Science 1998;282:754.
22. Grayston JT, Kuo CC, Wang SP, et al. A new *Chlamydia psittaci* strain, TWAR, isolated in acute respiratory tract infections. N Engl J Med 1986;315:161.
23. Kern JM, Maass V, Maass M. Molecular pathogenesis of chronic *Chlamydia pneumoniae* infection: a brief overview. Clin Microbiol Infect 2009;15:36.
24. Chedid MB, Chedid MF, Ilha DO, et al. Community-acquired pneumonia by *Chlamydophila pneumoniae*: a clinical and incidence study in Brazil. Braz J Infect Dis 2007;11:75.
25. Reechaipichitkul W, Saelee R, Lulitanond V. Prevalence and clinical features of *Chlamydia pneumoniae* pneumonia at Srinagarind Hospital, Khon Kaen, Thailand. Southeast Asian J Trop Med Public Health 2005;36:151.
26. Marston BJ, Plouffe JF, File TM Jr, et al. Incidence of community-acquired pneumonia requiring hospitalization. Results of a population-based active surveillance study in Ohio. The Community-Based Pneumonia Incidence Study Group. Arch Intern Med 1997;157:1709.
27. Phares CR, Wangroongsarb P, Chantra S, et al. Epidemiology of severe pneumonia caused by *Legionella longbeachae*, *Mycoplasma pneumoniae*, and *Chlamydia pneumoniae*: 1-year, population-based surveillance for severe pneumonia in Thailand. Clin Infect Dis 2007;45:e147.
28. Arnold FW, Summersgill JT, Lajoie AS, et al. A worldwide perspective of atypical pathogens in community-acquired pneumonia. Am J Respir Crit Care Med 2007; 175:1086.
29. Gupta SK, Sarosi GA. The role of atypical pathogens in community-acquired pneumonia. Med Clin North Am 2001;85:1349.
30. Cunha BA. The atypical pneumonias: clinical diagnosis and importance. Clin Microbiol Infect 2006;12:12.

31. Ekman MR, Grayston JT, Visakorpi R, et al. An epidemic of infections due to *Chlamydia pneumoniae* in military conscripts. Clin Infect Dis 1993;17:420.
32. Johnson DH, Cunha BA. Atypical pneumonias. Clinical and extrapulmonary features of Chlamydia, Mycoplasma, and Legionella infections. Postgrad Med 1993;93:69.
33. Wadowsky RM, Castilla EA, Laus S, et al. Evaluation of *Chlamydia pneumoniae* and *Mycoplasma pneumoniae* as etiologic agents of persistent cough in adolescents and adults. J Clin Microbiol 2002;40:637.
34. Kauppinen MT, Saikku P, Kujala P, et al. Clinical picture of community-acquired *Chlamydia pneumoniae* pneumonia requiring hospital treatment: a comparison between chlamydial and *pneumococcal pneumonia.* Thorax 1996;51:185.
35. Daian CM, Wolff AH, Bielory L. The role of atypical organisms in asthma. Allergy Asthma Proc 2000;21:107.
36. Feldman C. Pneumonia in the elderly. Med Clin North Am 2001;85:1441.
37. Emre U, Bernius M, Roblin PM, et al. *Chlamydia pneumoniae* infection in patients with cystic fibrosis. Clin Infect Dis 1996;22:819.
38. Miller ST, Hammerschlag MR, Chirgwin K, et al. Role of *Chlamydia pneumoniae* in acute chest syndrome of sickle cell disease. J Pediatr 1991;118:30.
39. Heinemann M, Kern WV, Bunjes D, et al. Severe *Chlamydia pneumoniae* infection in patients with neutropenia: case reports and literature review. Clin Infect Dis 2000;31:181.
40. Cosentini R, Blasi F, Raccanelli R, et al. Severe community-acquired pneumonia: a possible role for *Chlamydia pneumoniae.* Respiration 1996;63:61.
41. Cunha BA, Ortega AM. Atypical pneumonia. Extrapulmonary clues guide the way to diagnosis. Postgrad Med 1996;99:123.
42. Kauppinen MT, Lahde S, Syrjala H. Roentgenographic findings of pneumonia caused by *Chlamydia pneumoniae.* A comparison with *streptococcus pneumonia.* Arch Intern Med 1996;156:1851.
43. McConnell CT Jr, Plouffe JF, File TM, et al. Radiographic appearance of *Chlamydia pneumoniae* (TWAR strain) respiratory infections. CBPIS Study Group. Community-based Pneumonia Incidence Study. Radiology 1994;192:819.
44. Kumar S, Hammerschlag MR. Acute respiratory infection due to *Chlamydia pneumoniae*: current status of diagnostic methods. Clin Infect Dis 2007;44:568.
45. Bartlett JG. Is activity against "atypical" pathogens necessary in the treatment protocols for community-acquired pneumonia? Issues with combination therapy. Clin Infect Dis 2008;47:S232.
46. Hvidsten D, Halvorsen DS, Berdal BP, et al. *Chlamydophila pneumoniae* diagnostics: importance of methodology in relation to timing of sampling. Clin Microbiol Infect 2009;15:42.
47. Dowell SF, Peeling RW, Boman J, et al. Standardizing *Chlamydia pneumoniae* assays: recommendations from the Centers for Disease Control and Prevention (USA) and the Laboratory Centre for Disease Control (Canada). Clin Infect Dis 2001;33:492.
48. Wang S. The microimmunofluorescence test for *Chlamydia pneumoniae* infection: technique and interpretation. J Infect Dis 2000;181(Suppl 3):S421.
49. Peeling RW, Wang SP, Grayston JT, et al. *Chlamydia pneumoniae* serology: interlaboratory variation in microimmunofluorescence assay results. J Infect Dis 2000;181(Suppl 3):S426.
50. Campbell LA, Perez Melgosa M, Hamilton DJ, et al. Detection of *Chlamydia pneumoniae* by polymerase chain reaction. J Clin Microbiol 1992;30:434.

51. Tong CY, Sillis M. Detection of *Chlamydia pneumoniae* and *Chlamydia psittaci* in sputum samples by PCR. J Clin Pathol 1993;46:313.
52. Gaydos CA, Quinn TC, Eiden JJ. Identification of *Chlamydia pneumoniae* by DNA amplification of the 16S rRNA gene. J Clin Microbiol 1992;30:796.
53. Madico G, Quinn TC, Boman J, et al. Touchdown enzyme time release-PCR for detection and identification of *Chlamydia trachomatis*, *C. pneumoniae*, and *C. psittaci* using the 16S and 16S–23S spacer rRNA genes. J Clin Microbiol 2000;38:1085.
54. Nolte FS. Molecular diagnostics for detection of bacterial and viral pathogens in community-acquired pneumonia. Clin Infect Dis 2008;47:S123.
55. Oosterheert JJ, van Loon AM, Schuurman R, et al. Impact of rapid detection of viral and atypical bacterial pathogens by real-time polymerase chain reaction for patients with lower respiratory tract infection. Clin Infect Dis 2005;41:1438.
56. Thom DH, Grayston JT, Campbell LA, et al. Respiratory infection with *Chlamydia pneumoniae* in middle-aged and older adult outpatients. Eur J Clin Microbiol Infect Dis 1994;13:785.
57. Mandell LA, Wunderink RG, Anzueto A, et al. Infectious Diseases Society of America/American Thoracic Society consensus guidelines on the management of community-acquired pneumonia in adults. Clin Infect Dis 2007;44(Suppl 2):S27.
58. Lipsky BA, Tack KJ, Kuo CC, et al. Ofloxacin treatment of *Chlamydia pneumoniae* (strain TWAR) lower respiratory tract infections. Am J Med 1990;89:722.
59. Block S, Hedrick J, Hammerschlag MR, et al. *Mycoplasma pneumoniae* and *Chlamydia pneumoniae* in pediatric community-acquired pneumonia: comparative efficacy and safety of clarithromycin vs. erythromycin ethylsuccinate. Pediatr Infect Dis J 1995;14:471.
60. Roblin PM, Montalban G, Hammerschlag MR. Susceptibilities to clarithromycin and erythromycin of isolates of *Chlamydia pneumoniae* from children with pneumonia. Antimicrobial Agents Chemother 1994;38:1588.
61. Harris JA, Kolokathis A, Campbell M, et al. Safety and efficacy of azithromycin in the treatment of community-acquired pneumonia in children. Pediatr Infect Dis J 1998;17:865.
62. Roblin PM, Hammerschlag MR. Microbiologic efficacy of azithromycin and susceptibilities to azithromycin of isolates of *Chlamydia pneumoniae* from adults and children with community-acquired pneumonia. Antimicrobial Agents Chemother 1998;42:194.
63. Hammerschlag MR, Roblin PM. Microbiologic efficacy of moxifloxacin for the treatment of community-acquired pneumonia due to *Chlamydia pneumoniae*. Int J Antimicrob Agents 2000;15:149.
64. Hammerschlag MR, Chirgwin K, Roblin PM, et al. Persistent infection with *Chlamydia pneumoniae* following acute respiratory illness. Clin Infect Dis 1992;14:178.
65. Robenshtok E, Shefet D, Gafter-Gvili A, et al. Empiric antibiotic coverage of atypical pathogens for community acquired pneumonia in hospitalized adults. Cochrane Database Syst Rev 2008;1:CD004418.
66. Bratzler DW, Ma A, Nsa W. Initial antibiotic selection and patient outcomes: observations from the National Pneumonia Project. Clin Infect Dis 2008;47(Suppl 3):S193.
67. Nicks BA, Manthey DE, Fitch MT. The Centers for Medicare and Medicaid Services (CMS) community-acquired pneumonia core measures lead to unnecessary antibiotic administration by emergency physicians. Acad Emerg Med 2009;16:184.

Legionnaires' Disease: Clinical Differentiation from Typical and Other Atypical Pneumonias

Burke A. Cunha, MD, MACP[a,b,*]

KEYWORDS

- Clinical syndromic diagnosis • Relative bradycardia
- Ferritin levels • Hypophosphatemia

HISTORY

An outbreak of a severe respiratory illness occurred in Washington, DC, in 1965 and another in Pontiac, Michigan, in 1968. Despite extensive investigations following these outbreaks, no explanation or causative organism was found. In July 1976 in Philadelphia, Pennsylvania, an outbreak of a severe respiratory illness occurred at an American Legion convention. The US Centers for Disease Control and Prevention (CDC) conducted an extensive epidemiologic and microbiologic investigation to determine the cause of the outbreak. Dr Ernest Campbell of Bloomsburg, Pennsylvania, was the first to recognize the relationship between the American Legion convention in 3 of his patients who attended the convention and who had a similar febrile respiratory infection. Six months after the onset of the outbreak, a gram-negative organism was isolated from autopsied lung tissue. Dr McDade, using culture media used for rickettsial organisms, isolated the gram-negative organism later called *Legionella*. The isolate was believed to be the causative agent of the respiratory infection because antibodies to *Legionella* were detected in infected survivors. Subsequently, CDC investigators realized the antecedent outbreaks of febrile illness in Philadelphia and in Pontiac were caused by the same organism. They later demonstrated increased *Legionella* titers in survivors' stored sera. The same organism was responsible for the pneumonias that occurred after the American Legionnaires' Convention in Philadelphia in 1976.

[a] Infectious Disease Division, Winthrop-University Hospital, 259 First Street, Mineola, Long Island, NY 11501, USA
[b] State University of New York School of Medicine, Stony Brook, NY, USA
* Infectious Disease Division, Winthrop-University Hospital, 259 First Street, Mineola, Long Island, NY 11501.

Infect Dis Clin N Am 24 (2010) 73–105
doi:10.1016/j.idc.2009.10.014
id.theclinics.com

Legionnaires' disease had existed before the outbreaks but was never recognized as a cause of community-acquired pneumonia (CAP). Clustering of cases and outbreaks is useful in recognizing common epidemiologic and clinical features and is helpful in initiating investigative efforts to determine the cause of such outbreaks. Without the large number of cases in the Philadelphia 1976 outbreak, the eventual identification of *Legionella pneumophila* as the cause of legionnaires' disease would have taken longer. A key clinical finding in legionnaires' disease (ie, relative bradycardia) was noted in early descriptions. Subsequently, because the criteria for relative bradycardia was not defined, the clinical importance of relative bradycardia has been overlooked and underestimated (**Fig. 1**).[1,2]

Pneumonia caused by any *Legionella* species is termed legionnaires' disease. The outbreak in Pontiac, Michigan, known as "Pontiac fever," had an acute febrile illness but did not have pneumonia as in the Philadelphia outbreak. The isolation of *Legionella* was the first crucial step in understanding legionnaires' disease. The initial isolation of *Legionella pneumophila* paved the way for ecological/epidemiologic studies, various direct and indirect diagnostic tests, and refining our therapeutic approach to legionnaires' disease.

MICROBIOLOGY

The family Legionellae consists of more than 70 serogroups. *Legionella pneumophila* serotypes 1 to 6 account for most human infections. *Legionella* organisms are small obligate aerobic gram-nonfermenting gram-negative bacilli. *Legionella* are motile by bipolar flagella and stain poorly by Gram stain. *Legionella* seem to be filamentous in culture, but in tissue appear as small gram-negative coccobacilli. *Legionella* grow on buffered charcoal yeast extract (BCYE) and do not grow on standard media. *Legionella* require L-cysteine, and iron salts enhance their growth. BCYE is supplemented with L-cysteine, α-ketoglutarate and ferric pyrophosphate. *Legionella* colonies on BCYE develop a "ground glass" appearance with magnification. *Legionella* may be inhibited on artificial media by 0.6% sodium chloride peroxidides. Optimal pH for growth is 6.7 to 6.9. Colonies appear to be grayish white after 72 hours' incubation at 35°C with 5% CO_2.[3]

Legionella are better seen on Giemsa stain than Gram stain. Silver stains (ie, Dieterle and Warthin-Starry silver stains) demonstrate *Legionella* in fixed tissue preparations. The best way to demonstrate *Legionella* is by monoclonal or polyclonal immunofluorescent antibody staining. *Legionella micdadei* is weakly acid fast using Ziehl-Nielsen staining. *Legionella* may be extracellular or intracellular. In the lung, *Legionella* cells infect mononuclear cells (eg, alveolar macrophages). To demonstrate *Legionella* in respiratory secretions, monoclonal antibody staining is preferred to polyclonal antibody staining. With polyclonal antibodies, false positives (ie, cross-reactions with *Pseudomonas aeruginosa, Pseudomonas fluorescens, Bordetella pertussis, Staphylococcus aureus, Bacteroides fragilis,* and *Bacillus* sp) may occur. Cross-reactions with a monoclonal antibody are infrequent but may occur with *S aureus* or *Bacillus* species. Colonies of *Legionella* appear on *Legionella* solid culture media after approximately 3 days but some *Legionella* species may require 2 weeks to develop visible colonies. Between days 1 and 3, *Legionella* colonies are best detected on plates using magnification.[4,5]

Legionnaires' disease may be diagnosed by *Legionella* or acute/convalescent high rising titers. Seroconversion usually take 4–6 weeks. Monoclonal direct fluorescence assay (DFA) staining respiratory secretions/lung is diagnostic, but DFA positivity decreases rapidly with anti-*Legionella* therapy. *Legionella* antigenuria detects

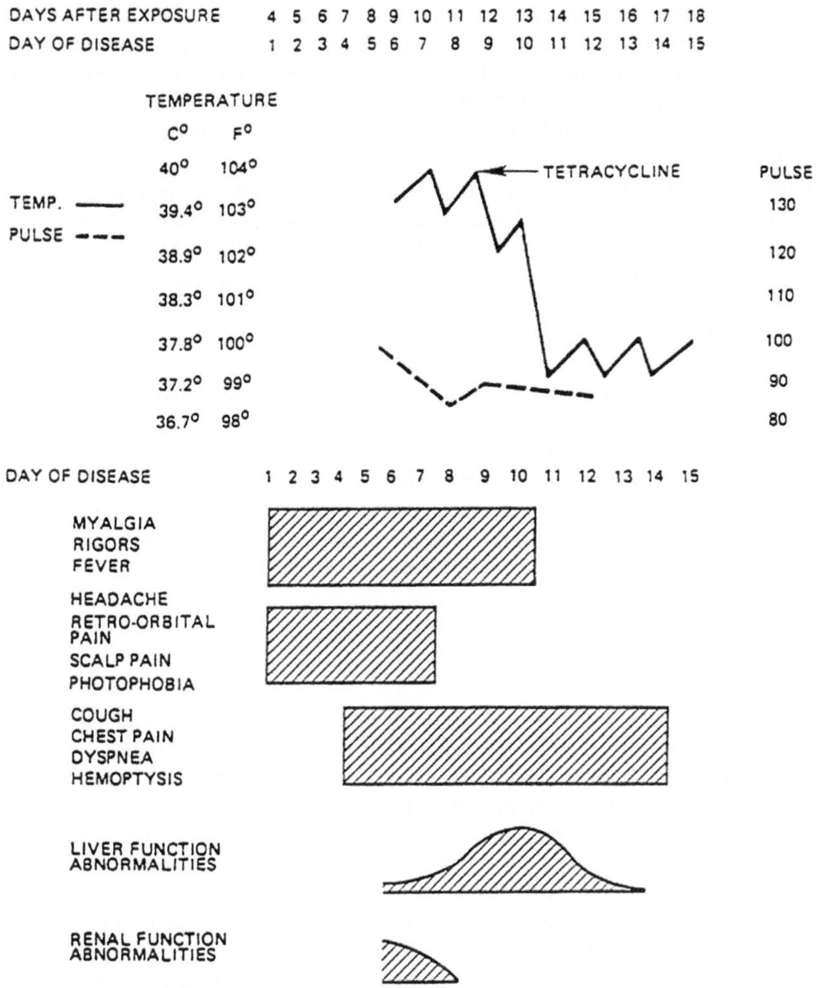

Fig. 1. Relative bradycardia, an early clinical clue, from an early case of Legionnaires' disease. (*Reprinted from* Lattimer GL, Ormsbee RA. Legionnaires' disease. New York: Marcel Dekker; 1981; with permission.)

L pneumophila serogroups 1 to 6 only. Seroconversion occurs in less than 50% of patients within 2 weeks of the onset of legionnaires' disease.[4–8]

Antimicrobial susceptibility testing of *L pneumophila* should not be performed because the organism is an intracellular alveolar macrophage pathogen. In vitro susceptibility tests of *Legionella* must be used in an intracellular model (eg, alveolar macrophage) that takes into account pH and intracellular concentrations of the antimicrobials being tested.[2,9,10]

EPIDEMIOLOGY

The natural habitat of *Legionella* species is fresh water. With *Legionella* CAP, there is a seasonal peak in the late summer and early fall. Sporadic cases occur throughout the year. Sporadic cases and outbreaks of *Legionella* CAP are often related to exposure to water colonized by *Legionella* (eg, during air travel or in water puddles, excavation, or construction sites).[1,2] Outbreaks of *Legionella* nosocomial pneumonia (NP) are related to exposure of water sources containing *Legionella* sp (eg, ice cubes, shower water). *Legionella* CAP occurs in all age groups but is most common in adults more than 50 years of age.[1,4,5]

Epidemiologically, the distribution of *Legionella* is reflective of the presence or absence of *Legionella* sp in local aquatic sources. Because *Legionella* sp are intracellular pathogens, patients with impaired cellular immunity (CMI) are particularly predisposed to legionnaires' disease (eg, patients infected with the human immunodeficiency virus [HIV]).[11,12] *Legionella* CAP caused by various *Legionella* spp has been described in transplant patients. Less commonly, legionnaires' disease may cause CAP in non-transplant immunocompromised hosts with impaired CMI. Patients on immunomodulating/immunosuppressive agents (eg, G-CSF) have an increased incidence and increased severity of legionnaires' disease.[13–16] Epidemiologic investigations of CAP outbreaks, like *Legionella* NP, have had in common a water source colonized by *Legionella* (eg, legionnaires' disease following gardening or hot tub exposure). Legionnaires' disease is endemic in some areas but not in others if *Legionella* is not in the water supply.[17–19] There has been an unexplained increase in legionnaires' disease during the swine influenza (H1N1) pandemic.[20]

CLINICAL PRESENTATION

Overview

Legionella CAP and NP have the same clinical features.[21–23] Like other atypical pulmonary pathogens, legionnaires' disease is associated with extrapulmonary manifestations. Legionnaires' disease, like other causes of atypical CAP, is characterized by its own pattern of extrapulmonary organ involvement.[22–30] Individual findings or specific organ involvement may occur with other atypical CAPs but it is the pattern of extrapulmonary organ involvement rather than individual findings characteristic of legionnaires' disease which permits a syndromic clinical diagnosis. The syndromic diagnosis of *Legionella* CAP is based on recognizing, when present, a constellation of key clinical findings that are suggestive of *Legionella* CAP. In legionnaires' disease, extrapulmonary clinical and laboratory findings have different clinical significance or diagnostic importance. By appreciating the relative diagnostic importance of various signs, symptoms, and laboratory tests, clinicians can apply these principles using a weighted diagnostic point score system that permits a rapid presumptive clinical diagnosis. With this approach, the clinicians can not only differentiate legionnaires' disease from typical bacterial CAPs but can also differentiate legionnaires' disease from other atypical CAPs.

Legionnaires' disease may present subacutely for days or a week but more commonly presents acutely. In normal hosts, *Legionella* often presents as severe CAP. Legionnaires' disease is in the differential diagnosis of atypical CAP and severe CAP. In the nosocomial setting, legionnaires' disease, although it has the same clinical findings as sporadic *Legionella* CAP, usually presents in clusters or outbreaks caused by exposure to contaminated water in the hospital.[24–27] Except for *C pneumoniae* outbreaks occurring in chronic care facilities or nursing homes (ie, nursing home-acquired pneumonia [NHAP]), legionnaires' disease is the most common atypical CAP pathogen in hospital outbreaks or in intensive care units.[24–27] The radiographic and nonspecific laboratory findings that accompany legionnaires' disease overlap with typical and atypical pulmonary pathogens.[28–37] The pulmonary manifestations of *Legionella* CAP (ie, productive cough, shortness of breath, rales, sometimes accompanied by consolidation or pleural effusion) are nonspecific. In legionnaires' disease pleuritic chest pain may be present if the infiltrates are pleural based.[2,3,34,38]

Radiologic Manifestations

Chest film findings

Chest radiograph (CXR) findings in legionnaires' disease are not specific.[35,36] However, certain radiological features may suggest the diagnosis or argue against the diagnosis. Although virtually every radiological manifestation of legionnaires' disease has been described, certain findings argue strongly against the diagnosis of *Legionella* CAP (ie, rapid cavitation within 72 hours, hilar adenopathy, or massive or bloody pleural effusion). Cavitation or abscess formation is rare with legionnaires' disease. Most characteristic of legionnaires' disease radiographically are rapidly progressive asymmetrical patchy infiltrates on CXR.[39,40] The rapid asymmetric progression of CXR infiltrates even with appropriate anti-*Legionella* sp therapy is usual with legionnaires' disease. When *Legionella* presents as severe CAP, the CXR is important in limiting/eliminating other diagnostic possibilities. Severe CAP with no/minimal infiltrates and profound hypoxemia should suggest a viral cause (eg, influenza [human, avian, swine], hantavirus pulmonary syndrome [HPS], severe acute respiratory syndrome [SARS], or cytomegalovirus [CMV]). The differential diagnosis of severe CAP with focal segmental/lobar infiltrates includes *Streptococcus pneumoniae* (in patients with impaired splenic function), legionnaires' disease and zoonotic atypical pathogens (eg, Q fever, tularemia, or adenovirus).[35] Because rapid asymmetrical progression of infiltrates on CXR may occur despite appropriate anti-*Legionella* therapy, the unwary clinician may be misled into thinking that the CAP is not caused by legionnaires' disease.[28–30,32–35]

Chest computed tomography findings

Frequently, chest computed tomography (CT) scans are performed when there is a discordance between radiological and clinical findings or when the CXR features would benefit from the enhanced definition of a chest CT scan.

Chest CT: *S pneumoniae* If *S pneumoniae* is in the differential diagnosis of CAP, the typical findings of *S pneumoniae* CAP on chest CT include peribronchovesicular/centrilobular nodules or bronchovascular bundle thickening. With *S pneumoniae*, the hallmark finding on CXR/chest CT is consolidation (present on chest CT in 90%). These findings are less frequently found on chest CT with *Chlamydophila pneumoniae* or *Mycoplasma pneumoniae* CAP.[41]

In general, atypical CAP pathogens often show centrilobular/acinar infiltrates with air space consolidation and "ground glass" attenuation in a lobar distribution. *Streptococcus pneumoniae* bronchopneumonia radiologically may resemble *Legionella* CAP. Although *S pneumoniae* CAP may, like legionnaires' disease, have consolidation with "ground glass" opacification/attenuation, the "ground glass" attenuation occurs only in the peripheral portions of the consolidation. The consolidation with *S pneumoniae* is usually not sharply demarcated in contrast to legionnaires' disease with sharp demarcation of consolidation.[42]

Chest CT: legionnaires' disease The characteristic appearance of *Legionella* CAP often shows chest CT multiple foci of sharply demarcated areas of consolidation intermingled with "ground glass" opacities. Another differential diagnostic point on chest CT is that the segmental/subsegmental consolidation in legionnaires' disease is more prominent in the perihilar areas rather than the peripheral regions of the lung. Other chest CT *Legionella* CAP findings include a bilateral diffuse interstitial pattern mimicking acute pulmonary edema/noncardiogenic pulmonary edema. Another specific feature of legionnaires' disease on chest CT is the "reversed halo sign." Although not apparent on CXR, legionnaires' disease on chest CT may show unilateral hilar or mediastinal minimal adenopathy. The "bulging fissure sign" is a manifestation of an increase in lobar volume and is typically associated with *Klebsiella pneumoniae* CAP but is not an infrequent finding with *S pneumoniae* CAP and may also occur rarely in legionnaires' disease. With legionnaires' disease, small pleural effusions may be present on chest CT that were not visible on CXR.[41–43]

Chest CT: *M pneumoniae* The advantage of chest CT is to demonstrate more accurately "ground glass" opacities and thickening/nodules of bronchovascular bundles. These findings are important in the differential diagnosis of atypical CAP. Clinically, *M pneumoniae* CAP is often in the differential diagnosis of *Legionella* CAP. Radiologically, both may have bilateral patchy infiltrates on CXR, but chest CT demonstrates differential radiographic features on legionnaires' disease compared with *M pneumoniae*. In nearly all patients with *M pneumoniae* CAP, diffuse bronchial wall thickening is the most characteristic finding on chest CT. Although the most common radiological feature of *M pneumoniae* CAP is central lobular nodules, the finding of generalized bronchial wall thickening is characteristic of *M pneumoniae* CAP.[35,41–44]

Chest CT: *C pneumoniae* Although the typical bacterial CAPs present with unilateral radiographic findings, bilateral infiltrates are common in CAP caused by *C pneumoniae*, *M pneumoniae*, and legionnaires' disease. Although bronchovesicular thickening is the hallmark of *M pneumoniae* CAP, it may also be present in *C pneumoniae* CAP. The chest CT finding that differentiates *C pneumoniae* from *M pneumoniae* CAP is airway dilatation. Diffuse bronchovesicular bundle thickening may be present with either *C pneumoniae* or *M pneumoniae* but the presence of peripheral airway dilatation favors the diagnosis of *C pneumoniae* CAP.[44,45]

Branching central lobular nodules are usually reported as having a "tree-in-bud" appearance is a nonspecific finding. "Tree-in-bud" appearance may be seen with *C pneumoniae* and *M pneumoniae* CAP but argues against the diagnosis of legionnaires' disease.[41–45]

Many radiological features of CAP are common to typical and atypical organisms on CXR. Enhanced definition visible of chest CT scans can help to further limit differential diagnostic possibilities, particularly with *M pneumoniae*, *C pneumoniae*, and legionnaires' disease. However, the presumptive diagnosis of *Legionella* CAP must be based on clinical and not radiologic criteria.[41–46]

Clinical Extrapulmonary Features

As with all atypical causes of CAP, presumptive diagnosis is based on the pattern of extrapulmonary findings, which is distinctive for each atypical CAP pathogen.[33–35] The zoonotic atypical CAP pathogens (ie, tularemia, psittacosis, and Q fever) may be eliminated from further diagnostic consideration by a negative history of recent contact with a zoonotic vector. In patients with CAP with extrapulmonary findings and a negative history of contact with a zoonotic vector, differential diagnostic possibilities are limited to the nonzoonotic atypical CAP pathogens (ie, *M pneumoniae, C pneumoniae,* and legionnaires' disease) (**Tables 1–3**).[47–49]

Table 1
Diagnostic features of the nonzoonotic atypical pneumonias

Key Characteristics	*M pneumoniae*[a]	Legionnaires' Disease	*C pneumoniae*
Signs			
• Rash	±[b]	–	–
• Nonexudative pharyngitis	+	–	+
• Hemoptysis	–	±	–
• Wheezing	–	–	+
• Lobar consolidation	–	±	–
• Cardiac involvement	±[c]	–[d]	–
• Splenomegaly	–	–	–
• Relative bradycardia	–	+	–
Laboratory abnormalities			
• WBC count	↑/N	↑	N
• Acute thrombocytosis	±	–	–
• Hyponatremia	–	+	–
• Hypophosphatemia	–	+	–
• ↑ AST/ALT	–	+	–
• ↑ CPK	–	+	–
• ↑ CRP (>30)	–	+	–
• ↑ Ferritin (>2 × n)	–	+	–
• ↑ Cold agglutinins (≥1:64)	+	–	–
• Microscopic hematuria	–	±	–
Chest radiograph			
• Infiltrates	Patchy	Patchy or consolidation	"Circumscribed" lesions
• Bilateral hilar adenopathy	–	–	–
• Pleural effusion	± (small)	±	–
Diagnostic tests			
• Direct isolation (culture)	±	+	±
• Serology (specific)	CF	IFA	CF
• *Legionella* IFA titers	–	↑↑↑	–
• *Legionella* DFA	–	+	–
• *Legionella* urinary antigen	–	+[e]	–

Abbreviations: CF, complement fixation; CPK, creatinine phosphokinase; CRP, C-reactive protein; CYE, charcoal yeast agar; DFA, direct fluorescent antibody; IFA, indirect fluorescent antibody; N, normal; WBC, white blood cell; +, usually present; ±, sometimes present; –, usually absent; ↑, increased; ↓, decreased; ↑↑↑, markedly increased.

[a] Mental confusion only if meningoencephalitis.

[b] Erythema multiforme.

[c] Myocarditis, heart block, or pericarditis.

[d] Unless endocarditis.

[e] Often not positive early, but antigenuria persists for weeks. Useful only to diagnose *L pneumophila*. (serogroups 01–06), not other species/serogroups.

Adapted from Cunha BA, editor. Pneumonia essentials. 3rd edition. Sudbury (MA): Jones & Bartlett; 2010.

Table 2
Diagnostic features of the zoonotic atypical pneumonias

Key Characteristics	Psittacosis	Q fever	Tularemia
Symptoms			
Mental confusion	−	±	−
Prominent headache	+	+	+
Meningismus	−	−	−
Myalgias	+	+	+
Ear pain	−	−	−
Pleuritic pain	±	±	±
Abdominal pain	−	−	−
Diarrhea	−	−	−
Signs			
Rash	±[a]	−	−
Nonexudative pharyngitis	−	−	±
Hemoptysis	−	−	±
Lobar consolidation	+	+	+
Cardiac involvement	±[b]	±[c]	−
Splenomegaly	+	+	−
Relative bradycardia	+	+	−
Chest radiograph			
Infiltrates	Patchy or consolidation	Patchy or consolidation	"Ovoid" or round infiltrates
Bilateral hilar adenopathy	−	−	±
Pleural effusion	−	−	Bloody
Laboratory abnormalities			
WBC count	↓	↑/N	↑/N
Acute thrombocytosis	−	+	−
↓ Na^+	±	±	±
Hypophosphatemia	−	−	−
↑ AST/ALT	+	+	−
↑ Cold agglutinins	−	±	−
ASM antibodies	−	±	−
Microscopic hematuria	−	−	−
Diagnostic tests			
Direct isolation (culture)	−	−	−
Serology (specific)	CF	CF	TA

Abbreviations: ASM, anti-smooth muscle; CF, complement fixation; N, normal; TA, tube agglutinins; WBC, white blood cells; +, usually present; ±, sometimes presents; −, usually absent; ↑, increased; ↓, decreased; ↑↑↑, markedly increased.

[a] Horder's spots (facial spots) resemble the abdominal rash of typhoid fever (Rose spots).

[b] Myocarditis.

[c] Endocarditis.

Adapted from Cunha BA, editor. Pneumonia essentials. 3rd edition. Sudbury (MA): Jones & Bartlett; 2010.

Table 3
Clinical features of legionnaires' disease

Organ Involvement	Common Features	Uncommon Features	Argues Against Legionnaires' Disease
CNS	Mental confusion encephalopathic, headache	Lethargy, stupor, dizziness	Meningeal signs, seizures, CN palsies
Upper respiratory tract	None	Vertigo	Sore throat, ear pain, bullous myringitis, otitis media
Cardiac	Relative bradycardia	Myocarditis, endocarditis[a]	Pericarditis, no relative bradycardia
GI	Loose stools/watery diarrhea	Abdominal pain	Hepatomegaly, hepatic tenderness, peritoneal signs
Renal	Microscopic hematuria, renal insufficiency	Decreased urine output, acute renal failure	CVA tenderness, chronic renal failure
Laboratory tests			
Gram stain (sputum)	Few mononuclear cells, few/no bacteria	PMN predominance, mixed flora	Purulent sputum, single predominant organism
WBC count	Leukocytosis, relative lymphopenia	Lymphocytosis	Leukopenia, atypical lymphocytes, thrombocytosis, thrombocytopenia
Pleural fluid	Exudative	↑ WBCs	RBCs, ↓ pH, ↓ glucose
AST/ALT	Mildly increased (2–5 × n)	Moderately increased (5–10 × n)	Markedly increased (>10 × n)
Serum phosphorus	Decreased transiently (early)	Decreased (later)	Increased/normal
CPK	Increased (early)	Rhabdomyolysis	Normal levels do not rule out legionnaires' disease
CRP	↑ >35 (early)	↓ >35 (later)	Normal levels does not rule out legionnaires'
Ferritin	Highly increased (>2 × n)	Moderately increased (<2 × n)	Normal ferritin levels early
CSF	Normal	Mild pleocytosis	RBCs, ↓ glucose, ↑ lactic acid
Urine analysis	RBCs	Myoglobinuria, gross hematuria	Pyuria, hemoglobinuria

Abbreviations: CN, cranial nerve; CNS, central nervous system; CPK, creatinine phosphokinase; CRP, C-reactive protein; CSF, cerebrospinal fluid; CVA, costovertebral angle; GI, gastrointestinal; PMN, polymorphonuclear leukocyte (neutrophil); RBC, red blood cell; WBC, white blood cell.

[a] Culture negative.

Adapted from Cunha BA, editor. Pneumonia essentials. 3rd edition. Sudbury (MA): Jones & Bartlett; 2010.

Diagnostic significance of relative bradycardia

As mentioned earlier, some clinical findings have more diagnostic importance than others and therefore have more diagnostic value when present. The specificity of findings is enhanced when key findings are combined in a syndromic diagnosis. In a patient with CAP with extrapulmonary findings and a negative history of recent zoonotic contact, the presence or absence of a pulse temperature (ie, relative bradycardia) is a key diagnostic sign. This key sign was present in early reports on legionnaires' disease (see **Fig. 1**). Most physicians are unaware of the criteria of relative bradycardia. In normal hosts, a temperature of 102°F should be accompanied by an appropriate pulse response of 110/min. In such a patient, if the pulse is less than 100/min, relative bradycardia is said to be present. Pulse-temperature relationships for different degrees of fever and the pulse diagnostic of relative bradycardia for given temperatures are presented in **Table 4**.[35,50] If the patient with nonzoonotic CAP is not on β-blockers, diltiazem, or verapamil, or does not have a pacemaker or heartblock, relative bradycardia points to legionnaires' disease. None of the typical bacterial

Table 4
Differential diagnosis of relative bradycardia

Temperature-pulse Relationships

Temperature °F (°C)	Appropriate pulse response (beats/min)	Relative bradycardia (pulse deficit) pulse (beats/min)
106 (41.1)	150	<140
105 (41.1)	140	<130
104 (41.1)	130	<120
103 (41.1)	120	<110
102 (41.1)	110	<100

Criteria for relative bradycardia

Inclusive	1. Patient must be an adult 2. Temperature ≥102°F 3. Pulse must be taken simultaneously with the temperature
Exclusive	1. Patient has normal sinus rhythm without arrhythmia, second/third-degree heart block or pacemaker-induced rhythm 2. Patient must not be on a β-blocker, verapamil, or diltiazem

Causes of Relative Bradycardia

Infectious	Noninfectious
• Legionnaires' disease	• β-blockers
• Psittacosis	• Verapamil
• Q fever	• Diltiazem
• Typhoid fever	• Central nervous system disorders
• Typhus	• Lymphomas
• Babesiosis	• Factitious fever
• Malaria	• Drug fever
• Leptospirosis	
• Yellow fever	
• Dengue fever	
• Viral hemorrhagic fevers	
• Rocky Mountain spotted fever	

Adapted from Cunha CB. Differential diagnosis of infectious disease. In: Cunha BA. Antibiotic essentials. 9th edition. Sudbury (MA): Jones & Bartlett; 2010; with permission.

CAPs are associated with relative bradycardia nor is *M pneumoniae* or *C pneumoniae* (**Fig. 2**).[35,49,50]

Central nervous system manifestations Some patients with CAP complain of headache, which is also the case with legionnaires' disease. However, among the atypical pathogens, *Legionella* is most likely to present with CAP with encephalopathy. Mental confusion may accompany headache in patients with legionnaires' disease. Among the nonzoonotic atypical pathogens, *M pneumoniae* (if CAP is accompanied by *M pneumoniae* meningoencephalitis) or Q fever CAP may rarely present with mental confusion. Such cases should be readily differentiated from legionnaires' disease by cold agglutinin titers. Increased cold agglutinin titers are not a feature of legionnaires' disease but may occur in low titer with various viral pathogens or with Q fever. *Mycoplasma pneumoniae* CAP may be accompanied by higher levels of cold agglutinins that when present are helpful diagnostically if the titer is 1:64 or higher. In CAP with mycoplasma meningoencephalitis, the cold agglutinin titers are usually high (ie, >1:512 and not uncommonly >1:1052). Excluding encephalopathy and headache, there are no other neurologic manifestations that suggest legionnaires' disease.[32–35,51,52]

Head, eyes, ears, nose, and throat manifestations There are no head, eyes, ears, nose, and throat (HEENT) manifestations of *Legionella* CAP. The presence of otitis/bullous myringitis or nonexudative pharyngitis should suggest *M pneumoniae* or less commonly *C pneumoniae* CAP.[33,35,49]

Cardiac manifestations The characteristic cardiac manifestation of legionnaires' disease is a pulse-temperature deficit, (ie, relative bradycardia). Diagnostic possibilities in patients who have otherwise unexplained relative bradycardia with CAP are limited to legionnaires' disease, Q fever, and psittacosis. Relative bradycardia is a nearly universal finding in legionnaires' disease and the absence of relative

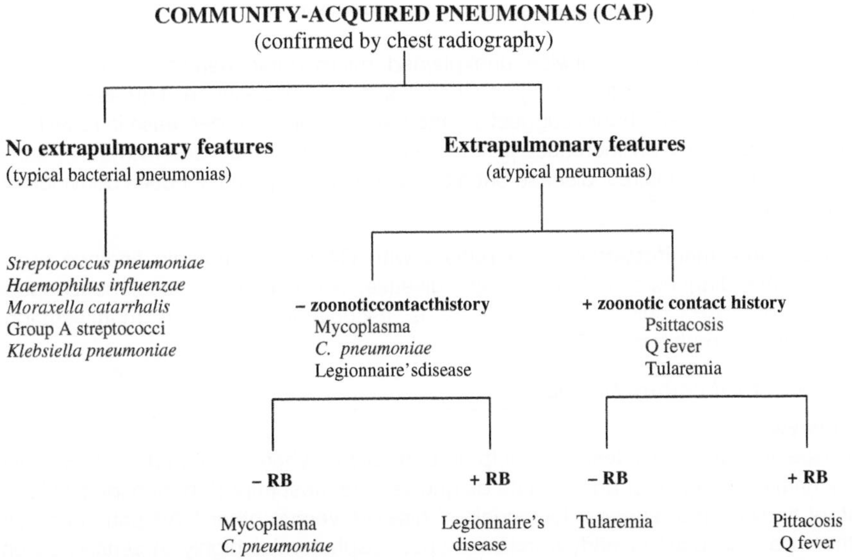

Fig. 2. Clinical approach to community-acquired pneumonias: the importance of the zoonotic contact history and relative bradycardia.

bradycardia should prompt the clinician to question the diagnosis. Relative bradycardia is a characteristic feature of legionnaires' disease but may be found less frequently in patients with Q fever or psittacosis CAP. Rarely, legionnaires' disease may present as "culture-negative" endocarditis. Culture-negative endocarditis may occur on normal or prosthetic heart valves. Myocarditis is rare with legionnaires' disease.[35,50,53–55]

Hepatic manifestations The hepatic manifestations of legionnaires' disease are mildly transiently increased serum transaminase (aspartate aminotransferase [AST]/alanine aminotransferase [ALT]) levels. The alkaline phosphatase level is occasionally increased in legionnaires' disease but is much less frequent than increased serum transaminase levels, which are present in nearly all patients. Hepatic enlargement or tenderness is not a feature of legionnaires' disease. Hepatomegaly, if present in a patient with CAP, should suggest an underlying disorder or an alternate diagnosis. Similarly, splenomegaly is not a clinical feature of legionnaires' disease. In a CAP patient with splenomegaly, legionnaires' disease is effectively ruled out and alternate diagnoses (eg, Q fever or psittacosis) should be considered instead.[35,53–55]

Gastrointestinal manifestations Atypical CAP gastrointestinal manifestations are loose or watery stools with or without abdominal pain. Loose stools or watery diarrhea in a patient with atypical CAP should suggest *M pneumoniae* or legionnaires' disease. The presence of abdominal pain with or without watery diarrhea limits differential diagnostic possibilities to legionnaires' disease.[2,33,35]

Musculoskeletal manifestations Legionnaires' disease is usually accompanied by fever, often with chills. Myalgias may accompany fever and chills in legionnaires' disease, but are usually not severe. Myalgias may be present with typical or atypical pathogens and are diagnostically unhelpful.

Severe myalgias should suggest an alternate diagnosis (eg, human, avian, or swine influenza). Some patients with legionnaires' disease develop rhabdomyolysis. In this patient subgroup, myalgias are not only severe but may be the predominant extrapulmonary manifestation of legionnaires' disease.[20,35,39,47]

Renal manifestations Otherwise unexplained microscopic hematuria is the most frequent renal manifestation of legionnaires' disease. The presence of gross hematuria in a patient with CAP should suggest an alternate diagnosis. A decrease in renal function manifested by an increased in the serum creatinine has been noted in some patients with legionnaires' disease but a causal relationship has not been convincingly demonstrated.[35,39,49]

Dermatologic manifestations In a patient with CAP, dermatologic findings argue against the diagnosis of legionnaires' disease. Among the atypical nonzoonotic causes of CAP, only *M pneumoniae* is associated with skin manifestations (eg, erythema multiforme).[35,49]

Nonspecific Laboratory Findings

Overview

Nonspecific laboratory tests are helpful, particularly when combined, in suggesting legionnaires' disease or an alternate diagnosis. The most important nonspecific laboratory findings that suggest legionnaires' disease versus other CAP pathogens are otherwise unexplained early/transient hypophosphatemia, highly increased serum ferritin levels, mildly/transiently early increases of serum transaminases, and microscopic hematuria.[35,49]

Complete blood count

Leukocytosis is a standard feature in patients with legionnaires' disease. In a patient with CAP the presence of leukopenia should suggest an alternate diagnosis (eg, adenoviral CAP). Legionnaires' disease does not affect the platelet count. Therefore, in a patient with CAP with either thrombocytosis or thrombocytopenia, an alternate diagnosis besides legionnaires' disease should be considered.[33–35]

Relative lymphopenia

Otherwise unexplained relative lymphopenia is a nearly universal nonspecific laboratory finding in legionnaires' disease. However, there are many infectious and noninfectious disorders associated with relative lymphopenia. Before ascribing relative lymphopenia to legionnaires' disease, the clinician must be careful to exclude other disorders associated with relative lymphopenia. Relative lymphopenia may occur with other causes of CAP, particularly CMV, influenza (human, avian, swine) pneumonia, and *Pneumocystis (carinii) jiroveci* pneumonia (PCP). Because otherwise unexplained relative lymphopenia is such a frequent finding in legionnaires' disease, clinicians should question the diagnosis of legionnaires' disease in a patient with CAP if relative lymphopenia is not present. Relative lymphopenia in legionnaires' disease, if present, is often profound and prolonged and also has prognostic significance (**Table 5**).[35,36,49]

Erythrocyte sedimentation rate/C-reactive protein

The erythrocyte sedimentation rate (ESR) and the C-reactive protein (CRP) level are nonspecific indicators of inflammation, infection, or neoplasm. Most patients acutely ill with CAP have an increased ESR or CRP. The ESR and CRP levels tend to be highly increased in legionnaires' disease but are nonspecific findings. Highly increased ESR or CRP level is consistent with but not characteristic of the diagnosis of legionnaires' disease. With legionnaires' disease, the ESR may be high and in some cases exceed 100 mm/h, and CRP values may exceed 35. Other nonspecific laboratory tests are better indicators of legionnaires' disease than are a highly increased ESR or CRP.[2,5,35,49]

Hyponatremia

Hyponatremia is commonly associated with CAP of any cause, but is most frequently associated with *Legionella* CAP. Because hyponatremia is a nonspecific finding, it is an unhelpful discriminant parameter in differentiating *Legionella* from other causes of CAP. Hyponatremia secondary to the syndrome of inappropriate antidiuretic hormone (SIADH) may occur with various infectious and noninfectious pulmonary disorders. Although hyponatremia is a frequent but nonspecific finding in legionnaires' disease, if present in legionnaires' disease, it is usually greater than in other pulmonary conditions associated with hyponatremia.[1–4] Many physicians ascribe undue diagnostic significance to hyponatremia, which, in addition to being secondary to SIADH, may represent dilutional hyponatremia. With legionnaires' disease, hyponatremia is a less specific laboratory test than is otherwise unexplained hypophosphatemia. In a patient with CAP, otherwise unexplained hypophosphatemia should suggest the diagnosis of legionnaires' disease.[33–35,39,49]

Hypophosphatemia

In contrast to hyponatremia, hypophosphatemia, if present in CAP, limits diagnostic possibilities to legionnaires' disease. Most nonspecific laboratory markers of legionnaires' disease may occur (eg, highly increased ESR, highly increased CRP levels,

Table 5
Differential diagnosis of relative lymphopenia ≤21% (n = 21%–52%)

Infectious Causes	Noninfectious Causes
• CMV	• Cytoxic drugs
• HHV-6	• Steroids
• HHV-8	• Sarcoidosis
• HIV	• SLE
• Miliary tuberculosis	• Lymphoma
• Legionnaires' disease	• Rheumatoid arthritis
• Typhoid fever	• Radiation
• Q fever	• Wiskott-Aldrich syndrome
• Brucellosis	• Whipple's disease
• Malaria	• Severe combined immunodeficiency disease (SCID)
• Babesiosis	• Common variable immune deficiency (CVID)
• SARS	• DiGeorge's syndrome
• Influenza	• Nezelof's syndrome
• Avian influenza	• Intestinal lymphangiectasia
• Swine influenza	• Ataxia telangiectasia
• Rocky Mountain spotted fever	• Constrictive pericarditis
• Histoplasmosis	• Tricuspid regurgitation
• Dengue fever	• Kawasaki's disease
• Chikungunya fever	• Idiopathic CD4 cytopenia
• Ehrlichiosis	• Acute/chronic renal failure
• Parvovirus B19	• Hemodialysis
• HPS	• Myasthenia gravis
• WNE	• Celiac disease
• Viral hepatitis (early)	• Alcoholic cirrhosis
	• Coronary bypass
	• Wegener granulomatosis
	• CHF
	• Acute pancreatitis
	• Carcinomas (terminal)

Abbreviations: CHF, congestive heart failure; CLL, chronic lymphocytic leukemia; EBV, Epstein-Barr virus; HCV, hepatitis C virus; HHV, human herpesvirus; HPS, hantavirus pulmonary syndrome; SARS, severe acute respiratory syndrome; SLE, systemic lupus erythematosus; WNE, West Nile encephalitis.

Adapted from Cunha CB. Infectious disease differential diagnosis. In: Cunha BA, editor. Antibiotic essentials. 9th edition. Sudbury (MA): Jones & Bartlett; 2010.

mildly increased serum transaminase levels, highly increased serum ferritin levels) with other causes of CAP. Otherwise unexplained hypophosphatemia is an important nonspecific laboratory marker for legionnaires' disease because it is not associated with any other CAP pathogen. Hypophosphatemia occurs commonly with legionnaires' disease. Hypophosphatemia, when present in legionnaires' disease, may occur at any time during the in-hospital clinical course (**Table 6**). Although hypophosphatemia of legionnaires' disease may be prolonged in duration, more frequently it may be transiently present early and easily missed. It is not uncommon for the hypophosphatemia in legionnaires' disease to resolve spontaneously within the first day or 2 of hospitalization (**Fig. 3**). Unless serum phosphorus levels are obtained on admission or in the first few days of hospital admission, hypophosphatemia may be missed. Because serum phosphorus levels are not always ordered on admission by physicians in patients with CAP, an important clue to legionnaires' disease in a patient with CAP is often missed or its clinical significance overlooked (see **Fig. 3** and **Table 6**).[35,49,56]

Table 6
Differential diagnosis of hypophosphatemia

Infectious Causes	Noninfectious Causes
• Legionnaires' disease • Malaria (acute) • Burkitt's lymphoma	• Alcoholism • Diabetes mellitus • Primary hyperparathyroidism • Idiopathic hypercalciuria • Hypokalemia • Hypomagnesemia • Cushing's syndrome • Acute gout • Diabetes mellitus • RTA • Malabsorption • Hyperalimentation • Vitamin D deficiency • Malnutrition • Vomiting • Diarrhea • Alcoholism • Alkalosis (respiratory) • Acidosis • Nutritional recovery syndrome • Salicylate poisoning • Multiple myeloma • Dialysis • AML • Histiocytic lymphomas • Malignant neuroleptic syndrome • Burns (severe) • Drugs Diuretics Corticosteroids Phosphate binding antacids Cisplatin Acetaminophen toxicity Foscarnet

Abbreviations: AML, acute myeloid leukemia; RTA, renal tubular acidosis.

Adapted from Cunha CB. Differential diagnosis of infectious disease. In: Cunha BA, editor. Antibiotic essentials. 9th edition. Sudbury (MA): Jones & Bartlett; 2010; with permission.

Elevated serum transaminase levels

Mildly increased serum transaminase levels are a common and consistent finding in *Legionella* CAP. Hepatic involvement (ie, mild increases of the serum transaminases) is not a feature of *M pneumoniae* or *C pneumoniae* CAP. Atypical CAP with mildly increased AST/ALT levels are sufficient to effectively rule out *C pneumoniae* or *M pneumoniae* from further diagnostic consideration. Hepatic involvement is one of the usual extrapulmonary manifestations of legionnaires' disease. Because serum transaminase (eg, AST/ALT) levels are mildly or transiently increased early in the course of legionnaires' disease, the presence and clinical significance of this laboratory finding is often overlooked. Physicians often regard mild transient increases of AST/ALT levels as nonspecific and do not appreciate its clinical significance in the context of the patient with CAP. Patients with typical bacterial CAPs do not have increased AST/ALT levels. The atypical CAP pathogens with mild/transiently

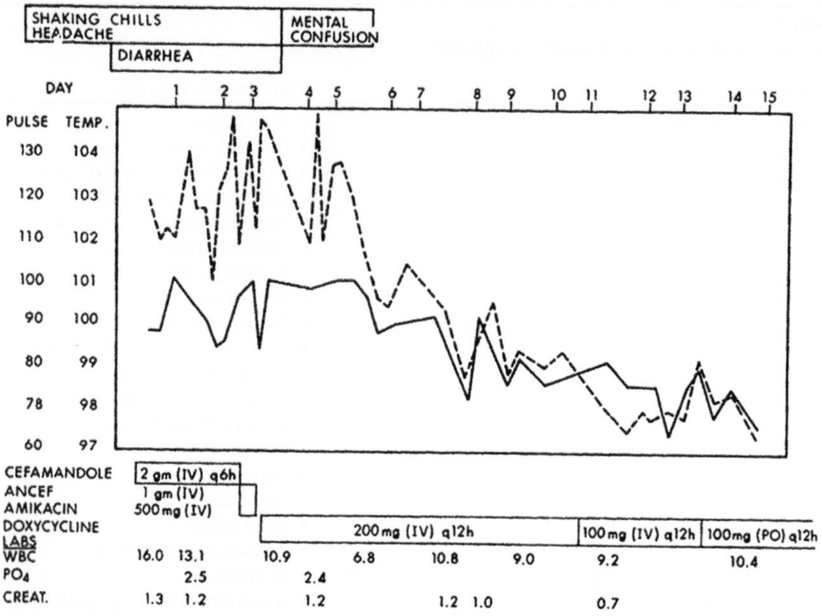

Fig. 3. Typical fever response (5–7 days) of legionnaires' disease to anti-*Legionella* antibiotic therapy with doxycycline (note lack of fever response to β-lactam therapy). (*Reprinted from* Cotton LM, Strampfer MJ, Cunha BA. Legionella and *Mycoplasma pneumonia*. A community hospital experience. Clin Chest Med 1987;8:441–53; with permission.)

increased AST/ALT levels are legionnaires' disease, Q fever, and psittacosis. From a differential diagnostic perspective liver involvement manifested by mildly increased serum transaminase levels is not a feature of tularemia or *M pneumoniae* or *C pneumoniae* CAP. Highly elevated AST/ALT levels should suggest a non-CAP diagnosis.[1–3,35,56–58]

Antismooth muscle antibodies

Antismooth muscle (ASM) antibodies are not ordinarily part of the laboratory tests ordered in a patient with CAP. The only cause of CAP associated with increased ASM antibody titers is Q fever. Because coinfections are rare, the finding of ASM antibodies in a patient with CAP argues against other diagnostic possibilities including legionnaires' disease and should suggest the diagnosis of Q fever CAP.[35,59]

Increased cold agglutinin titers

In a CAP patient there are nonspecific laboratory tests that, when present, should suggest a diagnosis other than legionnaires' disease. Because copathogens in CAP are rare, the presence of highly elevated cold agglutinin titers should suggest an alternative diagnosis to legionnaires' disease. Mildly increased cold agglutinin titers may occur with various viral respiratory infections. Increased cold agglutinin titers, excluding influenza (human, avian, swine), CMV, and adenovirus, are not associated with extrapulmonary clinical features. Being aware of the pattern of extrapulmonary organ involvement with various pulmonary pathogens, clinicians should have no difficulty in evaluating the clinical significance of mild/moderately increased serum cold agglutinin titers. Highly increased cold agglutinin titers in a patient with CAP points to the diagnosis of *M pneumoniae* CAP. Mild to moderate increases of cold agglutinins may also be present in patients with Q fever CAP. In a patient with CAP, the higher the cold agglutinin titer is over 1:64, the more likely it is that the patient has *M pneumoniae*. CAP with highly increased cold agglutinin titers (ie, >1:256) is virtually diagnostic of *M pneumoniae* CAP. Because coinfection in CAP is rare, cold agglutinin titers are important because increased cold agglutinins effectively rule out *Legionella* CAP (**Table 7**).[35,52,59]

Increased serum ferritin levels

Otherwise unexplained highly elevated serum ferritin levels are a characteristic laboratory finding in legionnaires' disease. In legionnaires' disease, highly elevated serum ferritin levels are usually, but not always, present on admission. However, during the course of legionnaires' disease, serum ferritin levels become highly and persistently elevated. Midly/transiently elevated serum ferritin may represent an acute phase reactant. However, the magnitude/duration of ferritin level elevations in legionnaires' disease is due to the infection and not an acute phase phenomenon. Highly elevated serum ferritin levels are such a consistent finding in legionnaires' disease, that with unelevated/minimally elevated serum ferritin levels the diagnosis of Legionnaires' disease should be questioned (**Table 8**).[35,60]

Increased serum creatinine phosphokinase levels

Creatinine phosphokinase (CPK) levels are often increased in patients with legionnaires' disease. Highly elevated CPK levels may also be a manifestation of

Table 7
Differential diagnosis of increased cold agglutinin titers

Infectious Causes	Non-infectious Causes
High cold agglutinin titers (≥1:64)	High cold agglutinin titers high (≥1:64)
• *Mycoplasma pneumoniae*	• Cold agglutinin disease
Elevated cold agglutinin titers (<1:64)	Elevated cold agglutinin titers (<1:64)
Respiratory pathogens	• SLE
• *M pneumoniae*	• Myeloma
• Adenovirus	• Waldenström's macroglobulinemia
• Influenza	• Lymphoma
Nonrespiratory pathogens	• CLL
• EBV	• Sinus histocytosis
• CMV	
• HCV	
• Malaria	
• Trypanosomiasis	
• Coxsackie viruses	
• Measles	
• Mumps	
• HIV	

Abbreviations: CLL, chronic lymphocytic leukemia; CMV, cytomegalovirus; EBV, Epstein-Barr virus; HCV, hepatitis C virus; HIV, human immuno deficiency virus; SLE, systemic lupus erythematosus.

Adapted from Cunha BA. The clinical diagnosis of *Mycoplasma pneumoniae*: the diagnostic importance of highly elevated serum cold agglutinins. Eur J Clin Microbiol Infect Dis 2008;27:1017–9.

Table 8
Differential diagnosis of highly increased serum ferritin levels (>2× normal)

Infectious Causes	Noninfectious Causes
Acute • Legionnaires' disease • WNE **Chronic** • HIV • CMV • TB	**Malignancies** • Preleukemias • Lymphomas • Multiple myeloma • Hepatomas • Breast cancer • Colon cancer • Prostate cancer • Lung cancer • Liver/CNS metastases **Myeloproliferative disorders** **Rheumatic/inflammatory disorders** • Rheumatoid arthritis • Adult Still's disease • SLE • TA **Renal disease** • Acute renal failure • Chronic renal failure **Liver disease** • Hemochromatosis • Cirrhosis • α_1-antitrypsin deficiency • CAH • Cholestatic jaundice **Miscellaneous** • Sickle cell anemia • Multiple blood transfusions

Abbreviations: CAH, chronic acute hepatitis; CNS, central nervous system; SLE, systemic lupus erythematosus; TA, temporal arteritis, TB, active tuberculosis; WNE, West Nile encephalitis.

Adapted from Cunha CB. Differential diagnosis of infectious disease. In: Cunha BA, editor. Antibiotic essentials. 9th edition. Sudbury (MA): Jones & Bartlett; 2010.

rhabdomyolysis. Mild to moderate increases of CPK may occur with various infectious and noninfectious disorders. Rhabdomyolysis may accompany various CAPs, particularly influenza (human, avian, swine) pneumonia and legionnaires' disease. In a CAP patient in whom influenza (human, avian, swine) is not a diagnostic consideration, the clinician should order *Legionella* sp diagnostic tests to confirm or rule out the diagnosis.[33,35]

Lactate dehydrogenase

Lactate dehydrogenase (LDH) levels are variably increased in legionnaires' disease. Mild increases in serum LDH levels may occur with various disorders and are diagnostically unhelpful in patients with CAP. Highly increased LDH levels in a patient with CAP and with shortness of breath/hypoxemia with a clear CXR or a CXR with bilateral patchy interstitial infiltrates should suggest the diagnosis of *Pneumocystis (carinii) jiroveci* CAP.[2–4,35]

Increased serum procalcitonin levels

Serum procalcitonin (PCT) levels have been used as a marker for bacterial CAP. Serum PCT levels are not increased in viral infections including influenza (human, avian, swine). In legionnaires' disease, serum PCT levels may be increased. Various disorders are associated with increased PCT levels. Like other nonspecific laboratory tests, the clinical significance of increased serum PCT must be interpreted in the appropriate clinical setting. With the exception of legionnaires' disease, serum PCT levels are not increased with the other atypical CAPs. Serum PCT levels offer no additional diagnostic information in diagnosing CAP other than what may be learned from the CXR. The CXR remains the best way to identify bacterial pneumonias and eliminate other disorders that may mimic radiologically bacterial CAPs. In CAPs, serum PCT levels are expensive and offer no additional diagnostic information than can be obtained by a CXR (**Table 9**).[35] Highly increased serum PCT levels may have prognostic significance in legionnaires' disease.[61]

Clinical Syndromic Diagnosis

In the clinical diagnosis of legionnaires' disease, individual clinical and nonspecific laboratory and radiologic findings have little diagnostic specificity. Studies reporting the inability clinically to differentiate typical from atypical CAP pathogens usually are based on comparing single parameters, such as fever or hyponatremia.[62–64] Such approaches do not work because critical parameters are not included (ie, hypophosphatemia, or relative bradycardia).[62–64] The diagnostic usefulness of selecting key nonspecific findings is enhanced when they are combined to increase diagnostic specificity, which is the basis of clinical syndromic diagnosis. In CAP patients with extrapulmonary findings and a negative history of zoonotic contact who present with relative bradycardia, hypophosphatemia, or increased serum ferritin levels, the

Table 9
Differential diagnosis of increased PCT levels

Infectious Disorders	Noninfectious Disorders
• Bacterial pneumonias	• Renal insufficiency
CAP	• Alcoholic hepatitis
NHAP	• Lung cancer (small cell)
NP	• Thyroid cancer
• Legionnaires' disease	• Surgery
• Bacteremias (gram-negative > gram-positive)	• Trauma
• TB	• Burns
• Bacterial meningitis	• Cardiogenic shock
• Fungal pneumonias	• Goodpasture syndrome shock
• Viral hepatitis	• GVHD
• Toxoplasmosis	• Hypotension
• Osteomyelitis	• Hemorrhagic/necrotic pancreatitis
• SBE	• Normal variant (elderly)
• Malaria (*Plasmodium falciparum*)	• Febrile neutropenia
	• Drug fever
	• HD (not PD)
	• Immunosuppression/steroids
	• BMT
	• Tumor fever

Abbreviations: BMT, bone marrow transplant; CAP, community acquired pneumonia; GVHD, graft-versus-host disease; HD, hemodialysis; NHAP, nursing home acquired pneumonia; NP, nosocomial pneumonia; PD, peritoneal dialysis; SBE, subacute bacterial endocarditis; TB, tuberculosis.

Data from Cunha CB. Differential diagnosis of infectious disease. In: Cunha BA, editor. Antibiotic essentials. 9th edition. Sudbury (MA): Jones & Bartlett; 2010.

likelihood of legionnaires' disease is high. Clinically, given these findings in a CAP patient, there is no alternative diagnosis that would be readily confused with legionnaires' disease (**Tables 10** and **11**).[35,65–67]

Legionnaires' disease often progresses within 2 to 3 days despite anti-*Legionella* antimicrobial therapy. This progress may be related to the intracellular location of *Legionella* in the alveolar macrophage. If the clinical syndromic diagnosis suggests legionnaires' disease based preferably on a weighted diagnostic index, clinicians should not add another antimicrobial therapy or consider alternative diagnoses. As the patient begins to improve, usually after 3 to 5 days, a decrease in temperature is accompanied by a disappearance of relative bradycardia (**Fig. 4**). Most clinical and laboratory abnormalities resolve quickly but fever and mental confusion may persist for 2 to 3 days. CXR may show legionnaires' disease infiltrates for weeks after clinical improvement (**Figs. 5–10**).[35]

Differential Diagnosis

Mimics of legionnaires' disease

Legionella CAP may resemble any one of the typical bacterial CAP pathogens radiologically. On CXR, *Legionella pneumophila* often presents with a lobar infiltrate that may or may not be accompanied by consolidation or pleural effusion, which are the radiological hallmarks of typical bacterial CAP pathogens. Radiologically, *Legionella* may also resemble some of the zoonotic atypical pulmonary pathogens, particularly Q fever and psittacosis. Psittacosis and Q fever, like legionnaires' disease, may present with lobar infiltrates with or without consolidation/pleural effusion. In patients with an appropriate history of recent epidemiologic or vector contact, either Q fever or psittacosis should be included in the differential diagnosis of CAP. The viral CAPs that may be confused with legionnaires' disease are adenoviral and swine influenza (H1N1) pneumonias. Adenovirus radiologically may present with lobar infiltrates with or without pleural effusion, resembling a typical bacterial CAP or legionnaires' disease. Mimics of legionnaires' disease may be diagnosed by ordering specific acute/convalescent serology appropriate to the pathogens that are clinically relevant in the differential diagnosis.[35,53,56]

Mycoplasma pneumoniae CAP

Clinically, legionnaires' disease and *M pneumoniae* CAP are the commonest nonzoonotic atypical CAP pathogens. Atypical CAP pathogens may be clinically differentiated from typical CAP pathogens by the presence or absence of extrapulmonary clinical and laboratory findings. Similarly, among the atypical CAPs a presumptive clinical diagnosis based on the characteristic pattern of extrapulmonary organ involvement of each individual pathogen is relatively straightforward. The zoonotic atypical CAP pathogens may be eliminated from consideration with a negative recent zoonotic contact history. If the patient has CAP and extrapulmonary findings ie, has an atypical CAP with zoonotic atypical pathogens eliminated by history, the differential diagnosis is limited to the nonzoonotic atypical CAP pathogens. Mycoplasma and legionnaires' disease are often in the differential diagnosis of non-zoonotic atypical CAPs, not because they resemble each other but because the *M pneumoniae* CAP is so common. Clinically, in terms of pattern of organ involvement and nonspecific laboratory tests, legionnaires' disease and *M pneumoniae* CAP are easily differentiated. The key cardinal findings that serve to differentiate legionnaires' disease from *M pneumoniae* are relative bradycardia, mildly increased serum transaminase levels, early/transient hypophosphatemia, highly increased ferritin levels, and microscopic hematuria. Although all of these findings are not present in every patient with *Legionella* CAP,

Table 10
Winthrop-University Hospital Infectious Disease Division's diagnostic weighted point score system for diagnosing legionnaires' disease in adults (modified)

Presentation	Qualifying Conditions[b]	Point Score
Clinical features		
• Temperature >102°F[a]	With relative bradycardia[a]	+5
• Headache[a]	Acute onset	+2
• Mental confusion/lethargy[a]	Not drug-induced or toxic/metabolic	+4
• Ear pain	Acute onset	−3
• Nonexudative pharyngitis	Acute onset	−3
• Hoarseness	Acute not chronic	−3
• Sputum (purulent)	Excluding AECB	−3
• Hemoptysis[a]	Mild/moderate	−3
• Chest pain	Pleuritic	−3
• Loose stools/watery diarrhea[a]	Not drug induced	+3
• Abdominal pain[a]	With/without diarrhea	+5
• Renal failure[a]	Acute (not chronic)	+3
• Shock/hypotension[a]	Excluding cardiac/pulmonary causes	+1
• Splenomegaly[a]	Excluding non-CAP causes	−5
• Lack of response to β-lactam antibiotics	after 72 h	+5
Laboratory tests		
• Chest radiograph	Rapidly progressive asymmetric infiltrates[a] (excluding influenza, CMV, HPS, SARS)	+3
• Severe hypoxemia (↑ A-a gradient >35)[a]	Acute onset (excluding influenza HPS, SARS)	−2
• Hyponatremia[a]	Acute onset	+1
• Hypophoshatemia[a]	Acute onset	+5
• ↑ AST/ALT (early/mild/transient)[a]	Acute onset	+2
• ↑ Total bilirubin	Acute onset	+1
• ↑ LDH (>400)[a]	Acute onset	−5
• ↑ CPK[a]	Acute onset	+3
• ↑ CRP >35[a]	Acute onset	+5
• ↑Cold agglutinin titers (≥1:64)[a]	Acute onset	−5
• Severe relative lymphopenia (<10%)[a]	Acute onset	+5
• ↑ Ferritin (>2 × n)[a]	Sustained elevations	+5
• Microscopic hematuria[a]	Excluding trauma, BPH, Foley catheter, bladder/renal neoplasms	+2
Likelihood of *Legionella*		
Total point score	>15 Legionnaires' disease **very likely** 5–15 Legionnaires' disease **likely** <5 Legionnaires' disease **unlikely**	

Abbreviations: AECB, acute exacerbation of chronic bronchitis; BPH, benign prostatic hyperplasia; LDH, lactate dehydrogenase.

[a] Otherwise unexplained.

[b] In adults, otherwise unexplained, acute and associated with the pneumonia.

Adapted from Cunha BA, editor. Pneumonia essentials. 3rd edition. Sudbury (MA): Jones & Bartlett; 2010; with permission.

Table 11
Rapid clinical diagnosis of legionnaires' disease: *Legionella* diagnostic triad

Entry Criteria	Key Clinical Features	Key Laboratory Features (any 3)
• Signs and symptoms of CAP plus • New infiltrate on chest radiograph[a] • Negative recent/close zoonotic vector contact history	Fever >102°F with relative bradycardia[a]	• Hypophosphatemia[a] • Highly increased serum ferritin levels[a] (>2 × n) • Mildly/transiently increased serum transaminases[a] • Relative lymphopenia[a]

[a] Otherwise unexplained.

From Cunha BA, Mickail N, Syed U, et al. The rapid clinical diagnosis of Legionnaires' disease during the "herald wave" of the swine influenza (H1N1) pandemic: the Legionnaires' disease triad. Heart Lung 2010;39; in press; with permission.

sufficient findings will be present to permit a presumptive clinical diagnosis, and prompt specific laboratory testing for *Legionella*. *Mycoplasma pneumoniae* CAP has none of these features. Because *M pneumoniae* CAP is not accompanied by a pulse-temperature deficit (eg, relative bradycardia, hypophosphatemia, highly increased ferritin levels, or renal involvement), the presence of several of these findings eliminates *M pneumoniae* CAP from further diagnostic consideration. Conversely, the hallmark laboratory abnormality present in approximately 75% of *M pneumoniae* patients is increased cold agglutinin titers. Although low titers of cold agglutinins may be associated with some viral infections and may be associated with a variety of medical disorders. Highly increased cold agglutinin titers should suggest the possibility of *M pneumoniae* in a patient with CAP. The only other pathogens that could be confused with *M pneumoniae* CAP are Q fever and adenovirus. Excluding other causes of highly increased cold agglutinins (eg, cold agglutinin disease) with CAP patients with highly increased cold agglutinin titers (ie, ≥1:64) should be considered as having *M pneumoniae* CAP until proven otherwise. The cold agglutinin titers with *M pneumoniae* may not be present on clinical presentation but may be elevated in the course of the infection. Although the diagnosis of *M pneumoniae* is likely in a patient with CAP and highly increased cold agglutinin titers, (ie, >1:64); elevated cold agglutinin titers occur in only 75% of patients. The diagnosis of *M pneumoniae*

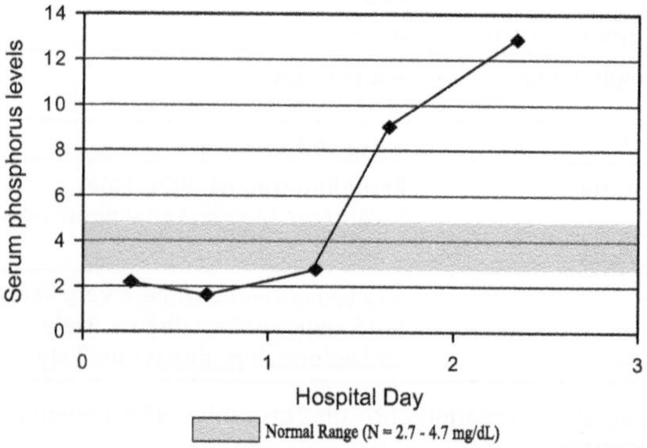

Fig. 4. Typical time course of early transient hypophosphatemia with legionnaires' disease. *From* Cunha BA. Hypophosphatemia: diagnostic significance in legionnaires' disease. Am J Med 2006;119:5–6.

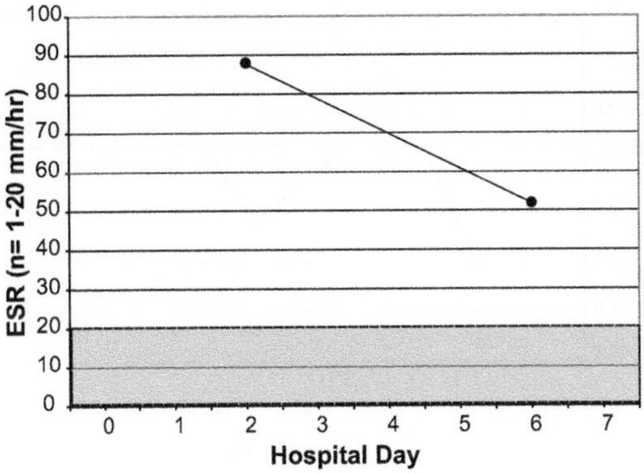

Fig. 5. Serial ESRs in a patient with *Legionella* CAP. (*From* Cunha BA, Mickail N, Syed U, et al. The rapid clinical diagnosis of Legionnaires' disease during the "herald wave" of the swine influenza (H1N1) pandemic: the Legionnaires' disease triad. Heart Lung 2010;39; in press; with permission.)

CAP is confirmed by demonstrating elevated *M pneumoniae* IgM titers acutely and increasing IgG titers during convalescence.[33,35,50,68,69]

Q fever CAP

Q fever is an uncommon cause zoonotic atypical CAP. CAP in patients with a recent history of close contact with a zoonotic vector is often overlooked or not appreciated. An initial history regarding zoonotic contact vectors is often not elicited in patients presenting with Q fever CAP. Although patients can recall contact with sheep, they often overlook the potential clinical significance of a neighbor with a parturient cat. Q fever may mimic legionnaires' disease in onset of clinical presentation. Although legionnaires' disease may have a subacute onset, legionnaires' disease onset is acute when presenting as severe CAP. Q fever CAP usually has a subacute onset, as with most cases of legionnaires' disease. Relative bradycardia may be present with Q

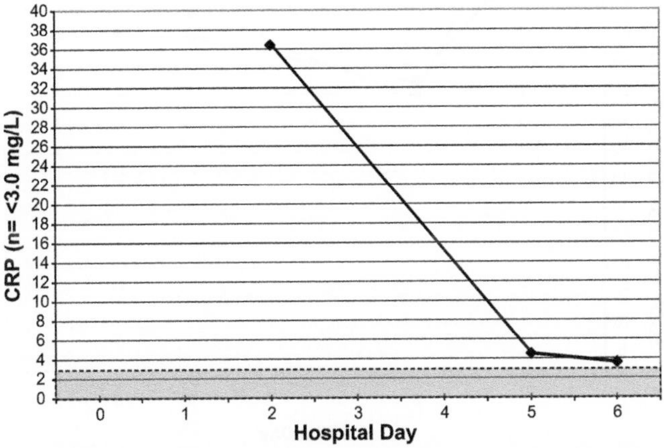

Fig. 6. Serial CRP levels in a patient with *Legionella* CAP. (*From* Cunha BA, Mickail N, Syed U, et al. The rapid clinical diagnosis of Legionnaires' disease during the "herald wave" of the swine influenza (H1N1) pandemic: the Legionnaires' disease triad. Heart Lung 2010;39; in press; with permission.)

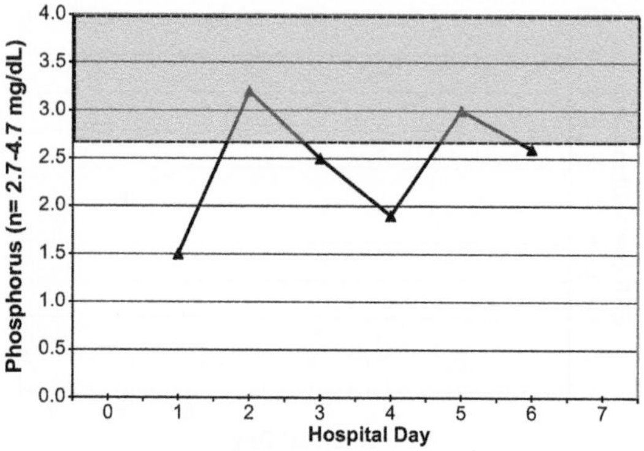

Fig. 7. Serial serum phosphorus levels in a patient with *Legionella* CAP. (*From* Cunha BA, Mickail N, Syed U, et al. The rapid clinical diagnosis of Legionnaires' disease during the "herald wave" of the swine influenza (H1N1) pandemic: the Legionnaires' disease triad. Heart Lung 2010;39; in press; with permission.)

fever, as with legionnaires' disease. Among the extrapulmonary manifestations that overlap with legionnaires' disease are headache and less commonly mental confusion. The cardinal clinical finding in Q fever CAP is the presence of splenomegaly. In a patient with CAP and splenomegaly, Q fever is the most likely diagnostic possibility; alternatively, psittacosis should be considered in those with a recent exposure to psitticine birds. Splenomegaly is not a feature of legionnaires' disease but may be easily overlooked or may not yet be detectable on physical examination. In patients with CAP, splenomegaly is usually detected as an incidental finding if the abdomen is included in the CXR or chest CT. Among the nonspecific laboratory tests, mild increases of the serum transaminase levels occur with Q fever, legionnaires' disease,

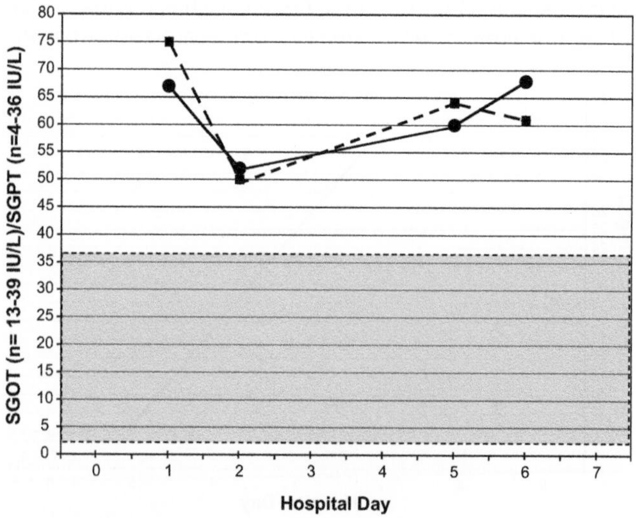

Fig. 8. Serial serum transaminase levels in a patient with *Legionella* CAP. (*From* Cunha BA, Mickail N, Syed U, et al. The rapid clinical diagnosis of Legionnaires' disease during the "herald wave" of the swine influenza (H1N1) pandemic: the Legionnaires' disease triad. Heart Lung 2010;39; in press; with permission.)

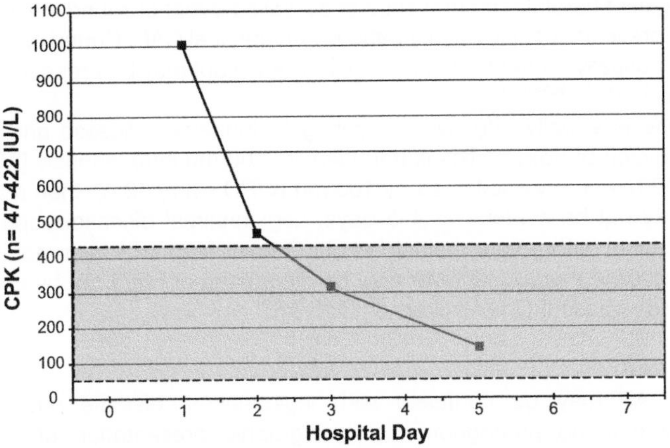

Fig. 9. Serial CPK levels in a patient with *Legionella* CAP. (*From* Cunha BA, Mickail N, Syed U, et al. The rapid clinical diagnosis of Legionnaires' disease during the "herald wave" of the swine influenza (H1N1) pandemic: the Legionnaires' disease triad. Heart Lung 2010;39; in press; with permission.)

and psittacosis. Increased serum ferritin levels may also occur with Q fever CAP, although they are less frequent and not as highly elevated as with legionnaires' disease. If ASM antibodies are present in a patient with atypical CAP, it points to the diagnosis of Q fever. In patients with an atypical CAP, otherwise unexplained thrombocytosis occurring during hospitalization is an important clue to Q fever CAP. Although thrombocytosis may occur with *M pneumoniae* CAP, it is more common, pronounced, and prolonged with Q fever CAP. Other nonspecific laboratory features (ie, increased serum transaminases) readily differentiate Q fever from *M pneumoniae* CAP. Although there are no pathognomonic radiologic features that clearly differentiate legionnaires' disease from Q fever, round opacities or infiltrates, if

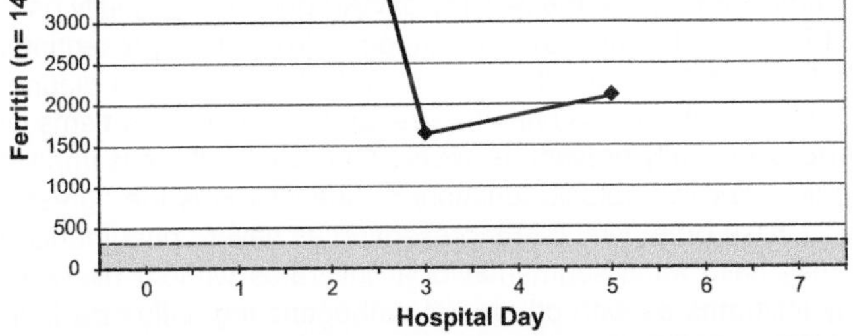

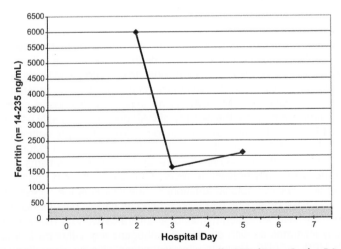

Fig. 10. Serial ferritin levels in a patient with *Legionella* CAP. (*From* Cunha BA, Mickail N, Syed U, et al. The rapid clinical diagnosis of Legionnaires' disease during the "herald wave" of the swine influenza (H1N1) pandemic: the Legionnaires' disease triad. Heart Lung 2010;39; in press; with permission.)

present, are most helpful. The presence of so-called ovoid or round infiltrates should suggest the presence of Q fever in a patient with atypical CAP. Round or nodular infiltrates are not usually present in legionnaires' disease but may be present with *Legionella micdadei* CAP.[35,53–55,69]

Doxycycline is equally effective in treating legionnaires' disease and Q fever. If a loading regimen of doxycycline is not used (ie, 200 mg intravenously [IV]/by mouth [PO] every 12 h × 3 days, followed by 100 mg IV/PO every 12 h), then a therapeutic response may not be evident for 4–5 days. Legionnaires' disease responds in 2–3 days to treatment with a fluoroquinolone but Q fever responds less rapidly and less well to doxycycline therapy. Q fever may be diagnosed or ruled out by acute/convalescent phase I phase II Q fever titers.[28,35,53–55,59]

Adenovirus CAP

Adenoviral CAP may be confused with legionnaires' disease radiographically. Although there is no pathognomonic radiographic presentation of legionnaires' disease, the radiographic behavior of the infiltrates is characteristic. Rapidly asymmetrical progression of infiltrates is characteristic of legionnaires' disease on CXR, which is not usual with adenoviral CAP. Adenoviral CAP often presents with a focal segmental/lobar infiltrate mimicking legionnaires' disease, Q fever, psittacosis, or typical bacterial CAPs. Although adenoviral CAP is not accompanied by relative bradycardia, many of the nonspecific laboratory findings associated with legionnaires' disease may be present in patients with adenoviral CAP. Most commonly, adenoviral CAP may be accompanied by a mild increase of AST/ALT levels, most commonly mimicking legionnaires' disease and less commonly, Q fever or psittacosis. Increased CPK levels are also frequently present in adenoviral CAP and legionnaires' disease. The key nonspecific markers of legionnaires' disease (ie, increased serum ferritin levels, hypophosphatemia, microscopic hematuria) are not features of adenoviral CAP. Of course, adenoviral CAP does not respond to anti-*Legionella* antibiotic therapy. Mild increases of cold agglutinin titers may be present, which would argue against the diagnosis of legionnaires' disease. Diagnosis is confirmed or ruled out by acute/convalescent adenoviral titers.[35,70]

Severe CAP

Legionnaires' disease not infrequently presents as severe CAP. In the differential diagnosis of severe CAP, common diagnostic considerations include influenza (human, avian, swine), SARS, HPS, CMV, and adenovirus. In compromised hosts (eg, patients with impaired CMI), *Pneumocystis (carinii) jiroveci* may present as severe CAP. Similarly, in transplant patients, CMV CAP is an important diagnostic consideration. Excluding zoonotic pathogens, the severity of CAP depends primarily on host factors rather than to the inherent virulence of the pathogen. In a patient presenting with severe CAP with focal segmental/lobar infiltrates on CXR, the differential diagnosis is often between legionnaires' disease, *S pneumoniae*, and adenovirus. Patients with *S pneumoniae* CAP do not usually present as severe CAP unless there is impaired humoral immunity (HI) (ie, impaired splenic function).[35] Adenovirus is the "great imitator" of bacterial CAP. Unlike other viral CAPs presenting as severe pneumonia, adenovirus on the CXR may have focal segmental/lobar infiltrates without bilateral symmetric diffuse patchy infiltrates as with other viral pathogens (eg, influenza [human, avian, swine], CMV, HPS, or SARS). Patients with legionnaires' disease presenting with severe CAP, like patients with adenovirus, may be accompanied by various degrees of hypoxemia. Legionnaires' disease should always be considered in the differential diagnosis of severe CAP. The likelihood of legionnaires' disease in patients presenting as severe

CAP is enhanced with otherwise unexplained relative bradycardia, hypophosphatemia, increased AST/ALT levels, or highly increased ferritin levels.[35,71–78]

In patients with severe CAP with these nonspecific laboratory features, clinicians should order specific tests to rule in or rule out legionnaires' disease. Initial *Legionella* sp titers (indirect fluorescent antibody [IFA]) are usually negative and serial determinations are usually needed to demonstrate an increase in *Legionella* sp IFA titers. DFA techniques may be used if the patient has sputum; although they are not often positive, they are most likely to be positive early in the course of the illness. Sputum DFA positivity for *Legionella* sp decreases rapidly with effective anti-*Legionella* antimicrobial therapy. *Legionella* antigen testing is also useful but may be negative early. *Legionella* antigenuria becomes progressively positive over time and antigenuria continues for weeks after the infection. Legionella urinary antigen testing only detects *Legionella pneumophila* serotypes 01–06.[2,5,35]

In patients with nonsevere CAP when *Legionella* is a reasonable diagnostic consideration, atypical pathogen coverage should be included in empiric antimicrobial therapy. Patients presenting with severe CAP and focal infiltrates with one or more of the extrapulmonary findings characteristic of legionnaires' disease should be treated for legionnaires' disease.[35,75–78]

THERAPY

Overview

When legionnaires' disease was recognized as an infectious disease after the Philadelphia outbreak in 1978, it was quickly appreciated that cell wall active antibiotics were ineffective against the causative organism of the disease. Subsequently, it was realized that legionnaires' disease was caused by an intracellular pathogen in alveolar macrophages. The organism responsible for legionnaires' disease was found to be susceptible in vivo to macrolides and tetracyclines.[1,2,9,35,79–82]

Macrolides

In the years following the Philadelphia outbreak, sporadic cases of legionnaires' disease were treated with variable effectiveness with macrolides. However, tetracycline was more consistently effective against *Legionella* sp than macrolides. Tetracycline for treatment of legionnaires' disease has been gradually replaced by doxycycline. There have been reports of erythromycin failures in legionnaires' disease. Although erythromycin, like other macrolides, concentrates to supraserum concentrations in alveolar macrophages, treatment failures are not infrequent, even with parenteral erythromycin.[35,81–85]

Doxycycline

Prior to the quinolones, doxycycline was the mainstay of anti-*Legionella* therapy and remains highly effective against *Legionella pneumophila* as well as other *Legionella* species causing legionnaires' disease. Rifampin has in vitro activity against *Legionella* sp and has been used in combination with tetracycline with no demonstrable clinical advantage compared to doxycycline monotherapy. When doxycycline is used for any serious systemic infection (eg, legionnaires' disease), optimally it should be administered using a loading regimen (not a loading dose). Because doxycycline is highly lipid soluble and has a long half-life ($t_{1/2}$ = 21–24 hours), it takes 4 to 5 days with IV/PO dosing to achieve steady state concentrations. Therefore, doxycycline therapy should be instituted using a 200 mg (IV/PO) dose every 12 hours for 72 hours, followed by 100 mg (IV/PO) every 12 hours for the remainder of therapy. Using a loading regimen provides rapid therapeutic concentrations of doxycycline in serum and lung. Like the fluoroquinolones, doxycycline has excellent bioavailability and may be administered with equal efficacy IV or PO.[35,86–88]

Tigecycline

Tigecycline is active against typical CAP pathogens and legionnaires' disease. Tigecycline concentrates well in lung tissue and alveolar macrophages and is useful for treating legionnaires' disease in patients intolerant to fluoroquinolone.[35,89,90]

Rifampin

Although rifampin concentrates in alveolar macrophages, it should not be used as monotherapy. Combination therapy with rifampin plus erythromycin or doxycycline is no more effective than erythromycin or doxycycline monotherapy. There are few studies on the effectiveness of erythromycin plus rifampin to base any potential benefit of rifampin compared to the activity of erythromycin or erythromycin/rifampin combination therapy.[35,91,92]

Quinolones

After doxycycline, the next most important therapeutic advance in the therapy of legionnaires' disease was the introduction of the fluoroquinolones. All quinolones are highly active in vitro and in vivo against all *Legionella* species. Although doxycycline is highly active against the common typical CAP pathogens (ie, *S pneumoniae, H influenzae*, and *M catarrhalis*), the "respiratory quinolones" have even higher activity against these pathogens. Doxycycline is highly active against penicillin-resistant *S pneumoniae* and most strains of multidrug-resistant (MDR) *S pneumoniae*, but "respiratory quinolones" are preferred for MDR *S pneumoniae*. Like doxycycline, quinolones are effective against typical and atypical CAP pathogens (eg, *Legionella* sp). "Respiratory quinolones," like macrolides and doxycycline, penetrate well into alveolar macrophages and concentrate intracellularly to supraserum concentrations. "Respiratory quinolones" provide optimal monotherapy for CAP caused by either typical or atypical pathogens. In patients who are quinolone intolerant doxycycline remains a highly effective agent for all *Legionella* species that cause legionnaires' disease. "Respiratory quinolones" have excellent bioavailability (ie, more than 90% absorption) and are ideal for PO or IV to PO switch therapy for CAP. Because of their excellent absorption, even in seriously ill patients, "respiratory quinolones" may be used to treat legionnaires' disease entirely by the oral route.[35,70,93–97]

Duration of Therapy

The duration of therapy for legionnaires' disease initially was 2 to 4 weeks. Relapse was common with erythromycin therapy, and for this reason the duration of therapy was extended to prevent relapse. Currently, the duration of therapy with doxycycline or respiratory quinolones is usually 2 weeks. Normal hosts with good cardiopulmonary function and mild to moderate legionnaires' disease may be treated with shorter courses of therapy but those with severe disease, impaired CMI, or severely limited cardiopulmonary function may require longer courses of therapy. With properly dosed anti-*Legionella* therapy with doxycycline or respiratory quinolones, relapses are rare.[35,95–97]

COMPLICATIONS AND PROGNOSIS

Because legionnaires' disease occurs primarily in older individuals, the prognosis in patients depends largely on the host's underlying cardiopulmonary function and disorders that impair CMI (T-lymphocyte function). Prognosis with *Legionella* CAP is also directly related to inoculum size, and early administration of effective anti-*Legionella* antibiotic therapy. Legionnaires' disease may be fatal in compromised hosts with impaired T-cell function and in those on immunosuppressive therapy, particularly monoclonal antibody or anti-tumor necrosis factor agents. If cardiopulmonary function is good, early treatment of *Legionella* CAP, even in compromised hosts, has a good prognosis.[14–16,35]

REFERENCES

1. Lattimer GL, Ormsbee RA. Legionnaires' disease. New York: Marcel Dekker, Inc; 1981.
2. Edelstein PH. *Legionella*. In: Murray PR, editor. Manual of clinical microbiology. 9th edition. Washington, DC: ASM Press; 2007. p. 835–49.
3. Forbes BA, Sahm DF, Weissfeld AS. *Legionella*. Bailey & Scott's diagnostic microbiology. 12th edition. St. Louis (MO): Mosby Elsevier; 2007. p. 424–8.
4. Edelstein PH. State of the art lecture. Laboratory diagnosis of legionnaire's disease. In: Thornsberry C, Balows A, Feeley JC, et al, editors. *Legionella*: proceedings of the 2nd international symposium. Washington, DC: ASM Press; 1984. p. 3–5.
5. Luck PC, Helbig JH, von Baum H, et al. Diagnostics and clinical disease treatment: usefulness of microbiological diagnostic methods for detection of *Legionella* infections. In: Cianciotto NP, Kwaik YA, Edelstein PH, et al, editors. *Legionella:* state of the art 30 years after its recognition. Washington, DC: ASM Press; 2006. p. 15–21.
6. Mykietiuk A, Carratal J, Fernandex-Sabe N, et al. Clinical outcomes for hospitalized patients with *Legionella* pneumonia in the antigenuria era: the influence of levofloxacin therapy. Clin Infect Dis 2005;15(40):794–9.
7. Marlow E, Whelan C. *Legionella* pneumonia and use of the *Legionella* urinary antigen test. J Hosp Med 2009;4(3):E1–2.
8. Olsen CW, Elverdal P, Jørgensen CS, et al. Comparison of the sensitivity of the *Legionella* urinary antigen EIA kits from Binax and Biotest with urine from patients with infections caused by less common serogroups and subgroups of *Legionella*. Eur J Clin Microbiol Infect Dis 2009;287:817–20.
9. Baltch AL, Bopp LH, Smith RP, et al. Antibacterial activities of gemifloxacin, levofloxacin, gatifloxacin, moxifloxacin and erythromycin against intracellular *Legionella pneumophila* and *Legionella micdadei* in human monocytes. J Antimicrob Chemother 2005;56:104–9.
10. Pedro-Botet L, Yu VL. *Legionella*: macrolides or quinolones? Clin Microbiol Infect 2006;12:25–30.
11. Hendrickson SE, Neil M. *Legionella* pneumonia and HIV infection: a case report. AIDS Read 2004;14:267–70.
12. Pedro-Botet ML, Sopena N, Garcia-Cruz A, et al. Community acquired pneumonia in human immunodeficiency virus-infected patients: comparative study of *Streptococcus pneumoniae* and *Legionella pneumophila* serogroup 1. In: Cianciotto NP, Kwaik YA, Edelstein PH, et al, editors. *Legionella*: state of the art 30 years after its recognition. Washington, DC: ASM Press; 2006. p. 30–2.
13. Hamid NS, Mohan SS, Cunha BA. Fatal disseminated *Legionella* pneumonia in a neonate with severe combined immunodeficiency (SCID). Infect Dis Clin Pract 2006;14:116–8.

14. Albert C, Vandenbos F, Brocq O, et al. Legionellosis in patient treated with infliximab. Rev Med Interne 2004;25:167–8.
15. Wondergem MJ, Voskuyl AE, van Agtmael MA. A case of legionellosis during treatment with a TNF-alpha antagonist. Scand J Infect Dis 2004;36:310–1.
16. Li Gobbi F, Benucci M, Del Rosso A. Pneumonitis caused by *Legionella pneumoniae* in a patient with rheumatoid arthritis treated with anti-TNF alpha therapy (infliximab). J Clin Rheumatol 2005;11:119–20.
17. Dubrou S, Guillotin L, Cabon S. Cooling towers and legionellosis: a large urban area experience. In: Marre R, Kwaik YA, Bartlett C, et al, editors. *Legionella*. Washington, DC: ASM Press; 2002. p. 291–4.
18. Nguyen TM, Ilef D, Harraud S, et al. A community-wide outbreak of legionnaires' disease linked to industrial cooling towers – how far can contaminated aerosols spread? J Infect Dis 2006;193:102.
19. Levy PY, Teysseire N, Etienne J, et al. A nosocomial outbreak of *Legionella pneumophila* caused by contaminated transesophageal echocardiography probes. Infect Control Hosp Epidemiol 2004;24:619–22.
20. Cunha BA, Mickail N, Syed U. Unexplained increase in legionnaires' disease during the "Herald Wave" of the swine influenza (H1N1) pandemic. Hosp Epidemiol Infect Control 2010;31, in press.
21. Forgie S, Marrie TJ. Healthcare-associated atypical pneumonia. Semin Respir Crit Care Med 2009;30:67–85.
22. Beaty HN. State of the art lecture. Clinical features of legionellosis. In: Thornsberry C, Balows A, Feeley JC, et al, editors. Legionella: proceedings of the 2nd international symposium. Washington, DC: ASM Press; 1984. p. 6–10.
23. Diederen BMW. *Legionella* spp. and Legionnaires' disease. J Infect 2008;56:1–12.
24. Phares CR, Russell E, Thigpen MC, et al. Legionnaires' disease among residents of a long-term care facility: the sentinel event in a community outbreak. Am J Infect Control 2007;5:319–23.
25. Carbonara S, Monno L, Longo B, et al. Legionella is often overlooked as a cause of NHAP outbreaks. Curr Opin Pulm Med 2009;15:261–73.
26. Nakashima K, Tanaka T, Kramer MH, et al. Outbreak of *Chlamydia pneumoniae* infection in a Japanese nursing home, 1999–2000. Infect Control Hosp Epidemiol 2006;27:1171–7.
27. Roig J, Aguilar X, Ruiz Z, et al. Comparative study of *Legionella pneumophila* and other nosocomial-acquired pneumonias. Chest 1991;99:344–50.
28. Cunha BA, Quintiliani R. The atypical pneumonias, a diagnostic and therapeutic approach. Postgrad Med 1979;66:95–102.
29. Cunha BA, Ortega AM. Atypical pneumonia. Extrapulmonary clues guide the way to diagnosis. Postgrad Med 1996;99:123–8.
30. Cunha BA. The extrapulmonary manifestations of community-acquired pneumonias. Chest 1998;112:945.
31. Cotton LM, Strampfer MJ, Cunha BA. *Legionella* and *Mycoplasma pneumonia*: community hospital experience. Clin Chest Med 1987;8:441–53.
32. Cunha BA. The atypical pneumonias: clinical diagnosis and importance. Clin Microbiol Infect 2006;12:12–24.
33. Cunha BA. Atypical pneumonias: current clinical concepts focusing on Legionnaires' disease. Curr Opin Pulm Med 2008;14:183–94.
34. Cunha BA. Clinical diagnosis of Legionnaires' disease. Semin Respir Infect 1998;13:116–27.

35. Cunha BA, editor. Pneumonia essentials. 3rd edition. Sudbury (MA): Jones & Bartlett; 2010.
36. Edelstein PH. Legionnaires' disease. Clin Infect Dis 1993;16:741–9.
37. Sugihara E, Dambara T, Aiba M, et al. Clinical characteristics of 8 sporadic cases of community-acquired Legionella pneumonia in advanced age. Intern Med 2007;46:461–5.
38. Pedro-Botet ML, Mateu L, Sopena N, et al. Hospital and community acquired Legionella pneumonia: two faces of the same disease. In: Cianciotto NP, Kwaik YA, Edelstein PH, et al, editors. *Legionella:* state of the art 30 years after its recognition. Washington, DC: ASM Press; 2006. p. 22–4.
39. Macfarlane JT, Miller AC, Morris AH, et al. Comparative radiologic features of Legionnaires' disease and other sporadic community-acquired pneumonias. In: Thornsberry C, Balows A, Feeley JC, et al, editors. *Legionella*: proceedings of the 2nd international symposium. Washington, DC: ASM Press; 1984. p. 12.
40. Coletta FS, Fein AM. Radiological manifestation of *Legionella/Legionella*-like organisms. Semin Respir Infect 1998;13:109–15.
41. Boermsa WG, Daniels JM, Lowernberg A, et al. Reliability of radiographic findings and the relation to etiologic agents in community-acquired pneumonia. Respir Med 2006;100:926–32.
42. Nambu A, Saito A, Araki T, et al. *Chlamydia pneumoniae*: comparison with findings of *Mycoplasma pneumoniae* and *Streptococcus pneumoniae* at thin-section CT. Radiology 2006;238:330–8.
43. Sakai F, Tokuda H, Goto H. Computed tomographic features of *Legionella pneumophilia* pneumonia in 38 cases. J Comput Assist Tomogr 2007;31:125–31.
44. Lee I, Kim TS, Yoon HK. *Mycoplasma pneumoniae* pneumonia: CT features in 16 patients. Eur Radiol 2006;16:719–25.
45. Okada F, Ando Y, Wakisaka M, et al. *Chlamydia pneumoniae* pneumonia and *Mycoplasma pneumoniae* pneumonia: comparison of clinical findings and CT findings. J Comput Assist Tomogr 2005;29:626–32.
46. Cunha BA, Pherez FM. Bilateral spontaneous pneumothoraces at the presenting finding in legionnaires' disease. Heart Lung 2008;37:238–41.
47. Sopena N, Sabria-Leal M, Pedro-Botet, et al. Comparative study of the clinical presentation of Legionella pneumonia and other community-acquired pneumonias. Chest 1998;113:1195–200.
48. Schneeberger PM, Dorigo-Zetsma JW, van der Zee A, et al. Diagnosis of atypical pathogens in patients hospitalized with community-acquired respiratory infection. Scand J Infect Dis 2004;36:269–73.
49. Strampfer MJ, Cunha BA. Legionnaires' disease. Semin Respir Infect 1987;2:228–34.
50. Cunha BA. Diagnostic significance of relative bradycardia. Clin Microbiol Infect 2000;6:633–4.
51. Sotgiu S, Pugliatti M, Rosati G, et al. Neurological disorders associated with *Mycoplasma pneumoniae* infection. Eur J Neurol 2003;10:165–8.
52. von Baum H, Welte T, Marre R, et al. *Mycoplasma pneumoniae* pneumonia revisited within the German Competence Network for Community-acquired pneumonia (CAPNETZ). BMC Infect Dis 2009;9:62.
53. Marrie TJ. Q fever pneumonia. Curr Opin Infect Dis 2004;17:137–42.
54. Cutler SJ, Bouzid M, Cutler RR. Q fever. J Infect 2007;54:313–8.
55. Parker NR, Barralet JH, Bell AM. Q fever. Lancet 2006;367:679–88.
56. Gregory DW, Schaffner W. Psittacosis. Semin Respir Infect 1997;12:7–11.
57. Cunha BA. Hypophosphatemia: diagnostic significance in legionnaires' disease. Am J Med 2006;119:5–6.

58. Cunha BA. Elevated serum transaminases in patients with *Mycoplasma pneumoniae* pneumonia. Clin Microbiol Infect 2005;11:1051–2.
59. Cunha BA, Nausheen S, Busch L. Severe Q fever mimicking Legionella community acquired pneumonia (CAP): the diagnostic importance of cold agglutinins, anti-smooth muscle antibodies, and thrombocytosis. Heart Lung 2009;38:354–62.
60. Cunha BA. Serum ferritin levels in *Legionella* community-acquired pneumonia. Clin Infect Dis 2008;46:1789–91.
61. Franzin L, Cabodi D. *Legionella* pneumonia and serum procalcitonin. Curr Microbiol 2005;50:43–6.
62. Miyashita N, Fukano H, Yoshid K, et al. Is it possible to distinguish between atypical pneumonia and bacterial pneumonia? Evaluation of the guidelines for community acquired pneumonia in Japan. Respir Med 2004;98:952–60.
63. Fiumefreddo R, Zaborsky R, Haeuptle J, et al. Clinical predictors for Legionella in patients presenting with community-acquired pneumonia to the emergency department. BMC Pulm Med 2009;9:4–7.
64. Masiá M, Gutiérrez F, Padilla S, et al. Clinical characterisation of pneumonia caused by atypical pathogens combining classic and novel predictors. Clin Microbiol Infect 2007;13:153–61.
65. Cunha BA. The clinical diagnosis of legionnaires' disease: diagnostic value of combining non-specific laboratory tests. Infection 2008;6:395–7.
66. Cunha BA. Severe legionella pneumonia: rapid diagnosis with Winthrop-University-Hospital's weighted point score system (modified). Heart Lung 2008;37:312–21.
67. Cunha BA, Mickail N, Syed U, et al. The rapid clinical diagnosis of Legionnaires' disease during the "herald wave" of the swine influenza (H1N1) pandemic: the Legionnaires' disease triad. Heart Lung 2010;39, in press.
68. Cunha BA, Pherez FM. *Mycoplasma pneumoniae* community acquired pneumonia (CAP) in the elderly: the diagnostic importance of acute thrombocytosis. Heart Lung 2009;38:444–9.
69. Cunha BA. Ambulatory community-acquired pneumonia: the predominance of atypical pathogens. Eur J Clin Microbiol Infect Dis 2003;2:579–83.
70. Cunha BA. Severe adenovirus community-acquired pneumonia mimicking Legionella. Eur J Clin Microbiol Infect Dis 2009;28:313–5.
71. Cunha BA, Klein NC, Strollo S, et al. Legionnaire's disease mimicking swine influenza (H1N1). Heart & Lung 2010;39, in press.
72. Lewis PF, Schmidt MA, Lu X, et al. A community-based outbreak of severe respiratory illness caused by human adenovirus serotype 14. J Infect Dis 2009;199:1427–34.
73. Cunha BA. Severe community acquired pneumonia. Crit Care Clin 1998;8:105–17.
74. Cunha BA, Gouzhva O, Nausheen S. Severe cytomegalovirus (CMV) community acquired pneumonia (CAP) precipitating a systemic lupus erythematosis (SLE) flare. Heart Lung 2009;38:249–52.
75. Sanford JP. Tularemia. JAMA 1983;250:3225–6.
76. Teutsch SM, Martone WJ, Brink EW, et al. Pneumonic tularemia on Martha's vineyard. N Engl J Med 1979;301:826–8.
77. Murdoch DR, Chambers ST. Atypical pneumonia–time to breathe new life into a useful term? Lancet Infect Dis 2009;9:512–9.
78. Cunha BA. Severe community acquired pneumonia in the CCU. In: Cunha BA, editor. Infectious diseases in critical care medicine. 3rd edition. New York: Informa Healthcare; 2010. p. 164–77.

79. Birteksoz AS, Zeybek Z, Cotuk A. In vitro activities of various antibiotics against *Legionella pneumophila*. In: Cianciotto NP, Kwaik YA, Edelstein PH, et al, editors. *Legionella*: state of the art 30 years after its recognition. Washington, DC: ASM Press; 2006. p. 43–6.
80. Cunha BA. Antibiotic pharmacokinetic considerations in pulmonary infections. Semin Respir Infect 1991;6:168–82.
81. Smith RP, Baltch AL, Franke M, et al. Effect of levofloxacin, erythromycin or rifampin pretreatment on growth of *Legionella pneumophila* in human monocytes. Antimicrob Agents Chemother 1997;40:673–8.
82. Baltch AL, Smith RP, Franke MA, et al. Antibacterial effects of levofloxacin, erythromycin, and rifampin in a human monocyte system against *Legionella pneumophila*. Antimicrob Agents Chemother 1998;42:3153–6.
83. Rudin JE, Evans TL, Wing EJ. Failure of erythromycin in treatment of *Legionella micdadei* pneumonia. Am J Med 1984;76:318–20.
84. Parker MM, Macher AM, Shelhamer JH, et al. Unresponsiveness of *Legionella bozemanii* pneumonia to erythromcyin administration despite in vitro sensitivity. Am Rev Respir Dis 1983;182:955–6.
85. Sabria M, Pedro-Botet ML, Gomez J, et al. Fluoroquinolones vs macrolides in the treatment of Legionnaires' disease. Chest 2005;128:1401–5.
86. Cunha BA, Sibley CM, Ristuccia AM. Doxycycline. Ther Drug Monit 1982;4:115–35.
87. Cunha BA. Doxycycline re-revisited. Arch Intern Med 1999;159:1006–7.
88. Cunha BA. Doxycycline for community acquired pneumonia. Clin Infect Dis 2003;37:870.
89. Dartois N, Castaing N, Gandjini H, et al. Tigecycline versus levofloxacin for the treatment of community-acquired pneumonia: European experience. J Chemother 2008;20:28–35.
90. Tanaseanu C, Milutinovic S, Calistru PI, et al. Efficacy and safety of tigecycline versus levofloxacin for community-acquired pneumonia. BMC Pulm Med 2009;9:44.
91. Mercatello A, Frappaz D, Robert D, et al. Failure of erythromycin/rifampicin treatment of Legionella pneumonia. J Infect 1985;10:282–3.
92. Amsden GW. Treatment of Legionnaires' disease. Drugs 2005;65:605–14.
93. Cunha BA. Fluoroquinolones in the treatment of Legionnaires' disease. Penetration 2000;3:32–9.
94. Ludlam HA, Enoch DA. Doxycycline or moxifloxacin for the management of community-acquired pneumonia in the UK? Int J Antimicrob Agents 2008;32:101–5.
95. Mandell LA, Wunderink RG, Anzueto A, et al. Infectious Diseases Society of America/American Thoracic Society consensus guidelines on the management of community-acquired pneumonia in adults. Clin Infect Dis 2007;1(44 Suppl 2):S27–72.
96. Cunha BA. Empiric antibiotic therapy for community-acquired pneumonia: guidelines for the perplexed? Chest 2004;125:1913–21.
97. Pedreo Botet ML, Yu VL. Treatment strategies for *Legionella* infection. Expert Opin Pharmacother 2009;10:1109–21.

Pneumocystis jirovecii Pneumonia

Emilie Catherinot, MD, PhD[a,b], Fanny Lanternier, MD, MSc[a], Marie-Elisabeth Bougnoux, MD, PhD[c], Marc Lecuit, MD, PhD[a], Louis-Jean Couderc, MD, PhD[b], Olivier Lortholary, MD, PhD[a,d,*]

KEYWORDS

- *Pneumocystis jirovecii* • AIDS • Pulmonary infections
- Chemoprophylaxis

Pneumocystis has gained attention during the last decade in the context of the AIDS epidemic and the increasing use of cytotoxic and immunosuppressive therapies. The accumulation of knowledge about this curious fungus is continuous. This article summarizes current knowledge on biology, pathophysiology, epidemiology, diagnosis, prevention, and treatment of pulmonary *Pneumocystis jirovecii* infection, with a particular focus on the evolving pathophysiology and epidemiology.

HISTORICAL BACKGROUND OF *PNEUMOCYSTIS* SPP

Members of the fungal genus now known as *Pneumocystis* were first identified in 1909 by Chagas in the lung of guinea pigs that had been experimentally infected with *Trypanosoma cruzi*. Chagas thought he had identified a new trypanosomal life form. In 1910, Carini noted morphologically similar organisms in the lung of rats infected with *Trypanosoma lewisi*, and likewise thought they were a new type of trypanosome. In 1912, Delanoe and Delanoe, working at the Institut Pasteur, Paris, reviewed Carini's data and observed the cysts in the lung of Parisian sewer rats. Delanoe and Delanoe realized this was a unique organism and a separate species from *Trypanosoma*, and named it *Pneumocystis carinii*, *Pneumocystis* highlighting the pulmonary tropism and pathogenesis of the organism, *carinii* in honor of A. Carini.[1]

[a] Université Paris Descartes, Service de Maladies Infectieuses et Tropicales, 149 Rue de Sèvres, Centre d'Infectiologie Necker-Pasteur, Hôpital Necker-Enfants Malades, Paris 75015, France
[b] Université Versailles-Saint Quentin, Hôpital Foch, Service de Pneumologie, Suresnes, France
[c] Université Paris Descartes, Hôpital Necker-Enfants Malades, Service de Microbiologie, Paris 75015, France
[d] Institut Pasteur, Centre National de Référence Mycologie et antifongiques, Paris, France
* Corresponding author. Université Paris Descartes, Hôpital Necker-Enfants Malades, Centre d'Infectiologie Necker-Pasteur, Service de Maladies Infectieuses et Tropicales, 149 Rue de Sèvres, Paris 75015, France.
E-mail address: olivier.lortholary@nck.aphp.fr (O. Lortholary).

Infect Dis Clin N Am 24 (2010) 107–138
doi:10.1016/j.idc.2009.10.010
id.theclinics.com

Just before World War II, German physicians described an epidemic form of interstitial plasma cell pneumonitis of unknown etiology occurring in malnourished infants.[2] A first relationship between *Pneumocystis* infection and disease was suggested in 1942, when Van der Meer and Brug observed *Pneumocystis* in lung sections from infants with plasma cell pneumonitis.[3] This observation was largely ignored. In 1951 and 1952, the Czech pathologists Vanek and Jirovec reported the association of *Pneumocystis* in the lung among premature and malnourished children with interstitial plasma cell pneumonitis housed in nursing homes of Central and Eastern Europe.[4] By the end of 1980, starvation and premature birth were important causes of *Pneumocystis* pneumonia (PCP). Among 3346 cases of PCP reported worldwide, 2281 (68%) occurred among infants whose predisposition was either malnutrition or prematurity.[5]

In 1955, Weller observed that prolonged high-dose dexamethasone corticosteroid treatment of rats resulted in pneumocystosis.[6] In the 1960s, *Pneumocystis* started to be recognized as an opportunistic pathogen in immunosuppressed children with acute leukemia or with congenital immunodeficiency impairing T-lymphocyte function.[7,8] In 1981, PCP was the first opportunistic infection reported in homosexual men in the United States, presenting with what was idiomatically coined the "Gay's syndrome," subsequently known as the acquired immunodeficiency syndrome (AIDS).[9,10] With the extent of the AIDS epidemic, there was a dramatic increase in the incidence of pneumocystosis. During the 1980s PCP was the AIDS-defining illness for more than half of adults and adolescents with AIDS in the United States.[11] The introduction of pneumocystosis prophylaxis in 1989 and potent combination antiretroviral therapy in 1996 have led to substantial declines in the incidence of PCP in human immunodeficiency virus (HIV)-infected persons.[12,13] However, PCP remains a leading cause of opportunistic infection, morbidity, and mortality in HIV-infected persons who either are not receiving or are not responding to highly active antiretroviral treatment (HAART) and among those who are unaware of their HIV status.[14] PCP is also of clinical importance in non-HIV immunocompromised persons, such as patients receiving immunosuppressive treatment or antineoplastic chemotherapy.

TAXONOMY

Pneumocystis organisms were considered to form a unique taxonomic entity (designated as *P carinii*). Recent research has demonstrated that the genus *Pneumocystis* is in fact a complex group with numerous species. Based on morphologic criteria and response of the infection to treatment with the antiprotozoan drug pentamidine, it was initially thought that *P carinii* was a protozoan. In 1988, Edman and Stringer independently showed that the ribosomal RNA sequences of *P carinii* were related to those of fungus and completely unrelated to those of other parasites.[15,16] All recent phylogenetic analyses place *Pneumocystis* within the fungal kingdom. *Pneumocystis* species are currently classified within the phylum Ascomycota, in a unique class, order, and family (Pneumocystidomycetes, Pneumocystidales, and Pneumocystidacae, respectively).[17] However, *Pneumocystis* organisms are atypical fungal microorganisms: (1) they are unable to grow in vitro in fungal culture media; (2) they respond to antiparasitic agents like pentamidine and cotrimoxazole; (3) their cell wall contains cholesterol rather than ergosterol—this difference explains why amphotericin B is inactive against *Pneumocystis* spp.

In 1976, Frenkel noted phenotypic differences between *Pneumocystis* from different mammals and proposed to elevate the organism that infects humans as a different species.[18] He named it *Pneumocystis jiroveci*, in recognition to the pathologist Jirovec who early reported the organism in humans. The name did not gain acceptance at this time. The first indication of a molecular difference between *Pneumocystis* organisms from humans and laboratory animals came from analyses of protein sizes.[19] However, demonstration that differences observed in protein sizes resulted from interspecies variability was difficult to establish because of possible confounding factors such as possible host-mediated modification of *Pneumocystis* proteins, presence of dead organisms, or contamination with host proteins.

DNA analysis provided further evidence of genetic divergence between *Pneumocystis* organisms.[20] The 18S rRNA sequences from human-derived *Pneumocystis* and rat-derived *Pneumocystis* differ by 5%. Several other genes or gene fragments have been analyzed.[21–28] In all cases, the gene sequence differed between host species. In addition, experiments with rats, mice, ferrets, and nonhuman primates have demonstrated host-species specificity.[29–31]

At the 2001 International Workshop on Opportunistic Protists in Cincinnati, the group of researchers discussed the nomenclature of *Pneumocystis* and proposed to rename the organisms currently named as special forms of *P carinii* as species in the genus *Pneumocystis*, and drew up guidelines for the creation of a new species name.[32] *Pneumocystis jiroveci* was chosen to deign the form that infects humans and *Pneumocystis carinii* to deign 1 of the 2 the species that infect rats, in which it was first recognized. DNA analysis further demonstrated that DNA sequence polymorphisms were often observed in isolates of *P jiroveci*, suggesting that multiple strains exist.[20] The correct and valid name according to the international code of zoologic nomenclature (ICBU) is *P jirovecii* with a double "i." To date, taxonomy and nomenclature for these organisms is a focus of continuing controversy.[33–35]

BASIC BIOLOGY AND IMMUNOPATHOGENESIS

Life Cycle

Many investigators have attempted to cultivate *Pneumocystis* using a variety of techniques, but have had limited success, impeding studies of *Pneumocystis*. Studies of the life cycle of *Pneumocystis* have been based mainly on light and electron microscopic analysis of forms seen in infected lungs or short-term culture.[36] There are 2 predominant life cycle forms, the trophic form and the cyst form. The trophic form is small (1–4 μm) and predominate over the cyst form during infection by approximately 10 to 1. The mature cyst is 8 to 10 μm in diameter. Three intermediate cyst stages (early, intermediate, and late precysts) have been visualized. It has been hypothesized that the trophic form can conjugate and develop into cysts that undergo maturation, then the mature cyst, containing 8 intracystic nuclei, produce trophic forms as it ruptures. This model is compatible with the life cycle of other ascomyceteous fungi. Whether encystment stage is an obligate step for the replication of the trophic forms remains a matter of controversy.[37]

Interaction with Host Cells

In an infected host, *Pneumocystis* exists almost exclusively within the alveoli of the lung. The trophic forms attach to the alveolar epithelium, through interdigitation of their cell membranes with those of the host cells. Ultrastructural analysis has shown that the adherence is characterized by close apposition of the cell surfaces without fusion of the membranes or changes in the intramenbranous particles.[38,39] Studies using cultured lung epithelial cells showed that adherence of *Pneumocystis* alone does not disrupt alveolar epithelial cell structure or the barrier function.[36] *Pneumocystis* maintains an extracellular existence within alveoli, and probably obtains essential nutrients from the alveolar fluid or living cells.[39]

Binding of *Pneumocystis* to alveolar epithelial cell is facilitated by both fibronectin and vitronectin that are present in alveolar lung fluid. These proteins coat the surface of *Pneumocystis* and subsequently mediate attachment, presumably working through cognate integrins, as well as through mannose binding receptors on the host cells.[37] Interaction of *Pneumocystis* with alveolar epithelial cell and alveolar macrophages initiates cascades of cellular response in both *Pneumocystis* organism and lung cells. It has been demonstrated that attachment of *Pneumocystis* to lung epithelial cells enhances *Pneumocystis* proliferation by activation of selective kinase signaling pathways.[37] The adherence of *Pneumocystis* also inhibits the growth of lung epithelial cells through cyclin-dependent kinase regulatory pathways.[39–41]

Alveolar macrophages are the primary resident phagocytes that mediate the clearance of the organisms from the lung. Cultured rodent alveolar macrophages can bind and take up *Pneumocystis*, through the interactions of macrophage mannose receptors with the *Pneumocystis* major surface glycoprotein termed Msg as well as through interaction of macrophage dectin-1 receptors interacting with the β-glucan moiety of the organisms. IgG may facilitate the uptake process by opsonization of the organisms.[36] Once internalized, *Pneumocystis* is incorporated into phagolysosomes and subsequently degraded.[36] The essential role of macrophages in the control of PCP has been demonstrated in animal models. Clearance of *Pneumocystis* is markedly impaired in macrophage-depleted animals.[42] Blocking *Pneumocystis*-induced macrophage apoptosis enhances host defense to the infection and prolongs survival in an animal model.[43] Phagocytosis, respiratory burst, and inflammatory activation of alveolar macrophages in response to *Pneumocystis* are impaired in HIV-infected persons, and may contribute to the pathogenesis of infection.[44,45]

Immune control of *Pneumocystis* also involves production of chemokines and inflammatory cytokines by alveolar macrophages and epithelial cells.[36] Accumulating evidence indicates that β-glucan molecules, which are abundant in the cell wall of *Pneumocystis*, are important components that drive the initiation of inflammatory response during PCP. Macrophages expresses several β-glucan receptors, including dectin-1, Toll-like receptor 2, and the CD11b/CD18 (CR3) integrin, whose binding initiate signaling cascades result in nuclear factor (NF) κB activation and subsequently stimulation of inflammatory gene expression such as tumor necrosis factor, and chemokines such as interleukin (IL)-8.[36] The dectin-1 and CR3 β-glucan receptors are absent from alveolar epithelial cells. In these cells, lactosylceramide and other receptors, including Toll-like receptors, trigger inflammatory signaling in response to β-glucans.[36]

Immune Response to Pneumocystis Pneumonia

Ultimately, pattern recognition induces chemokines and inflammatory cytokine production, which promote neutrophils and T-lymphocyte recruitment and activation. CD4+ T cells are essential for the control of *Pneumocystis* infection. Indeed, specific depletion of CD4+ T cells in mice induces susceptibility to *Pneumocystis*, and infection resolves when mice are repopulated with sensitized or naive splenic CD4+ T cells.[37,46] Reconstitution with CD4+ T cells clears *Pneumocystis* infection in severe combined immune deficiency (SCID) mice.[37,47–49] CD4+ T cells coordinate the host inflammatory response by recruiting and activating additional immune effector cells including monocytes and macrophages, which are responsible for elimination of the organism. In contrast to CD4+ T cells, the role of CD8+ T cells in host defense against *Pneumocystis* is more controversial. Reconstitution of SCID mice with CD8+ T cells does not protect them against infection, and wild-type mice depleted of CD8+ T cells alone are resistant.[37,47–49] However, CD8+ T cells may have some beneficial effect, particularly in a situation of chronic CD4+ depletion. For example, mice depleted of both CD4+ and CD8+ T cells develop more intense infection than mice depleted of CD4+ T cells alone.[47,50]

However, proinflammatory responses to *Pneumocystis* may be detrimental to the host. For example, *Pneumocystis* infected SCID mice have preserved oxygenation and lung function until the late stage of the disease.[36] Reconstitution of these mice with intact spleen cells results in an intense T-cell mediated inflammatory response, consisting of both CD4+ and CD8+ T cells, causing impaired lung compliance and gas exchange.[51] Both CD4+ and CD8+ T cells may result in deleterious lung inflammation. Reconstitution with CD4+ T cells of SCID mice can result in hyperinflammatory responses, resulting in the death of the host.[48] Other investigators have demonstrated that the lung damage and hypoxia in mouse models depend on the presence of CD8+ T cells in the lung.[51,52]

In addition to T cells, neutrophils, recruited by CXCL2 and IL-8, also participate in lung inflammation during PCP. Neutrophil recruitment seems to closely correlate with lung injury in humans.[53] Furthermore, IL-8 production is correlated with neutrophil infiltration and impaired gas exchange during severe PCP in humans.[54,55] The level of IL-8 in the bronchoalveolar lavage fluid could be a predictor of lung impairment and death from PCP.[55] Recruited neutrophils release protease and reactive oxygen species that directly injure alveolar epithelial cells and capillary endothelial cells. However, in CD4+ T-cell depleted mice, *Pneumocystis* infection induces similar lung injury in mice with or without normal neutrophil function, suggesting that CD8+ T-cell mediated inflammation might be more directly responsible for pulmonary injury than neutrophil-mediated inflammation during PCP in mouse models.[56]

EPIDEMIOLOGY

In this section the possible reservoirs of *Pneumocystis* spp and data on human colonization are discussed, and groups at risk of PCP are addressed.

Although *Pneumocystis* DNA has been identified in the air surrounding apple orchards and the surface of pond water, the existence of an environmental niche for *Pneumocystis* is uncertain.[57–60] However, exposure to *P jirovecii* is common early during life, as demonstrated by a high seroprevalence of anti-*Pneumocystis* antibodies in immunocompetent children. In a Spanish study conducted in 3 rural villages, the overall seroprevalence was 73% among 233 children aged 6 to 13 years.[61] An age-related increase in seroprevalence was observed, from 52% at age 6 years to 66% at 10 years and 80% at 13 years. International seroepidemiologic surveys have shown that *Pneumocystis* had a worldwide distribution, but that the prevalence of antibodies varies among different geographic areas. Indeed, in a study conducted in the urban area of Santiago, Chile, the seroprevalence of anti-*Pneumocystis* antibodies reached 85% by 20 months of age.[62] This primary infection is probably asymptomatic, although careful analysis has not been performed to determine if subtle clinical manifestations do occur. Indeed, a recent study suggests that *P jirovecii* may manifest itself as a self-limiting upper respiratory tract infection in infants aged 9 months or less, predominantly those between 1,5 and 4 months old.[63]

For decades, the theory of the reactivation of a latent *Pneumocystis* infection acquired during infancy was popular. However, some epidemiologic and experimental evidence argues against the reactivation of latent PCP. Geographic clustering of cases of PCP in the urban setting has been observed,[64,65] and genotypes found in patients with PCP are similar to those found in the current patient's environment but not those from his or her place of birth.[66,67] Some experimental evidence also argues against a reactivation of a previously acquired latent infection. Indeed, healthy adult mice inoculated with *Pneumocystis* clear the infection from the lung within 3 weeks, whereas the process takes slightly longer in neonates.[67] Mice that have cleared the infection do not develop PCP once they are rendered CD4+ T-cell deficient.[68]

At present, animal and human studies favor an airborne transmission model for PCP. Animal model studies have shown that *Pneumocystis* spp is communicable and that the principal mode of transmission is the airborne route. Indeed, exposure of animals colonized with *Pneumocystis* led to colonization of healthy animals and to development of clinical disease in immunocompromised animals.[69–71] In addition, the presence of *Pneumocystis* DNA has been demonstrated (by using nested polymerase chain reaction [PCR]) on filters from cages housing *Pneumocystis* infected Wistar rats,[72] and transmission of *Pneumocystis* without physical contact from infected conventional rats to germ-free rats has also been demonstrated.[73]

Several outbreaks of PCP have been reported, mainly among renal transplant recipients.[74–79] Molecular analyses of *Pneumocystis* in some of these studies demonstrated nosocomial acquisition of the infection.[80–82] Although human and animal reports favor an airborne transmission pattern for *Pneumocystis* infection, the mode of transmission, that is, direct person-to-person spread or common environmental source, is still unknown.

As PCP seems to succeed to a dynamic process of infection, the role of colonization in humans should be of major importance in *Pneumocystis* transmission. A permanent colonization/clearance cycle of *Pneumocystis* has been demonstrated in humans much like that observed in animal models.[71,83] Many reports indicate that *Pneumocystis* DNA can be detected in the respiratory tract without clinical disease. These situations have been described as *Pneumocystis* colonization or carriage. The prevalence of *Pneumocystis* colonization among healthy adults is low, although varying between studies from 0% to 20%.[84,85] However, it should be recognized that various PCR techniques and samples were used: nested or heminested PCR; autopsy lung specimens, bronchoalveolar lavage fluid (BAL), oral washing samples, induced sputum, or nasal-swab samples could explain the discrepancies between results among studies. Another explanation could be the varying occupational or geographic exposures of the targeted populations.

Some groups of adult patients are at higher risk of *Pneumocystis* colonization. *Pneumocystis* colonization is more prevalent in the HIV-infected population. *Pneumocystis* colonization, versus infection, has been demonstrated by nested PCR analysis: (1) on induced sputum or BAL fluid of patients who had clinical and laboratory diagnoses other than PCP[86–88]; and (2) on lung tissue from patients who died of other causes.[89] Using these various respiratory samples, the prevalence of *Pneumocystis* colonization was 31% to 68%, including patients who were receiving anti-*Pneumocystis* prophylaxis and patients with CD4 cell counts of less than 200/μL.

Pneumocystis airway colonization is also more prevalent in patients with chronic lung diseases.[90–92] Among chronic lung disease, chronic obstructive pulmonary disease (COPD) was associated with the highest prevalence of *Pneumocystis* colonization, reaching 37% to 55%.[93–95] Frequency of *Pneumocystis* colonization is correlated with more severe stages of COPD, regardless of smoking history, suggesting a role of *Pneumocystis* colonization in the progression of disease.[94] Smoking increases the risk of *Pneumocystis* colonization. Indeed, in patients with interstitial lung disease, smokers have a higher risk of *Pneumocystis* colonization than nonsmokers.[96] Within HIV-infected individuals, smoking increased the risk of *Pneumocystis* colonization[89] and infection.[97,98]

Pneumocystis colonization also occurs in other patients with various underlying conditions. Among 82 patients with diabetes mellitus, multiple myeloma, chronic lymphoid leukemia, or sarcoidosis, 13 (16%) were colonized with *Pneumocystis* on BAL using heminested PCR.[99] Corticosteroid treatment may also favor *Pneumocystis* colonization. In a study of 93 subjects undergoing diagnostic bronchoscopy with BAL and PCR to detect *Pneumocystis*, 8 (44%) of 18 patients receiving more than 20 mg/d prednisolone were colonized, compared with 9 (12%) of the 75 not receiving such prednisolone dosage.[100] Pregnancy also seems to be a risk factor of colonization; with one study reporting up to 16% of third-trimester pregnant women being colonized, suggesting that physiologic immunosuppression associated with pregnancy may favor *Pneumocystis* colonization.[101]

High seroprevalence of anti-*Pneumocystis* antibody in children suggests that *Pneumocystis* colonization occurs frequently in children, who could be a reservoir for *Pneumocystis*. *Pneumocystis* colonization has been demonstrated by nested and real-time PCR on nasopharyngeal aspirate in 15% to 32% of children aged 1 month to 2 years hospitalized with bronchiolitis or acute respiratory infection and without evidence of PCP.[62,63,102,103] *Pneumocystis* organisms have also been found by immunohistochemical or Gomori methenamine silver stain on autopsy lung of 9% to 32% of infants aged 5 days to 1 year dying of sudden infant death syndrome or other causes (including medical condition or injuries).[104] The observation of *Pneumocystis* colonization early in life, in human neonates, has suggested vertical transmission of *Pneumocystis* as an additional route of transmission. A recent study supports this hypothesis, demonstrating *Pneumocystis* DNA by PCR from 11 lung and 8 placenta samples of 20 aborted fetuses from immunocompetent women who had miscarriages.[105] These data provide, for the first time, molecular evidence of *P jirovecii* transplacental transmission in humans.

The consideration of possible nosocomial transmission of *Pneumocystis* prompted studies about *Pneumocystis* colonization among health care workers (HCW). *Pneumocystis* colonization has been found more frequently in immunocompetent HCW in close occupational contact with patients with PCP than in HCW who had no occupational exposure.[106,107] In contrast, a previous study failed to find *Pneumocystis* colonization by PCR on oropharyngeal washings obtained from 20 exposed and 20 unexposed HCW.[108] In addition, Miller and colleagues[106] demonstrated that strains were different between patients and HCW by genotype analysis. Further studies should assess the impact of asymptomatic carriers in the dynamic of *Pneumocystis* transmission.

In conclusion, various host populations may be susceptible to *Pneumocystis* colonization, with several clinical consequences. Individuals colonized with *Pneumocystis* may be at risk of development of PCP.[109,110] These populations may also serve as a reservoir for maintenance and transmission of the organism. In patients with COPD, *Pneumocystis* colonization might favor progression of the disease by sustained inflammation, as has been suggested by animal studies.[95,111] Animal models of simian immunodeficiency virus–infected macaques also suggests that *Pneumocystis* colonization may favor development of chronic lung disease in HIV-infected patients.[112] An association between *Pneumocystis* colonization and sudden infant death syndrome has been evoked, although it remains unclear.[62,104,113] However, further evaluation of the impact of *Pneumocystis* colonization is warranted.

GROUPS AT RISK FOR *PNEUMOCYSTIS* PNEUMONIA

HIV Infection

During HIV infection, the level and percentage of circulating CD4+ cells and the control of viral replication have been found to be predictive of the risk of pneumocystosis. Indeed, PCP develops predominantly in persons whose CD4+ cell count is less than 200 cells/μL or 15% of T cells, and whose viral replication is not controlled.[114–116] Early in the epidemic, the incidence of PCP was almost 20 cases per 100 person-years among HIV-infected patients with CD4+ cell counts of less than 200 cells/μL.[115] There is a gradient of risk, however, as the CD4+ cell count approaches this level. Approximately 10% to 15% of cases of PCP occur in patients with CD4+ T-cell counts of more than 200/μL, but the incidence of such cases is very low given the large number if HIV-infected patients who belong to this category.[117] It has also been noted that HIV-infected infants tend to develop PCP with a CD4+ cell count well above 200/μL. These observations suggest that CD4 cell depletion is not entirely responsible for *Pneumocystis* disease susceptibility. At present, most HIV-infected patients who develop PCP are unaware of their HIV infection or are outside of medical care.[118] In this situation, pneumocystosis is still the most frequent opportunistic infection in developed areas.[119]

Non-HIV Immunocompromised Hosts

Since the routine use of PCP prophylaxis and HAART in HIV-infected patients, patients without HIV infection account now for the majority of cases of PCP in industrialized countries.[120,121] In addition, incidence of PCP has been shown to increase in these patients.[122,123] Non-HIV immunocompromised hosts at risk for PCP include some patients with primary immunodeficiency, patients with secondary immunodeficiency such as hematological malignancies and solid tumors (especially brain tumor), solid organ and bone marrow transplant recipients, and patients with collagen-vascular disorders (especially Wegener granulomatosis). There is no biologic quantitative marker clearly correlated with the risk of *Pneumocystis* infection in these immunodeficiencies as CD4+ cell count is in HIV infection. Indeed, PCP is encountered in patients with normal CD4+ cell count.[124] The most common treatment-related risk factors are steroid and cytotoxic therapy.[122,125]

Primary Immunodeficiencies

Infants with primary immunodeficiency (PID) may be at increased risk of PCP. In this setting, PCP occurs mainly before 1 year of age and often reveals the immunologic disorder. Most of the cases have been reported in PID impairing T-cell function.[8,126–131] Severe combined immunodeficiency and X-linked hyper-IgM syndrome are at higher risk.[8,126–129] In some instances, PCP has been observed in the setting of X-linked agammaglobulinemia.[8,132–134] B cells in *Pneumocystis* have a role experimentally in the generation of anti-*Pneumocystis* CD4+ memory T cells, though susceptibility seems to be cellular-mediated[135] and immunoglobulin therapy does not prevent the disease.[133,136] However, PCP in pure B-cell deficiency is rare and occurs in infants a few months old, and does not justify primary prophylaxis. PCP is extremely uncommon in primary immunodeficiencies of phagocytes such as chronic granulomatous disease.[137–139]

Hematologic Malignancies

Hematologic malignant disorders, especially leukemias and lymphomas, are the most common underlying immunosuppressive conditions at the time of PCP diagnosis in HIV negative patients.[123,124,139,140] Patients with acute lymphoblastic leukemia were historically at higher risk of PCP. With the routine use of PCP prophylaxis in these patients, the attack rate for PCP, which was 1.1% to 21%, markedly decreased to 0.17% for 2929 patients in a study conducted in the 1980s.[123] Thus, attack rates for patients with other hematological malignancies are now higher. The attack rate in large groups of patients was 0.31% to 0.34% for lymphoma patients, and 0.32% for patients with leukemia other than acute lymphoblastic leukemia.[123,125]

Some specific therapeutic regimens received for the underlying hematologic disease are associated with an increased level of cellular immunosuppression and a consequent increased risk of PCP. Most of the patients received corticosteroids at the time of PCP diagnosis.[124,125,139–141] Indeed, difference in attack rate observed historically in patients with acute lymphoblastic leukemia in comparison with acute myeloid leukemia resulted from high-dose steroids they received. Purine analogues, commonly used in chronic lymphoid malignancies, lead to severe and prolonged T-cell immunosuppression predisposing to opportunistic infections including PCP.[142–144] Thereby, the attack rate for PCP was 0.97% of 2969 patients with low-grade lymphoid malignancies who received fludarabine, most of whom had previously received alkylator agents or corticosteroids.[123] Other cytotoxic agents that have been found to be associated with an increased risk of PCP are cytarabine, vincristine, cyclophosphamide, and methotrexate.[123,124,145,146] Monoclonal antibody therapies are recently developed agents increasingly used for the treatment of lymphoid malignancies. Among them, alemtuzumab, which targets CD52, induces a global lymphocyte depletion resulting in profound and prolonged (12–18 months) cellular immunodeficiency, also predisposing to PCP.[147–150] Rituximab, which targets CD20+ B cells, increases the risk of PCP in patients receiving CHOP-14 and CHEOP-14 based chemotherapy.[151,152]

Solid Tumors

The incidence of PCP in patients with solid tumors seems to be increasing. At Memorial Sloan-Kettering Cancer Center, cases among patients with solid tumors increased from 14% during 1963 to 1975 to 47% in 1988 to 1992.[5] In patients with solid tumors, corticosteroid use seems to be the common predisposition. Indeed, half of the patients with solid tumor at the diagnosis of PCP had primary or metastatic brain tumors and had received high doses of corticosteroids.[153,154] The attack rate for this subpopulation was reported to be 1.3% to 1.7%.[123] PCP has also been rarely reported in patients with cancer treated with chemotherapy alone.[125,155] It is noticeable that most of the patients with metastatic brain lesions had primitive breast or lung cancer, and that most of the cases of PCP in patients without brain lesions are encountered in patients with lung or breast neoplasm.[125,140] The high frequency of these 2 neoplasms may explain this observation. Another hypothesis is the role of thoracic irradiation and smoking on lung damage, and the increased risk of *Pneumocystis* colonization and subsequent infection.

Inflammatory and Collagen-Vascular Disease

In one series, the overall incidence of PCP for patients with collagen-vascular disease was estimated to be 2% or less.[5] In a retrospective study of 34 cases of PCP in patients with various inflammatory or collagen-vascular diseases (Wegener granulomatosis, n = 12; systemic lupus erythematosus, n = 6; polyarteritis nodosa, n = 4; poly/dermatomyositis, n = 5, other, n = 7), most patients received corticosteroid therapy plus a second immunosuppressive agent.[156] Among patients receiving immunosuppressive therapy for inflammatory or collagen-vascular disease, patients with Wegener granulomatosis are at higher risk for the development of PCP: Incidence of PCP was 6% in a series of 180 patients followed between 1968 and 1992 receiving daily corticosteroid with additional immunosuppressive therapy.[157] All patients were lymphocytopenic, and PCP occurred during the tapering of steroid therapy in more than 90% of patients.

Among patients with systemic lupus, PCP has been observed before immunosuppressive therapy was initiated, and risk may be associated with a lymphocyte count of 0.4×10^9/L.[5] Patients with dermatomyositis or polymyositis and pulmonary involvement receiving high-dose corticosteroid therapy have a high risk of PCP.[158–160] In addition, cases of fulminant PCP have been reported in patients with dermatomyositis treated with corticosteroids who were lymphopenic before therapy.[161]

Patients with ulcerative colitis treated with corticosteroids with or without cyclosporine are also at some risk.[162,163] Infliximab therapy may increase the risk of PCP.[164] An attack rate of 0.4% was observed in 5000 patients with rheumatoid arthritis who received this treatment.[165] Other cases have been reported in patients receiving infliximab for inflammatory bowel disease, others inflammatory arthritis or collagen-vascular disease.[160,164,165] Median length of time from onset of infliximab infusion and development of PCP was short: 21 days to 8.5 weeks.[164,165]

Solid Organ Transplantation

Transplantation of solid organs is increasingly used, placing a growing number of patients at risk for PCP.

Among renal transplant recipients, incidence of PCP is 1% to 10%[5,166] in the absence of prophylaxis. The vast majority of PCP occurs 3 to 6 months after transplantation. Risk factors for the development of PCP, including previous treatment of rejection episodes, drugs used for maintenance of immunosuppression (cyclosporine, tacrolimus, sirolimus, and mycophenolate mofetil), have been identified in some studies but not confirmed by others.[77,78,167–173] However, practices in immunosuppressive therapy continually change and may modulate the risk of infection.[174,175] Indeed, increasing use of alemtuzumab and rituximab for rejection management will probably result in an increased incidence of opportunistic infection in solid organ transplant recipients. In addition to these risk factors, several groups have reported outbreaks of PCP among renal transplant recipients, suggesting that the risk of acquiring PCP is higher if the disease is prevalent in the local community.[75]

The reported attack rate among heart transplant recipients has varied widely, from 5% to 41%.[5] In studies among liver transplant recipients, 10% to 11% of patients developed PCP.[5,123] PCP is more frequent in the recipients of lung and heart-lung transplants than in other solid organ transplant recipients, with reported attack rates of 16% to 43% of heart-lung and lung transplant recipients in the absence of prophylaxis.[5,123] Similar to renal transplant recipients, PCP usually occurs before 6 months in the post-transplant period, and is unlikely to occur in patients compliant with prophylaxis.

Bone Marrow and Hematopoietic Stem Cell Transplantation

Allogenic bone marrow transplantation (BMT) and hematopoietic stem cell transplantation (HSCT) leads to severe immunosuppression, which extends in the post-transplant period for months to a more prolonged period if graft versus host disease (GVHD) requires continuous immunosuppressive therapy. The risk of development of PCP is also increased with the use of T-cell depleted graft.[125,176] Before the routine use trimethoprim-sulfamethoxazole prophylaxis, PCP developed in 9% to 16% of allogenic bone marrow transplant recipients.[5] Most bone marrow transplant recipients who developed PCP did not receive adequate prophylaxis.[177,178]

Miscellaneous Disorders

Besides these more common situations, *Pneumocystis* is an opportunistic pathogen in patients with idiopathic CD4+ T-cell lymphocytopenia.[179] Three cases of PCP have also been reported among 51 patients with Good syndrome.[180] In some instance, PCP has been reported in patients without predisposing conditions.[181] Some of these patients were elderly, and clustered cases have been reported. Pulmonary involvement was atypical in some of the patients. Localized lobar or focal infiltrate and pleural effusion were seen. An increasing recognition of infections that have been existent but not identified has been evoked.[182] The existence of an underlying unrecognized immunodeficiency in these patients remains possible.

The relationship of corticosteroids to *Pneumocystis* has been emphasized by the occurrence of pneumocystosis in patients with Cushing syndrome and in children receiving corticosteroid for asthma, a disease not known to predispose to any opportunistic infection.[183–185] In a study of patients with endogenous Cushing syndrome who developed opportunistic infections, the plasma cortisol levels were highest among patients who developed PCP compared with those who developed cryptococcosis, aspergillosis, or nocardiosis, suggesting that higher amounts of immunosuppression may be required to produce *P jirovecii* disease.[183]

CLINICAL PRESENTATION

PCP classically presents with fever, cough, and dyspnea. Physical examination is nonspecific, and the pulmonary auscultation is often normal, even in the presence of significant disease and hypoxemia. Discrete crackles may be present. Acute dyspnea with pleuritic chest pain may indicate the development of a pneumothorax, which has been described in 2% to 4% of patients.[186,187] In general, HIV-infected persons present with a subacute course and longer symptom duration than other immunocompromised persons, respectively 25 to 28 and 5 to 6 days.[123,139] Respiratory involvement is usually less severe in HIV-infected persons, with a high arterial oxygen tension and a lower respiratory rate.[123,139] Reflecting severity of the lung inflammation, their BAL specimens contain significantly fewer neutrophils compared with patients without HIV infection.[188]

RADIOLOGICAL PRESENTATION

On chest radiograph, PCP usually presents with bilateral, diffuse, reticular, or granular opacities. Chest radiograph may be normal at diagnosis in as many as 39% of cases.[189] High-resolution computed tomography (CT) scanning is more sensitive than chest radiograph for detection of PCP (**Fig. 1**; for a review, see Boiselle and colleagues.[189]). A CT scan typically shows ground-glass opacities with patchy distribution, predominating in perihilar regions of lungs. Thickened septal lines and areas of consolidation may be present. Multiple and bilateral cysts are observed in 10% to 34% of cases. Cyst formation increases the risk of pneumothorax. Other atypical manifestations include multiple thick-walled cavitary nodules and noncavitary nodules. Lymphadenopathy and effusions are less frequent.[190] In the setting of *Pneumocystis* prophylaxis with aerosolized pentamidine, patients are more likely to present with predominantly upper lobe disease, pneumothorax, or cyst formation.[187,191]

MICROBIOLOGICAL DIAGNOSIS

As *Pneumocystis* cannot readily be cultured in the laboratory, the diagnosis of PCP continues to mostly rely on the microscopic demonstration of the characteristic organisms in respiratory specimens such as BAL fluid or induced sputum. Trophic forms can be detected with the use of certain stains, such as modified Papanicolaou, Giemsa, or Gram-Weigert. Cysts can be stained with Gomori-methenamine silver, cresyl echt

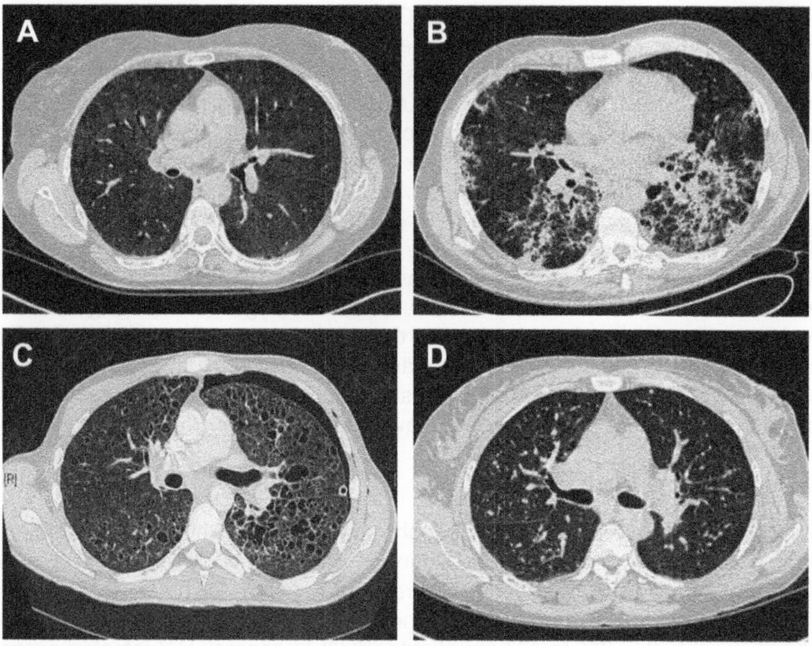

Fig. 1. *Pneumocystis* pneumonia appearances on high-resolution CT scan. (*A*) Diffuse ground-glass opacities. (*B*) Thickened septal lines and areas of consolidation. (*C*) Diffuse ground-glass opacities and multiple cysts. Left pneumothorax and chest-tube. (*D*) Multiple nodules in a granulomatous *Pneumocystis* pneumonia.

violet, and toluidine blue O or Calcofluor white (**Fig. 2**).[192] Fluorescein-labeled monoclonal anti-*Pneumocystis* antibodies are commercially available. An advantage of some immunofluorescent monoclonal antibodies is their ability to stain both trophic forms and cysts, which is important because the trophic forms are generally more abundant during PCP. In addition, monoclonal antibodies are more sensitive than the general stains and represent the "gold standard" technique for the diagnosis of PCP.

A variety of suitable specimens have been proposed for microbiological assessment. At this time, most centers use induced sputum and BAL for diagnosis. Sputum induction with hypertonic saline is a rapid and cost-effective method. Under optimal technical circumstances, sputum induction combined with conventional staining has a sensitivity range of 55% to 66% in HIV-infected patients.[193,194] Monoclonal antibodies for detecting *Pneumocystis* have a higher sensitivity and specificity in induced-sputum samples than conventional tinctorial stains. These antibodies increase the sensitivity of induced sputum to more than 90% in HIV-infected patients.[195]

PCP patients without AIDS have a lower burden of *P jiroveci* than those with AIDS, which leads to difficulty in detecting the organisms. In these patients, or in HIV-infected patients with early disease or those with breakthrough episodes while receiving aerosol pentamidine prophylaxis, sputum induction may be negative, and bronchoscopy with BAL is the preferred diagnostic procedure, with reported sensitivity from 89% to 98% using tinctorial or immunofluorescent monoclonal antibody staining.[37] In granulomatous *Pneumocystis*, an atypical form of PCP, BAL study is usually negative, requiring an open lung biopsy for diagnosis.[149]

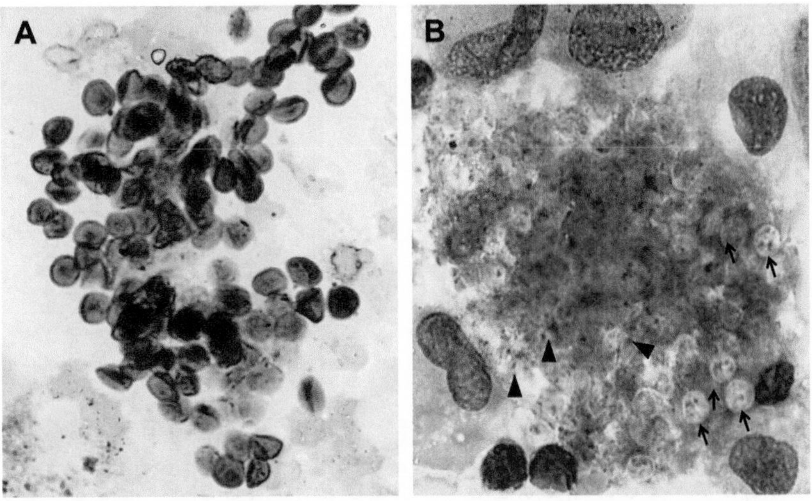

Fig. 2. Typical *Pneumocystis* forms in a bronchoalveolar lavage specimen stained with Gomori methamine silver (*A*) and Giemsa (*B*) (original magnification × 500). (*A*) Gomori methamine silver stains the cyst walls. Cysts are well recognizable as round, oval, or flat bodies of approximately 4–5 μm in diameter. (*B*) Giemsa staining showing trophic forms and cysts of *Pneumocystis jirovecii* within foamy exudates. Cyst structures containing intracystic bodies at their periphery (*arrows*); trophic forms are visible with dotlike nuclei and pale blue-gray cytoplasm (*arrowheads*).

In an attempt to improve diagnosis of PCP, PCR methods have been developed. Two types of PCR have been studied: conventional PCR (nested or heminested) and quantitative PCR. Conventional PCR has a higher sensitivity than microscopic observation but suffers from low specificity and low positive predictive value, limiting its utility in clinical practice.[196–198] The chief interest in conventional PCR may be in its high negative predictive value, allowing withdrawal of anti-PCP therapy.[199] Quantitative PCR is more promising, as a cut-off of clinical significance may be determined for differentiation between carriage and PCP.[196,198] However, most studies have used home-made PCR, precluding generalization of results. At this time, PCR is still a clinical research tool.

TREATMENT

Because of high efficacy and the availability of oral and parenteral forms, trimethoprim-sulfamethoxazole (TMP-SMX) is the first-line agent for the treatment of mild to severe PCP either in HIV and non-HIV-infected patients. Adverse reactions usually begin during the second week of treatment. These reactions are more frequent in HIV-infected patients. First-line and alternative therapies are summarized in **Table 1**. Parenteral pentamidine is the most studied drug as an alternative to TMP-SMX. Pentamidine is about as effective as TMP-SMX.[200–202] The principal limitation is its poor tolerability. Adverse drug reactions occur in 71% of patients, leading to drug withdrawal in 18%.[203] Nephrotoxicity, dysglycemia, hepatotoxicity, hyperkalemia, and pancreatitis account for 80% of adverse events. No clinical trials have been performed to compare atovaquone, clindamycin-primaquine, or dapsone-TMP with TMP-SMX in the treatment of moderate to severe PCP (defined by an arterial oxygen pressure of less than 70 mm Hg or an arterial-alveolar gradient of more than 35 mm Hg). More data are

Table 1
Treatment of *Pneumocystis* pneumonia

	Medication	Dose and Route	Comments	Adverse Events
First choice	Trimethoprim + sulfamethoxazole	15–20 mg/kg 75–100 mg/kg Intravenous or orally, divided into 3–4 doses daily	Contraindication in cases of allergy to sulfa drugs	Cytopenia Skin reactions (mild to severe: toxic epidermal necrolysis, Stevens-Johnson syndrome) Hepatitis, pancreatitis Gastrointestinal disturbance Renal insufficiency, hyperkalemia Anaphylaxis
Alternative choice Mild to moderate PCP	Dapsone + trimethoprime	100 mg/d orally 5 mg/kg 3 times daily	Contraindication in cases of G6PD deficiency Possible cross-reaction with sulfa allergy	Methemoglobinemia Skin rash Fever Gastrointestinal disturbance
	Atovaquone	750 mg 2–3 times daily orally	Bioavailability increased with high-fat meal	Skin rash Fever Gastrointestinal disturbance Hepatitis
	Clindamycin + primaquine	600 mg 4 times daily intravenous or 350–400 mg 4 times daily orally 30 mg daily orally	Contraindication in cases of G6PD	Skin rash Fever Neutropenia Gastrointestinal disturbance Methemoglobinemia
Alternative choice Moderate to severe PCP	Pentamidine	4 mg/kg daily intravenous		Hypotension, Cardiac arrhythmias (torsades de pointes) Hyperkalemia, hypomagnesemia, hypocalcemia Renal insufficiency Pancreatitis, hypoglycemia (early), diabetes mellitus (late) Neutropenia Hepatitis

available in the treatment of mild to moderate PCP (defined by an arterial-alveolar gradient of less than 35 mm Hg and between 35 and 45 mm Hg, respectively): Clindamycin-primaquine and dapsone-TMP exhibit comparable efficacy and toxicity to TMP-SMX[204–206]; atovaquone is less effective but better tolerated than TMP-SMX and as effective as pentamidine.[207,208] In addition to the classic alternative therapy, caspofungin may be a promising drug, although experience is limited. Two patients were treated successfully with caspofungin alone,[209,210] while 4 other patients had received caspofungin in addition to TMP-SMX.[211]

Available data of the pre-corticosteroid era suggest that patients generally improved after 4 to 8 days of therapy.[139] If progression is observed after 4 days, a second pathogen should be excluded and another treatment of PCP should be considered. The most studied second-line drugs are intravenous pentamidine and clindamycin-primaquine.[212–214] A recent systematic review showed that clindamycin-primaquine was associated with a better outcome of second-line treatment compared with pentamidine.[212] TMP-SMX was associated with a favorable outcome of second-line treatment for those failing another first-line regimen. More recently, caspofungin was successfully administered as a salvage therapy in 2 transplant-recipient patients in addition to TMP-SMX.[211]

No clear association between mutations in the dihydropteroate synthetase (DHPS), the target enzyme of sulfonamides, and TMP-SMX treatment failure or altered outcome has been demonstrated.[39,215,216] Mutations in the gene encoding cytochrome B, conferring potential atovaquone resistance, have also been described; however, their clinical impact on treatment failure has not been determined.[217] Recommended duration of treatment is 21 days in HIV-infected patients and 14 days in non-HIV immunocompromised hosts. Recommendation for longer treatment in HIV-infected patients is supported by a higher organism burden and a slower clinical response, leading to a higher risk of relapse after only 14 days of treatment. Subsequently, treatment should be extended in non-HIV infected patients when clinical improvement is prolonged.

Corticosteroids in HIV-Infected Patients

Inflammation is correlated to lung injury in animal models (see earlier discussion). Early in the AIDS epidemic, randomized trials accordingly had evaluated the efficacy of corticosteroid treatment to reduce morbidity and mortality of PCP. Benefit to survival on corticosteroid administration begins during the first 72 hours of treatment, and has been demonstrated in HIV-infected patients whose arterial oxygen pressure is equal or less than 70 mm Hg or whose alveolar-arterial oxygen gradient is of 35 mm Hg or more.[218] The United States recommended regimen is 40 mg prednisone twice daily for 5 days, then 40 mg once daily for 5 days, followed by 20 mg once daily for 11 days.[219]

Corticosteroids in Non-HIV Infected Patients

No randomized studies on the use of adjunctive corticosteroids have been conducted in non-HIV infected patients. The problems are that non-HIV immunocompromised hosts constitute a nonhomogeneous group of patients and that most of them have been on corticosteroids at the time they developed PCP. One retrospective study demonstrated an accelerated recovery among 16 patients with severe PCP who received 60 mg or more of prednisone daily in comparison with 14 patients maintained on a low-dose regimen.[220] Another study of 31 patients with severe PCP failed to demonstrate any benefit from corticosteroid adjunctive therapy.[221] There was a trend, however, among patients who received corticosteroid adjunctive therapy, to a lower mortality rate in the 8 patients with a high *Pneumocystis* burden in their BAL fluid compared with the 11 patients with fewer organisms (25% versus 63%, $P = .10$). However, routine use of adjunctive corticosteroid could not be recommended. Tapering of corticosteroid should probably be avoided, and whether doses should be increased must be individualized.

PROGNOSIS

Despite treatment, mortality of PCP still remains high. Some early studies showed similar poor survival between AIDS and non-AIDS patients of 50% to 64%.[11,123,139] However, most studies demonstrate a better survival (86%–92%) in AIDS patients[118,222,223] in comparison with non-AIDS patients with various underlying conditions (survival 51%–80%).[125,140,141,154,224–226] As PCP is a severe infection with a high mortality rate, prevention is essential in the groups at risk.

PREVENTION

Prevention of Nosocomial Transmission

As nosocomial acquisition of *Pneumocystis* infection has been demonstrated in some of the PCP outbreaks,[80–82] prevention of air transmission from hospitalized patients with PCP should be considered to avoid secondary cases. As person-to-person transmission has not been demonstrated, respiratory isolation is not currently recommended in national guidelines. However, mice-to-mice transmission has been demonstrated.[69–71] In the authors' practice, patients with PCP are hospitalized in single room.

CHEMOPROPHYLAXIS

Recommendation for HIV-Infected Patients

The Infectious Disease Society of America and the US Public Health Service had published guidelines for the prevention of opportunistic infection including PCP.[227] HIV-infected adults and adolescents, including pregnant women and those on HAART, should receive chemoprophylaxis against PCP if they have a CD4+ T-cell count of less than 200/μL or oropharyngeal candidiasis. Persons who have a CD4+ T-cell percentage of less than 14% should be considered for prophylaxis. Primary and secondary PCP prophylaxis can be safely discontinued in patients who have responded to HAART with an increased in CD4+ T-cell count to greater than 200/μL for at least 3 months.

Evidence in Non-HIV Immunocompromised Patients

As PCP is severe in non-HIV infected patients, prophylaxis should be discussed concerning any patient who receives immunosuppressive therapy. However, widespread routine prophylaxis may create problems. TMP-SMZ has many side effects such as rash, hematological toxicity, and hepatitis. In a recent meta-analysis, the number needed to harm (NNH) for severe adverse events that required discontinuation was 32.[228] Therefore, the number needed to treat to prevent one case of PCP was equal to the NNH when the risk of PCP was 3,5%. Indeed, the benefit of prophylaxis should be balanced with the risk of severe adverse events, and depends on the attack rate of PCP.

In cancer patients, PCP prophylaxis should be administered in those who receive high-dose steroid therapy. In patients with hematologic malignancies, TMP-SMX prophylaxis is recommended in patients with acute lymphoblastic leukemia or with hematologic malignancies treated with T-cell depleting agents[143,148]; it is also recommended for patients treated with CHOP-14 and CHEOP-14 regimens.[151] Routine prophylaxis is considered in patients with other regimens if they have other risk factors (chronic lung disease, corticotherapy).

Guidelines have been published in HSCT recipients.[229] (1) Allogenic HSCT patients should receive prophylaxis from engraftment until 6 months post HSCT in all cases, and throughout all periods of immunosuppression for those who are receiving immunosuppressive therapy or have chronic GVHD. (2) PCP prophylaxis should be considered for autologous HSCT patients who have underlying hematologic malignancies such as lymphoma or leukemia, are undergoing intense conditioning regimens or graft manipulation, or have recently received fludarabine or 2-CDA. Attention should be given to absorption of the drugs in patients with digestive GVHD, foe example, atovaquone, which requires a fatty meal for a good absorption.

PCP prophylaxis should be administered lifelong in lung, heart, and heart-lung transplant recipients.[230] PCP prophylaxis is administered to liver transplant recipients for 1 year in most transplant centers. However, it has been suggested that the low incidence of PCP in this population after the 6-month post-transplant period permits a shorter duration of prophylaxis.[231] In renal transplant recipients, PCP prophylaxis is recommended for a minimum of 4 months after transplantation and for another 3 to 4 months after a rejection episode.[232] However, prophylactic therapy should be extended (duration 6–12 months) in patients who received lymphocyte-depleting monoclonal antibody or antithymocyte globulin.[175] PCP prophylaxis merits consideration in patients who require a high level of immunosuppression for the treatment of organ rejection, and in patients with frequent opportunistic infection, including cytomegalovirus disease.[230]

PCP prophylaxis should be administered in patients with Wegener granulomatosis while they are receiving daily corticosteroids.[157,233] Although there are no published guidelines, PCP prophylaxis should be initiated in patients with dermatomyositis, polymyositis, or systemic lupus erythematosus who have known risk factors for the development of PCP, that is, high-dose corticosteroids, lymphopenia, and interstitial pulmonary disease.[158,159,161] TMP-SMX prophylaxis could be administered in patients treated with up to 25 mg of methotrexate per week. Such patients need to receive folate supplementation (1 mg per day) or leucovorin on the day after receiving methotrexate, as well as monitoring of blood cells count and liver function tests.[192]

Chemoprophylaxis Regimen

TMP-SMX is the most studied and the first-choice prophylaxis in HIV-infected and in non-HIV immunocompromised hosts. Protection rates are excellent, reaching 89% to 100%.[234–238] One double-strength tablet daily is the preferred regimen.[227] One single-strength tablet per day and one double-strength tablet 3 times per week are acceptable alternative regimens, associated with fewer side effects.[227] First-choice and alternative prophylaxis schemes are reported in **Table 2**. Aerosolized pentamidine given monthly is less effective, particularly in patients with low CD4+ cell count (protection rate 60%–90%).[234–240] Pentamidine must be administered in a Respigard nebulizer to a patient in decubitus, to optimize repartition of the drug throughout the lung. The major side effects are cough and bronchospasm.

Resistance and Prophylaxis Failure

Mutation prevalence in the DHPS gene has clearly increased during the past years. In one study conducted in the United States on 145 isolates, mutation prevalence was 0% in 1983 to 1993, 25% in 1994 to 1995, and 70% in 2000 to 2001.[241] Virtually all of the observed DHPS gene mutations are nonsynonymous point mutations at 2 amino

Table 2
Prophylactic regimen against *Pneumocystis* pneumonia

	Medication	Dose and Route	Comments
First choice	Trimethoprim + sulfamethoxazole	80–160 mg daily 400–800 mg daily orally or intravenous	Contraindication in cases of allergy to sulfa drugs
	Trimethoprim + sulfamethoxazole	160 mg 3 times a week 800 mg 3 times a week orally or intravenous	
Alternative choice	Dapsone	100 mg daily orally	Contraindication in cases of G6PD deficiency Possible cross-reaction with sulfa allergy
	Dapsone + pyrimethamine	50 mg daily orally 50 mg per week + leucovorin 25 mg per week	Contraindication in cases of G6PD deficiency Possible cross-reaction with sulfa allergy
	Atovaquone	750 mg 2 times daily orally	Bioavailability increased with high-fat meal
	Pentamidine	300 mg monthly	Administrate in decubitus to optimize lung distribution

Double-strength tablet daily dose of trimethoprim-sulfamethoxazole (TMP-SMX) and dapsone + pyrimethamine prophylactic regimen are also effective against toxoplasmosis. Atovaquone and single-strength tablet daily dose of TMP-SMX also can be considered.

acid positions in an active site involved in substrate binding.[37,242] DHPS mutations have been associated with failure of TMP-SMX and dapsone prophylaxis.[241–245] Mutations in the dihydrofolate reductase, the target enzyme of trimethoprim and pyrimethamine, have also been recognized.[246] Mutations in the atovaquone target gene, encoding cytochrome B, have been associated with prior exposure to atovaquone, although their clinical relevance is uncertain.[217]

SUMMARY

PCP still remains a severe opportunistic infection, associated with a high mortality rate. Despite a growing knowledge base on PCP, progress is desired in many directions. First, one is still not able to measure the level of risk of PCP in the non-HIV immunocompromised host. Biologic markers of immunodeficiency, such as CD4 levels in HIV-infected patients, are needed. It is hoped that such tools will exist in the future. Factors influencing colonization, such as previous lung disease or smoking habit, should be taken into consideration in immunocompromised patients with a low incidence risk of PCP. Second, treatment needs to be improved. Available anti-*Pneumocystis* drugs are associated with many side effects, and mutations have emerged. Although patients infected with *Pneumocystis* that contains DHPS mutations still respond to TMP-SMX treatment, new drugs with different mechanisms of action are needed. Caspofungin, which targets *Pneumocystis* glucans synthetase (GSC1), thereby inhibiting fungal cell wall synthesis, theoretically acts synergistically with TMP-SMX. Further clinical evaluation of this treatment is warranted. Finally, as mortality of PCP results from lung injury, progress in the management of the lung inflammatory response could improve prognosis.

REFERENCES

1. Delanoe P, Delanoe M. [Sur les rapports des kystes de carinii du poumon des rats avec le *Trypanosoma lewisi*]. CR Acad Sci 1912;155:658–60 [in French].
2. Ammich O. [Uber die nichtsyphilitische interstitielle pneumoniae des ersten kindersalters]. Virchows Arch Pathol Anat 1938;302:539–54 [in German].
3. Van der Meer G, Brug SL. [Infection par *Pneumocystis* chez l'homme et chez les animaux]. Annales de la Société Belge de Médecine Tropicale 1942;22:301–5 [in French].
4. Vanek J, Jirovec O. [Parasitaere pneumonie. Interstitielle plasmazellen pneumonie der fruehgeborenen verursacht durch *Pneumocytis carinii*]. Zentralbl Bakteriol 1952;158:120–7 [in German].
5. Sepkowitz KA, Brown AE, Armstrong D. *Pneumocystis carinii* pneumonia without acquired immunodeficiency syndrome. More patients, same risk. Arch Intern Med 1995;155(11):1125–8.
6. Ng VL, Yajko DM, Hadley WK. Extrapulmonary pneumocystosis. Clin Microbiol Rev 1997;10(3):401–18.
7. Excler JL, Mojon M, Guyonnet C, et al. [*Pneumocystis carinii* pneumonia in children. Apropos of 33 cases]. Pediatrie 1984;39(7):513–23 [in French].
8. Walzer PD, Schultz MG, Western KA, et al. *Pneumocystis carinii* pneumonia and primary immune deficiency diseases. Natl Cancer Inst Monogr 1976;43:65–74.
9. Gottlieb MS, Schroff R, Schanker HM, et al. *Pneumocystis carinii* pneumonia and mucosal candidiasis in previously healthy homosexual men: evidence of a new acquired cellular immunodeficiency. N Engl J Med 1981;305(24):1425–31.
10. Masur H, Michelis MA, Greene JB, et al. An outbreak of community-acquired *Pneumocystis carinii* pneumonia: initial manifestation of cellular immune dysfunction. N Engl J Med 1981;305(24):1431–8.
11. Jaffe HW, Bregman DJ, Selik RM. Acquired immune deficiency syndrome in the United States: the first 1,000 cases. J Infect Dis 1983;148(2):339–45.
12. Gebo KA, Fleishman JA, Moore RD. Hospitalizations for metabolic conditions, opportunistic infections, and injection drug use among HIV patients: trends between 1996 and 2000 in 12 states. J Acquir Immune Defic Syndr 2005; 40(5):609–16.
13. San-Andres FJ, Rubio R, Castilla J, et al. Incidence of acquired immunodeficiency syndrome-associated opportunistic diseases and the effect of treatment on a cohort of 1115 patients infected with human immunodeficiency virus, 1989-1997. Clin Infect Dis 2003;36(9):1177–85.
14. Bonnet F, Lewden C, May T, et al. Opportunistic infections as causes of death in HIV-infected patients in the HAART era in France. Scand J Infect Dis 2005; 37(6-7):482–7.
15. Edman JC, Kovacs JA, Masur H, et al. Ribosomal RNA sequence shows *Pneumocystis carinii* to be a member of the fungi. Nature 1988;334(6182):519–22.
16. Stringer SL, Stringer JR, Blase MA, et al. *Pneumocystis carinii*: sequence from ribosomal RNA implies a close relationship with fungi. Exp Parasitol 1989; 68(4):450–61.

17. Redhead SA, Cushion MT, Frenkel JK, et al. *Pneumocystis* and *Trypanosoma cruzi*: nomenclature and typifications. J Eukaryot Microbiol 2006;53(1):2–11.
18. Frenkel JK. *Pneumocystis jiroveci* n. sp. from man: morphology, physiology, and immunology in relation to pathology. Natl Cancer Inst Monogr 1976;43:13–30.
19. Walzer PD, Linke MJ. A comparison of the antigenic characteristics of rat and human *Pneumocystis carinii* by immunoblotting. J Immunol 1987;138(7): 2257–65.
20. Stringer JR, Beard CB, Miller RF, et al. A new name (*Pneumocystis jiroveci*) for *Pneumocystis* from humans. Emerg Infect Dis 2002;8(9):891–6.
21. Li J, Edlind T. Phylogeny of *Pneumocystis carinii* based on beta-tubulin sequence. J Eukaryot Microbiol 1994;41(5):97S.
22. Mazars E, Odberg-Ferragut C, Dei-Cas E, et al. Polymorphism of the thymidylate synthase gene of *Pneumocystis carinii* from different host species. J Eukaryot Microbiol 1995;42(1):26–32.
23. Ma L, Kovacs JA. Expression and characterization of recombinant human-derived *Pneumocystis carinii* dihydrofolate reductase. Antimicrob Agents Chemother 2000;44(11):3092–6.
24. Banerji S, Lugli EB, Miller RF, et al. Analysis of genetic diversity at the arom locus in isolates of *Pneumocystis carinii*. J Eukaryot Microbiol 1995;42(6):675–9.
25. Sinclair K, Wakefield AE, Banerji S, et al. *Pneumocystis carinii* organisms derived from rat and human hosts are genetically distinct. Mol Biochem Parasitol 1991;45(1):183–4.
26. Liu Y, Rocourt M, Pan S, et al. Sequence and variability of the 5.8s and 26s rRNA genes of *Pneumocystis carinii*. Nucleic Acids Res 1992;20(14):3763–72.
27. Denis CM, Mazars E, Guyot K, et al. Genetic divergence at the soda locus of six different formae speciales of *Pneumocystis carinii*. Med Mycol 2000;38(4): 289–300.
28. Shah JS, Pieciak W, Liu J, et al. Diversity of host species and strains of *Pneumocystis carinii* is based on rRNA sequences. Clin Diagn Lab Immunol 1996;3(1):119–27.
29. Aliouat EM, Mazars E, Dei-Cas E, et al. *Pneumocystis* cross infection experiments using SCID mice and nude rats as recipient host, showed strong host-species specificity. J Eukaryot Microbiol 1994;41(5):71S.
30. Gigliotti F, Harmsen AG, Haidaris CG, et al. *Pneumocystis carinii* is not universally transmissible between mammalian species. Infect Immun 1993;61(7): 2886–90.
31. Beard CB, Jennings VM, Teague WG, et al. Experimental inoculation of immunosuppressed owl monkeys with *Pneumocystis carinii* f. sp. hominis. J Eukaryot Microbiol 1999;46(5):113S–5S.
32. Stringer JR, Cushion MT, Wakefield AE. New nomenclature for the genus *Pneumocystis*. J Eukaryot Microbiol 2001;(Suppl):184S–9S.
33. Gigliotti F. *Pneumocystis carinii*: has the name really been changed? Clin Infect Dis 2005;41(12):1752–5.
34. Cushion MT, Stringer JR. Has the name really been changed? It has for most researchers. Clin Infect Dis 2005;41(12):1756–8.
35. Gigliotti F. *Pneumocystis carinii* nomenclature: response to cushion and stringer. Clin Infect Dis 2006;42(8):1208–9.
36. Thomas CF Jr, Limper AH. Current insights into the biology and pathogenesis of *Pneumocystis* pneumonia. Nat Rev Microbiol 2007;5(4):298–308.
37. Huang L, Morris A, Limper AH, et al. An official ATS workshop summary: recent advances and future directions in *Pneumocystis* pneumonia (PCP). Proc Am Thorac Soc 2006;3(8):655–64.

38. Yoneda K, Walzer PD. Attachment of *Pneumocystis carinii* to type I alveolar cells studied by freeze-fracture electron microscopy. Infect Immun 1983;40(2):812–5.
39. Walzer PD, Smulian AG. *Pneumocystis* species. In: Linvingstone C, editor, Principles and practice of infectious disease, vol. 2. Elsevier; 2004. p. 3080–94.
40. Limper AH, Martin WJ 2nd. *Pneumocystis carinii*: inhibition of lung cell growth mediated by parasite attachment. J Clin Invest 1990;85(2):391–6.
41. Limper AH, Edens M, Anders RA, et al. *Pneumocystis carinii* inhibits cyclin-dependent kinase activity in lung epithelial cells. J Clin Invest 1998;101(5):1148–55.
42. Limper AH, Hoyte JS, Standing JE. The role of alveolar macrophages in *Pneumocystis carinii* degradation and clearance from the lung. J Clin Invest 1997; 99(9):2110–7.
43. Lasbury ME, Durant PJ, Ray CA, et al. Suppression of alveolar macrophage apoptosis prolongs survival of rats and mice with *Pneumocystis* pneumonia. J Immunol 2006;176(11):6443–53.
44. Koziel H, Eichbaum Q, Kruskal BA, et al. Reduced binding and phagocytosis of *Pneumocystis carinii* by alveolar macrophages from persons infected with HIV-1 correlates with mannose receptor downregulation. J Clin Invest 1998;102(7): 1332–44.
45. Koziel H, Li X, Armstrong MY, et al. Alveolar macrophages from human immunodeficiency virus-infected persons demonstrate impaired oxidative burst response to *Pneumocystis carinii* in vitro. Am J Respir Cell Mol Biol 2000; 23(4):452–9.
46. Beck JM, Warnock ML, Kaltreider HB, et al. Host defenses against *Pneumocystis carinii* in mice selectively depleted of CD4+ lymphocytes. Chest 1993; 103(Suppl 2):116S–8S.
47. Bhagwat SP, Gigliotti F, Xu H, et al. Contribution of T cell subsets to the pathophysiology of *Pneumocystis*-related immunorestitution disease. Am J Physiol Lung Cell Mol Physiol 2006;291(6):L1256–66.
48. Roths JB, Sidman CL. Both immunity and hyperresponsiveness to *Pneumocystis carinii* result from transfer of CD4+ but not CD8+ T cells into severe combined immunodeficiency mice. J Clin Invest 1992;90(2):673–8.
49. Harmsen AG, Stankiewicz M. Requirement for CD4+ cells in resistance to *Pneumocystis carinii* pneumonia in mice. J Exp Med 1990;172(3):937–45.
50. Beck JM, Newbury RL, Palmer BE, et al. Role of CD8+ lymphocytes in host defense against *Pneumocystis carinii* in mice. J Lab Clin Med 1996;128(5): 477–87.
51. Wright TW, Gigliotti F, Finkelstein JN, et al. Immune-mediated inflammation directly impairs pulmonary function, contributing to the pathogenesis of *Pneumocystis carinii* pneumonia. J Clin Invest 1999;104(9):1307–17.
52. Beck JM, Warnock ML, Curtis JL, et al. Inflammatory responses to *Pneumocystis carinii* in mice selectively depleted of helper T lymphocytes. Am J Respir Cell Mol Biol 1991;5(2):186–97.
53. Azoulay E, Parrot A, Flahault A, et al. AIDS-related *Pneumocystis carinii* pneumonia in the era of adjunctive steroids: implication of BAL neutrophilia. Am J Respir Crit Care Med 1999;160(2):493–9.
54. Limper AH, Offord KP, Smith TF, et al. *Pneumocystis carinii* pneumonia. Differences in lung parasite number and inflammation in patients with and without AIDS. Am Rev Respir Dis 1989;140(5):1204–9.
55. Benfield TL, Vestbo J, Junge J, et al. Prognostic value of interleukin-8 in AIDS-associated *Pneumocystis carinii* pneumonia. Am J Respir Crit Care Med 1995; 151(4):1058–62.

56. Swain SD, Wright TW, Degel PM, et al. Neither neutrophils nor reactive oxygen species contribute to tissue damage during *Pneumocystis* pneumonia in mice. Infect Immun 2004;72(10):5722–32.
57. Wakefield AE. DNA sequences identical to *Pneumocystis carinii* f. sp. *carinii* and *Pneumocystis carinii* f. sp. hominis in samples of air spora. J Clin Microbiol 1996;34(7):1754–9.
58. Casanova-Cardiel L, Leibowitz MJ. Presence of *Pneumocystis carinii* DNA in pond water. J Eukaryot Microbiol 1997;44(6):28S.
59. Morris A, Beard CB, Huang L. Update on the epidemiology and transmission of *Pneumocystis carinii.* Microbes Infect 2002;4(1):95–103.
60. Wakefield AE. Detection of DNA sequences identical to *Pneumocystis carinii* in samples of ambient air. J Eukaryot Microbiol 1994;41(5):116S.
61. Respaldiza N, Medrano FJ, Medrano AC, et al. High seroprevalence of *Pneumocystis* infection in Spanish children. Clin Microbiol Infect 2004;10(11): 1029–31.
62. Vargas SL, Hughes WT, Santolaya ME, et al. Search for primary infection by *Pneumocystis carinii* in a cohort of normal, healthy infants. Clin Infect Dis 2001;32(6):855–61.
63. Larsen HH, von Linstow ML, Lundgren B, et al. Primary *Pneumocystis* infection in infants hospitalized with acute respiratory tract infection. Emerg Infect Dis 2007;13(1):66–72.
64. Morris AM, Swanson M, Ha H, et al. Geographic distribution of human immunodeficiency virus-associated *Pneumocystis carinii* pneumonia in San Francisco. Am J Respir Crit Care Med 2000;162(5):1622–6.
65. Dohn MN, White ML, Vigdorth EM, et al. Geographic clustering of *Pneumocystis carinii* pneumonia in patients with HIV infection. Am J Respir Crit Care Med 2000;162(5):1617–21.
66. Beard CB, Carter JL, Keely SP, et al. Genetic variation in *Pneumocystis carinii* isolates from different geographic regions: Implications for transmission. Emerg Infect Dis 2000;6(3):265–72.
67. Garvy BA, Qureshi MH. Delayed inflammatory response to *Pneumocystis carinii* infection in neonatal mice is due to an inadequate lung environment. J Immunol 2000;165(11):6480–6.
68. Chen W, Gigliotti F, Harmsen AG. Latency is not an inevitable outcome of infection with *Pneumocystis carinii.* Infect Immun 1993;61(12):5406–9.
69. An CL, Gigliotti F, Harmsen AG. Exposure of immunocompetent adult mice to *Pneumocystis carinii* f. sp. *muris* by cohousing: growth of *P. carinii* f. sp. *muris* and host immune response. Infect Immun 2003;71(4):2065–70.
70. Gigliotti F, Harmsen AG, Wright TW. Characterization of transmission of *Pneumocystis carinii* f. sp. *muris* through immunocompetent BALB/c mice. Infect Immun 2003;71(7):3852–6.
71. Chabe M, Dei-Cas E, Creusy C, et al. Immunocompetent hosts as a reservoir of *Pneumocystis* organisms: histological and RT-PCR data demonstrate active replication. Eur J Clin Microbiol Infect Dis 2004;23(2):89–97.
72. Olsson M, Sukura A, Lindberg LA, et al. Detection of *Pneumocystis carinii* DNA by filtration of air. Scand J Infect Dis 1996;28(3):279–82.
73. Hughes WT, Bartley DL, Smith BM. A natural source of infection due to *Pneumocystis carinii.* J Infect Dis 1983;147(3):595.
74. Arichi N, Kishikawa H, Mitsui Y, et al. Cluster outbreak of *Pneumocystis* pneumonia among kidney transplant patients within a single center. Transplant Proc 2009;41(1):170–2.

75. de Boer MG, Bruijnesteijn van Coppenraet LE, Gaasbeek A, et al. An outbreak of *Pneumocystis jiroveci* pneumonia with 1 predominant genotype among renal transplant recipients: interhuman transmission or a common environmental source? Clin Infect Dis 2007;44(9):1143–9.
76. Olsson M, Eriksson BM, Elvin K, et al. Genotypes of clustered cases of *Pneumocystis carinii* pneumonia. Scand J Infect Dis 2001;33(4):285–9.
77. Hennequin C, Page B, Roux P, et al. Outbreak of *Pneumocystis carinii* pneumonia in a renal transplant unit. Eur J Clin Microbiol Infect Dis 1995;14(2):122–6.
78. Branten AJ, Beckers PJ, Tiggeler RG, et al. *Pneumocystis carinii* pneumonia in renal transplant recipients. Nephrol Dial Transplant 1995;10(7):1194–7.
79. Singer C, Armstrong D, Rosen PP, et al. *Pneumocystis carinii* pneumonia: a cluster of eleven cases. Ann Intern Med 1975;82(6):772–7.
80. Hocker B, Wendt C, Nahimana A, et al. Molecular evidence of *Pneumocystis* transmission in pediatric transplant unit. Emerg Infect Dis 2005;11(2):330–2.
81. Schmoldt S, Schuhegger R, Wendler T, et al. Molecular evidence of nosocomial *Pneumocystis jirovecii* transmission among 16 patients after kidney transplantation. J Clin Microbiol 2008;46(3):966–71.
82. Rabodonirina M, Vanhems P, Couray-Targe S, et al. Molecular evidence of interhuman transmission of *Pneumocystis* pneumonia among renal transplant recipients hospitalized with HIV-infected patients. Emerg Infect Dis 2004;10(10):1766–73.
83. Montes-Cano MA, de la Horra C, Dapena FJ, et al. Dynamic colonisation by different *Pneumocystis jirovecii* genotypes in cystic fibrosis patients. Clin Microbiol Infect 2007;13(10):1008–11.
84. Morris A, Wei K, Afshar K, et al. Epidemiology and clinical significance of *Pneumocystis* colonization. J Infect Dis 2008;197(1):10–7.
85. Nevez G, Jounieaux V, Linas MD, et al. High frequency of *Pneumocystis carinii* sp.f. hominis colonization in HIV-negative patients. J Eukaryot Microbiol 1997; 44(6):36S.
86. Huang L, Crothers K, Morris A, et al. *Pneumocystis* colonization in HIV-infected patients. J Eukaryot Microbiol 2003;50(Suppl):616–7.
87. Wakefield AE, Lindley AR, Ambrose HE, et al. Limited asymptomatic carriage of *Pneumocystis jiroveci* in human immunodeficiency virus-infected patients. J Infect Dis 2003;187(6):901–8.
88. Rabodonirina M, Raffenot D, Cotte L, et al. Rapid detection of *Pneumocystis carinii* in bronchoalveolar lavage specimens from human immunodeficiency virus-infected patients: use of a simple DNA extraction procedure and nested PCR. J Clin Microbiol 1997;35(11):2748–51.
89. Morris A, Kingsley LA, Groner G, et al. Prevalence and clinical predictors of *Pneumocystis* colonization among HIV-infected men. AIDS 2004;18(5):793–8.
90. Sing A, Roggenkamp A, Autenrieth IB, et al. *Pneumocystis carinii* carriage in immunocompetent patients with primary pulmonary disorders as detected by single or nested PCR. J Clin Microbiol 1999;37(10):3409–10.
91. Sing A, Geiger AM, Hogardt M, et al. *Pneumocystis carinii* carriage among cystic fibrosis patients, as detected by nested PCR. J Clin Microbiol 2001; 39(7):2717–8.
92. Matos O, Costa MC, Correia I, et al. *Pneumocystis jirovecii* carriage in Portuguese immunocompetent patients: preliminary results. J Eukaryot Microbiol 2003;50(Suppl):647–8.
93. Probst M, Ries H, Schmidt-Wieland T, et al. Detection of *Pneumocystis carinii* DNA in patients with chronic lung diseases. Eur J Clin Microbiol Infect Dis 2000;19(8):644–5.

94. Morris A, Sciurba FC, Lebedeva IP, et al. Association of chronic obstructive pulmonary disease severity and *Pneumocystis* colonization. Am J Respir Crit Care Med 2004;170(4):408–13.
95. Calderon EJ, Rivero L, Respaldiza N, et al. Systemic inflammation in patients with chronic obstructive pulmonary disease who are colonized with *Pneumocystis jiroveci*. Clin Infect Dis 2007;45(2):e17–9.
96. Vidal S, de la Horra C, Martin J, et al. *Pneumocystis jirovecii* colonisation in patients with interstitial lung disease. Clin Microbiol Infect 2006;12(3):231–5.
97. Miguez-Burbano MJ, Ashkin D, Rodriguez A, et al. Increased risk of *Pneumocystis carinii* and community-acquired pneumonia with tobacco use in HIV disease. Int J Infect Dis 2005;9(4):208–17.
98. Miguez-Burbano MJ, Burbano X, Ashkin D, et al. Impact of tobacco use on the development of opportunistic respiratory infections in HIV seropositive patients on antiretroviral therapy. Addict Biol 2003;8(1):39–43.
99. Nevez G, Raccurt C, Vincent P, et al. Pulmonary colonization with *Pneumocystis carinii* in human immunodeficiency virus-negative patients: assessing risk with blood CD4+ T cell counts. Clin Infect Dis 1999;29(5): 1331–2.
100. Maskell NA, Waine DJ, Lindley A, et al. Asymptomatic carriage of *Pneumocystis jiroveci* in subjects undergoing bronchoscopy: a prospective study. Thorax 2003;58(7):594–7.
101. Vargas SL, Ponce CA, Sanchez CA, et al. Pregnancy and asymptomatic carriage of *Pneumocystis jiroveci*. Emerg Infect Dis 2003;9(5):605–6.
102. Nevez G, Totet A, Pautard JC, et al. *Pneumocystis carinii* detection using nested-PCR in nasopharyngeal aspirates of immunocompetent infants with bronchiolitis. J Eukaryot Microbiol 2001;(Suppl):122S–3S.
103. Totet A, Meliani L, Lacube P, et al. Immunocompetent infants as a human reservoir for *Pneumocystis jirovecii*: rapid screening by non-invasive sampling and real-time PCR at the mitochondrial large subunit rRNA gene. J Eukaryot Microbiol 2003;50(Suppl):668–9.
104. Vargas SL, Ponce CA, Galvez P, et al. *Pneumocystis* is not a direct cause of sudden infant death syndrome. Pediatr Infect Dis J 2007;26(1):81–3.
105. Montes-Cano MA, Chabe M, Fontillon-Alberdi M, et al. Vertical transmission of *Pneumocystis jirovecii* in humans. Emerg Infect Dis 2009;15(1):125–7.
106. Miller RF, Ambrose HE, Wakefield AE. *Pneumocystis carinii* f. sp. hominis DNA in immunocompetent health care workers in contact with patients with *P. carinii* pneumonia. J Clin Microbiol 2001;39(11):3877–82.
107. Vargas SL, Ponce CA, Gigliotti F, et al. Transmission of *Pneumocystis carinii* DNA from a patient with *P. carinii* pneumonia to immunocompetent contact health care workers. J Clin Microbiol 2000;38(4):1536–8.
108. Lundgren B, Elvin K, Rothman LP, et al. Transmission of *Pneumocystis carinii* from patients to hospital staff. Thorax 1997;52(5):422–4.
109. Wissmann G, Varela JM, Calderon EJ. Prevention of *Pneumocystis* pneumonia in patients with inflammatory bowel disease based on the detection of *Pneumocystis* colonization. Inflamm Bowel Dis 2008;14(12):1751–2.
110. Mori S, Cho I, Ichiyasu H, et al. Asymptomatic carriage of *Pneumocystis jiroveci* in elderly patients with rheumatoid arthritis in Japan: a possible association between colonization and development of *Pneumocystis jiroveci* pneumonia during low-dose MTX therapy. Mod Rheumatol 2008;18(3):240–6.
111. Christensen PJ, Preston AM, Ling T, et al. *Pneumocystis murina* infection and cigarette smoke exposure interact to cause increased organism burden,

development of airspace enlargement, and pulmonary inflammation in mice. Infect Immun 2008;76(8):3481–90.
112. Norris KA, Morris A, Patil S, et al. *Pneumocystis* colonization, airway inflammation, and pulmonary function decline in acquired immunodeficiency syndrome. Immunol Res 2006;36(1–3):175–87.
113. Vargas SL, Ponce CA, Hughes WT, et al. Association of primary *Pneumocystis carinii* infection and sudden infant death syndrome. Clin Infect Dis 1999;29(6): 1489–93.
114. Masur H, Ognibene FP, Yarchoan R, et al. CD4 counts as predictors of opportunistic pneumonias in human immunodeficiency virus (HIV) infection. Ann Intern Med 1989;111(3):223–31.
115. Phair J, Munoz A, Detels R, et al. The risk of *Pneumocystis carinii* pneumonia among men infected with human immunodeficiency virus type 1. Multicenter AIDS Cohort Study Group. N Engl J Med 1990;322(3):161–5.
116. D'Egidio GE, Kravcik S, Cooper CL, et al. *Pneumocystis jiroveci* pneumonia prophylaxis is not required with a CD4+ T-cell count <200 cells/microl when viral replication is suppressed. AIDS 2007;21(13):1711–5.
117. Kovacs JA, Masur H. Evolving health effects of *Pneumocystis*: one hundred years of progress in diagnosis and treatment. JAMA 2009;301(24):2578–85.
118. Walzer PD, Evans HE, Copas AJ, et al. Early predictors of mortality from *Pneumocystis jirovecii* pneumonia in HIV-infected patients: 1985–2006. Clin Infect Dis 2008;46(4):625–33.
119. Pillonel J. [Surveillance de l'infection par le VIH/SIDA en France, 2006]. Bull Épidémiol Hebd 2007;46–47:386–93 [in French].
120. Mikaelsson L, Jacobsson G, Andersson R. *Pneumocystis* pneumonia—a retrospective study 1991–2001 in Gothenburg, Sweden. J Infect 2006;53(4):260–5.
121. Hui M, Kwok WT. *Pneumocystis carinii* pneumonia in Hong Kong: a 10 year retrospective study. J Med Microbiol 2006;55(Pt 1):85–8.
122. Arend SM, Kroon FP, van't Wout JW. *Pneumocystis carinii* pneumonia in patients without AIDS, 1980 through 1993. An analysis of 78 cases. Arch Intern Med 1995;155(22):2436–41.
123. Russian DA, Levine SJ. *Pneumocystis carinii* pneumonia in patients without HIV infection. Am J Med Sci 2001;321(1):56–65.
124. Overgaard UM, Helweg-Larsen J. *Pneumocystis jiroveci* pneumonia (PCP) in HIV-1-negative patients: a retrospective study 2002-2004. Scand J Infect Dis 2007;39(6–7):589–95.
125. Sepkowitz KA, Brown AE, Telzak EE, et al. *Pneumocystis carinii* pneumonia among patients without AIDS at a cancer hospital. JAMA 1992;267(6):832–7.
126. Leggiadro RJ, Winkelstein JA, Hughes WT. Prevalence of *Pneumocystis carinii* pneumonitis in severe combined immunodeficiency. J Pediatr 1981; 99(1):96–8.
127. Walzer PD, Schultz MG, Western KA, et al. *Pneumocystis carinii* pneumonia and primary immune deficiency diseases of infancy and childhood. J Pediatr 1973; 82(3):416–22.
128. Levy J, Espanol-Boren T, Thomas C, et al. Clinical spectrum of X-linked hyper-IgM syndrome. J Pediatr 1997;131(1 Pt 1):47–54.
129. Winkelstein JA, Marino MC, Ochs H, et al. The X-linked hyper-IgM syndrome: clinical and immunologic features of 79 patients. Medicine (Baltimore) 2003; 82(6):373–84.
130. Imai K, Morio T, Zhu Y, et al. Clinical course of patients with wasp gene mutations. Blood 2004;103(2):456–64.

131. Elhasid R, Etzioni A. Major histocompatibility complex class II deficiency: a clinical review. Blood Rev 1996;10(4):242–8.
132. Richman DD, Zamvil L, Remington JS. Recurrent *Pneumocystis carinii* pneumonia in a child with hypogammaglobulinemia. Am J Dis Child 1973;125(1):102–3.
133. Dittrich AM, Schulze I, Magdorf K, et al. X-linked agammaglobulinaemia and *Pneumocystis carinii* pneumonia—an unusual coincidence? Eur J Pediatr 2003;162(6):432–3.
134. Burke BA, Good RA. *Pneumocystis carinii* infection. Medicine (Baltimore) 1973; 52(1):23–51.
135. Lund FE, Hollifield M, Schuer K, et al. B cells are required for generation of protective effector and memory CD4 cells in response to *Pneumocystis* lung infection. J Immunol 2006;176(10):6147–54.
136. Alibrahim A, Lepore M, Lierl M, et al. *Pneumocystis carinii* pneumonia in an infant with X-linked agammaglobulinemia. J Allergy Clin Immunol 1998;101(4 Pt 1):552–3.
137. Adinoff AD, Johnston RB Jr, Dolen J, et al. Chronic granulomatous disease and *Pneumocystis carinii* pneumonia. Pediatrics 1982;69(1):133–4.
138. Rosenszweig SD, Holland SM. Phagocyte immunodeficiencies and their infections. J Allergy Clin Immunol 2004;113(4):620–6.
139. Kovacs JA, Hiemenz JW, Macher AM, et al. *Pneumocystis carinii* pneumonia: a comparison between patients with the acquired immunodeficiency syndrome and patients with other immunodeficiencies. Ann Intern Med 1984;100(5):663–71.
140. Yale SH, Limper AH. *Pneumocystis carinii* pneumonia in patients without acquired immunodeficiency syndrome: associated illness and prior corticosteroid therapy. Mayo Clin Proc 1996;71(1):5–13.
141. Pagano L, Fianchi L, Mele L, et al. *Pneumocystis carinii* pneumonia in patients with malignant haematological diseases: 10 years' experience of infection in gimema centres. Br J Haematol 2002;117(2):379–86.
142. Cheson BD. Infectious and immunosuppressive complications of purine analog therapy. J Clin Oncol 1995;13(9):2431–48.
143. Byrd JC, Hargis JB, Kester KE, et al. Opportunistic pulmonary infections with fludarabine in previously treated patients with low-grade lymphoid malignancies: a role for *Pneumocystis carinii* pneumonia prophylaxis. Am J Hematol 1995; 49(2):135–42.
144. Morra E, Nosari A, Montillo M. Infectious complications in chronic lymphocytic leukaemia. Hematol Cell Ther 1999;41(4):145–51.
145. Roblot F, Imbert S, Godet C, et al. Risk factors analysis for *Pneumocystis jiroveci* pneumonia (PCP) in patients with haematological malignancies and pneumonia. Scand J Infect Dis 2004;36(11–12):848–54.
146. De Castro N, Pavie J, Lagrange-Xelot M, et al. [*Pneumocystis jiroveci* pneumonia in patients with cancer: is it unavoidable?]. Rev Mal Respir 2007;24(6): 741–50 [in French].
147. Martin SI, Marty FM, Fiumara K, et al. Infectious complications associated with alemtuzumab use for lymphoproliferative disorders. Clin Infect Dis 2006;43(1): 16–24.
148. Lundin J, Kimby E, Bjorkholm M, et al. Phase II trial of subcutaneous anti-CD52 monoclonal antibody alemtuzumab (Campath-1H) as first-line treatment for patients with B-cell chronic lymphocytic leukemia (B-CLL). Blood 2002;100(3): 768–73.
149. Otahbachi M, Nugent K, Buscemi D. Granulomatous *Pneumocystis jiroveci* pneumonia in a patient with chronic lymphocytic leukemia: a literature review and hypothesis on pathogenesis. Am J Med Sci 2007;333(2):131–5.

150. Morrison VA. Update on prophylaxis and therapy of infection in patients with chronic lymphocytic leukemia. Expert Rev Anticancer Ther 2001;1(1):84–90.
151. Kolstad A, Holte H, Fossa A, et al. *Pneumocystis jirovecii* pneumonia in B-cell lymphoma patients treated with the rituximab-CHOEP-14 regimen. Haematologica 2007;92(1):139–40.
152. Venhuizen AC, Hustinx WN, van Houte AJ, et al. Three cases of *Pneumocystis jirovecii* pneumonia (PCP) during first-line treatment with rituximab in combination with CHOP-14 for aggressive B-cell non-Hodgkin's lymphoma. Eur J Haematol 2008;80(3):275–6.
153. Varthalitis I, Meunier F. *Pneumocystis carinii* pneumonia in cancer patients. Cancer Treat Rev 1993;19(4):387–413.
154. Henson JW, Jalaj JK, Walker RW, et al. *Pneumocystis carinii* pneumonia in patients with primary brain tumors. Arch Neurol 1991;48(4):406–9.
155. Kulke MH, Vance EA. *Pneumocystis carinii* pneumonia in patients receiving chemotherapy for breast cancer. Clin Infect Dis 1997;25(2):215–8.
156. Godeau B, Coutant-Perronne V, Le Thi Huong D, et al. *Pneumocystis carinii* pneumonia in the course of connective tissue disease: report of 34 cases. J Rheumatol 1994;21(2):246–51.
157. Ognibene FP, Shelhamer JH, Hoffman GS, et al. *Pneumocystis carinii* pneumonia: a major complication of immunosuppressive therapy in patients with Wegener's granulomatosis. Am J Respir Crit Care Med 1995;151(3 Pt 1):795–9.
158. Kadoya A, Okada J, Iikuni Y, et al. Risk factors for *Pneumocystis carinii* pneumonia in patients with polymyositis/dermatomyositis or systemic lupus erythematosus. J Rheumatol 1996;23(7):1186–8.
159. Alarcon GS. Infections in systemic connective tissue diseases: systemic lupus erythematosus, scleroderma, and polymyositis/dermatomyositis. Infect Dis Clin North Am 2006;20(4):849–75.
160. Marie E. [Infections au cours des polymyosites et des dermatomyosites]. Presse Med 2009;38:303–16 [in French].
161. Bachelez H, Schremmer B, Cadranel J, et al. Fulminant *Pneumocystis carinii* pneumonia in 4 patients with dermatomyositis. Arch Intern Med 1997;157(13):1501–3.
162. Smith MB, Hanauer SB. *Pneumocystis carinii* pneumonia during cyclosporine therapy for ulcerative colitis. N Engl J Med 1992;327:497–8.
163. Bernstein CN, Kolodny M, Block E, et al. *Pneumocystis carinii* pneumonia in patients with ulcerative colitis treated with steroids. Am J Gastroenterol 1993;88:574–7.
164. Kaur N, Mahl TC. *Pneumocystis jiroveci* (*carinii*) pneumonia after infliximab therapy: a review of 84 cases. Dig Dis Sci 2007;52(6):1481–4.
165. Komano Y, Harigai M, Koike R, et al. *Pneumocystis jiroveci* pneumonia in patients with rheumatoid arthritis treated with infliximab: a retrospective review and case-control study of 21 patients. Arthritis Rheum 2009;61(3):305–12.
166. Gordon SM, LaRosa SP, Kalmadi S, et al. Should prophylaxis for *Pneumocystis carinii* pneumonia in solid organ transplant recipients ever be discontinued? Clin Infect Dis 1999;28(2):240–6.
167. Hardy AM, Wajszczuk CP, Suffredini AF, et al. *Pneumocystis carinii* pneumonia in renal-transplant recipients treated with cyclosporine and steroids. J Infect Dis 1984;149(2):143–7.
168. Lufft V, Kliem V, Behrend M, et al. Incidence of *Pneumocystis carinii* pneumonia after renal transplantation. Impact of immunosuppression. Transplantation 1996;62(3):421–3.

169. Sollinger HW. Mycophenolate mofetil for the prevention of acute rejection in primary cadaveric renal allograft recipients. U.S. Renal Transplant Mycophenolate Mofetil Study Group. Transplantation 1995;60(3):225–32.
170. Dominguez J, Mahalati K, Kiberd B, et al. Conversion to rapamycin immunosuppression in renal transplant recipients: report of an initial experience. Transplantation 2000;70(8):1244–7.
171. Radisic M, Lattes R, Chapman JF, et al. Risk factors for *Pneumocystis carinii* pneumonia in kidney transplant recipients: a case-control study. Transpl Infect Dis 2003;5(2):84–93.
172. Arend SM, Westendorp RG, Kroon FP, et al. Rejection treatment and cytomegalovirus infection as risk factors for *Pneumocystis carinii* pneumonia in renal transplant recipients. Clin Infect Dis 1996;22(6):920–5.
173. Neff RT, Jindal RM, Yoo DY, et al. Analysis of USRDS: incidence and risk factors for *Pneumocystis jiroveci* pneumonia. Transplantation 2009;88(1):135–41.
174. Shapiro R, Young JB, Milford EL, et al. Immunosuppression: evolution in practice and trends, 1993-2003. Am J Transplant 2005;5(4):874–86.
175. Issa NC, Fishman JA. Infectious complications of antilymphocyte therapies in solid organ transplantation. Clin Infect Dis 2009;48(6):772–86.
176. Anderson KC, Soiffer R, DeLage R, et al. T-cell-depleted autologous bone marrow transplantation therapy: analysis of immune deficiency and late complications. Blood 1990;76(1):235–44.
177. Tuan IZ, Dennison D, Weisdorf DJ. *Pneumocystis carinii* pneumonitis following bone marrow transplantation. Bone Marrow Transplant 1992;10(3):267–72.
178. De Castro N, Neuville S, Sarfati C, et al. Occurrence of *Pneumocystis jiroveci* pneumonia after allogeneic stem cell transplantation: a 6-year retrospective study. Bone Marrow Transplant 2005;36(10):879–83.
179. Duncan RA, von Reyn CF, Alliegro GM, et al. Idiopathic CD4+ T-lymphocytopenia—four patients with opportunistic infections and no evidence of HIV infection. N Engl J Med 1993;328(6):393–8.
180. Tarr PE, Sneller MC, Mechanic LJ, et al. Infections in patients with immunodeficiency with thymoma (good syndrome). Report of 5 cases and review of the literature. Medicine (Baltimore) 2001;80(2):123–33.
181. Al Soub H, Taha RY, El Deeb Y, et al. *Pneumocystis carinii* pneumonia in a patient without a predisposing illness: case report and review. Scand J Infect Dis 2004;36(8):618–21.
182. Hughes WT. *Pneumocystis carinii* infections in mothers, infants and non-AIDS elderly adults. In: Sattler FR, Walzer PD, editors, *Pneumocystis carinii* clinical infectious diseases, vol. 2. London: Bailliere Tindall; 1995. p. 461–70.
183. Graham BS, Tucker WS Jr. Opportunistic infections in endogenous Cushing's syndrome. Ann Intern Med 1984;101(3):334–8.
184. Abernathy-Carver KJ, Fan LL, Boguniewicz M, et al. *Legionella* and *Pneumocystis* pneumonias in asthmatic children on high doses of systemic steroids. Pediatr Pulmonol 1994;18(3):135–8.
185. Oosterhuis JK, van den Berg G, Monteban-Kooistra WE, et al. Life-threatening *Pneumocystis jiroveci* pneumonia following treatment of severe Cushing's syndrome. Neth J Med 2007;65(6):215–7.
186. Walzer PD, Perl DP, Krogstad DJ, et al. *Pneumocystis carinii* pneumonia in the United States. Epidemiologic, diagnostic, and clinical features. Ann Intern Med 1974;80(1):83–93.

187. Sepkowitz KA, Telzak EE, Gold JW, et al. Pneumothorax in AIDS. Ann Intern Med 1991;114(6):455–9.
188. Munoz P, Munoz RM, Palomo J, et al. *Pneumocystis carinii* infection in heart transplant recipients. Efficacy of a weekend prophylaxis schedule. Medicine (Baltimore) 1997;76(6):415–22.
189. Boiselle PM, Crans CA Jr, Kaplan MA. The changing face of *Pneumocystis carinii* pneumonia in AIDS patients. AJR Am J Roentgenol 1999;172(5): 1301–9.
190. Kennedy CA, Goetz MB. Atypical roentgenographic manifestations of *Pneumocystis carinii* pneumonia. Arch Intern Med 1992;152(7):1390–8.
191. Jules-Elysee KM, Stover DE, Zaman MB, et al. Aerosolized pentamidine: effect on diagnosis and presentation of *Pneumocystis carinii* pneumonia. Ann Intern Med 1990;112(10):750–7.
192. Thomas CF Jr, Limper AH. *Pneumocystis* pneumonia. N Engl J Med 2004; 350(24):2487–98.
193. Pitchenik AE, Ganjei P, Torres A, et al. Sputum examination for the diagnosis of *Pneumocystis carinii* pneumonia in the acquired immunodeficiency syndrome. Am Rev Respir Dis 1986;133(2):226–9.
194. O'Brien RF, Quinn JL, Miyahara BT, et al. Diagnosis of *Pneumocystis carinii* pneumonia by induced sputum in a city with moderate incidence of AIDS. Chest 1989;95(1):136–8.
195. Kovacs JA, Ng VL, Masur H, et al. Diagnosis of *Pneumocystis carinii* pneumonia: improved detection in sputum with use of monoclonal antibodies. N Engl J Med 1988;318(10):589–93.
196. Fujisawa T, Suda T, Matsuda H, et al. Real-time PCR is more specific than conventional PCR for induced sputum diagnosis of *Pneumocystis* pneumonia in immunocompromised patients without HIV infection. Respirology 2009; 14(2):203–9.
197. Ribes JA, Limper AH, Espy MJ, et al. PCR detection of *Pneumocystis carinii* in bronchoalveolar lavage specimens: analysis of sensitivity and specificity. J Clin Microbiol 1997;35(4):830–5.
198. Flori P, Bellete B, Durand F, et al. Comparison between real-time PCR, conventional PCR and different staining techniques for diagnosing *Pneumocystis jiroveci* pneumonia from bronchoalveolar lavage specimens. J Med Microbiol 2004;53(Pt 7):603–7.
199. Azoulay E, Bergeron A, Chevret S, et al. Polymerase chain reaction for diagnosing *Pneumocystis* pneumonia in non-HIV immunocompromised patients with pulmonary infiltrates. Chest 2009;135(3):655–61.
200. Wharton JM, Coleman DL, Wofsy CB, et al. Trimethoprim-sulfamethoxazole or pentamidine for *Pneumocystis carinii* pneumonia in the acquired immunodeficiency syndrome. A prospective randomized trial. Ann Intern Med 1986; 105(1):37–44.
201. Sattler FR, Cowan R, Nielsen DM, et al. Trimethoprim-sulfamethoxazole compared with pentamidine for treatment of *Pneumocystis carinii* pneumonia in the acquired immunodeficiency syndrome. A prospective, noncrossover study. Ann Intern Med 1988;109(4):280–7.
202. Klein NC, Duncanson FP, Lenox TH, et al. Trimethoprim-sulfamethoxazole versus pentamidine for *Pneumocystis carinii* pneumonia in AIDS patients: results of a large prospective randomized treatment trial. AIDS 1992;6(3):301–5.
203. O'Brien JG, Dong BJ, Coleman RL, et al. A 5-year retrospective review of adverse drug reactions and their risk factors in human immunodeficiency

virus-infected patients who were receiving intravenous pentamidine therapy for *Pneumocystis carinii* pneumonia. Clin Infect Dis 1997;24(5):854–9.
204. Safrin S, Finkelstein DM, Feinberg J, et al. Comparison of three regimens for treatment of mild to moderate *Pneumocystis carinii* pneumonia in patients with AIDS. A double-blind, randomized, trial of oral trimethoprim-sulfamethoxazole, dapsone-trimethoprim, and clindamycin-primaquine. ACTG 108 Study Group. Ann Intern Med 1996;124(9):792–802.
205. Toma E, Fournier S, Dumont M, et al. Clindamycin/primaquine versus trimethoprim-sulfamethoxazole as primary therapy for *Pneumocystis carinii* pneumonia in AIDS: a randomized, double-blind pilot trial. Clin Infect Dis 1993;17(2):178–84.
206. Leoung GS, Mills J, Hopewell PC, et al. Dapsone-trimethoprim for *Pneumocystis carinii* pneumonia in the acquired immunodeficiency syndrome. Ann Intern Med 1986;105(1):45–8.
207. Dohn MN, Weinberg WG, Torres RA, et al. Oral atovaquone compared with intravenous pentamidine for *Pneumocystis carinii* pneumonia in patients with AIDS. Atovaquone Study Group. Ann Intern Med 1994;121(3):174–80.
208. Rosenberg DM, McCarthy W, Slavinsky J, et al. Atovaquone suspension for treatment of *Pneumocystis carinii* pneumonia in HIV-infected patients. AIDS 2001;15(2):211–4.
209. Mu XD, Que CL, He B, et al. Caspofungin as salvage treatment of severe *Pneumocystis* pneumonia: case report and literature review. Chin Med J (Engl) 2009; 122(8):996–9.
210. Hof H, Schnulle P. *Pneumocystis jiroveci* pneumonia in a patient with Wegener's granulomatosis treated efficiently with caspofungin. Mycoses 2008;51(Suppl 1): 65–7.
211. Utili R, Durante-Mangoni E, Basilico C, et al. Efficacy of caspofungin addition to trimethoprim-sulfamethoxazole treatment for severe *Pneumocystis* pneumonia in solid organ transplant recipients. Transplantation 2007;84(6):685–8.
212. Benfield T, Atzori C, Miller RF, et al. Second-line salvage treatment of AIDS-associated *Pneumocystis jirovecii* pneumonia: a case series and systematic review. J Acquir Immune Defic Syndr 2008;48(1):63–7.
213. Toma E, Fournier S, Poisson M, et al. Clindamycin with primaquine for *Pneumocystis carinii* pneumonia. Lancet 1989;1(8646):1046–8.
214. Noskin GA, Murphy RL, Black JR, et al. Salvage therapy with clindamycin/primaquine for *Pneumocystis carinii* pneumonia. Clin Infect Dis 1992;14(1):183–8.
215. Navin TR, Beard CB, Huang L, et al. Effect of mutations in *Pneumocystis carinii* dihydropteroate synthase gene on outcome of *P carinii* pneumonia in patients with HIV-1: a prospective study. Lancet 2001;358(9281):545–9.
216. Crothers K, Beard CB, Turner J, et al. Severity and outcome of HIV-associated *Pneumocystis* pneumonia containing *Pneumocystis jirovecii* dihydropteroate synthase gene mutations. AIDS 2005;19(8):801–5.
217. Kazanjian P, Armstrong W, Hossler PA, et al. *Pneumocystis carinii* cytochrome b mutations are associated with atovaquone exposure in patients with AIDS. J Infect Dis 2001;183(5):819–22.
218. Briel M, Bucher HC, Boscacci R, et al. Adjunctive corticosteroids for *Pneumocystis jiroveci* pneumonia in patients with HIV-infection. Cochrane Database Syst Rev 2006;(3):CD006150.
219. Bozzette SA, Sattler FR, Chiu J, et al. A controlled trial of early adjunctive treatment with corticosteroids for *Pneumocystis carinii* pneumonia in the acquired immunodeficiency syndrome. California Collaborative Treatment Group. N Engl J Med 1990;323(21):1451–7.

220. Pareja JG, Garland R, Koziel H. Use of adjunctive corticosteroids in severe adult non-HIV *Pneumocystis carinii* pneumonia. Chest 1998;113(5):1215–24.
221. Delclaux C, Zahar JR, Amraoui G, et al. Corticosteroids as adjunctive therapy for severe *Pneumocystis carinii* pneumonia in non-human immunodeficiency virus-infected patients: retrospective study of 31 patients. Clin Infect Dis 1999;29(3): 670–2.
222. Mansharamani NG, Garland R, Delaney D, et al. Management and outcome patterns for adult *Pneumocystis carinii* pneumonia, 1985 to 1995: comparison of HIV-associated cases to other immunocompromised states. Chest 2000; 118(3):704–11.
223. Gerrard JG. *Pneumocystis carinii* pneumonia in HIV-negative immunocompromised adults. Med J Aust 1995;162(5):233–5.
224. Roblot F, Godet C, Le Moal G, et al. Analysis of underlying diseases and prognosis factors associated with *Pneumocystis carinii* pneumonia in immunocompromised HIV-negative patients. Eur J Clin Microbiol Infect Dis 2002;21(7): 523–31.
225. Roblot F, Le Moal G, Godet C, et al. *Pneumocystis carinii* pneumonia in patients with hematologic malignancies: a descriptive study. J Infect 2003;47(1):19–27.
226. Bollee G, Sarfati C, Thiery G, et al. Clinical picture of *Pneumocystis jiroveci* pneumonia in cancer patients. Chest 2007;132(4):1305–10.
227. Masur H, Kaplan JE, Holmes KK. Guidelines for preventing opportunistic infections among HIV-infected persons—2002. Recommendations of the U.S. Public Health Service and the Infectious Diseases Society of America. Ann Intern Med 2002;137(5 Pt 2):435–78.
228. Green H, Paul M, Vidal L, et al. Prophylaxis of *Pneumocystis* pneumonia in immunocompromised non-HIV-infected patients: systematic review and meta-analysis of randomized controlled trials. Mayo Clin Proc 2007;82(9):1052–9.
229. Dykewicz CA. Summary of the guidelines for preventing opportunistic infections among hematopoietic stem cell transplant recipients. Clin Infect Dis 2001;33(2): 139–44.
230. Fishman JA. Prevention of infection caused by *Pneumocystis carinii* in transplant recipients. Clin Infect Dis 2001;33(8):1397–405.
231. Trotter JF, Levi M, Steinberg T, et al. Absence of *Pneumocystis jiroveci* pneumonia in liver transplantation recipients receiving short-term (3-month) prophylaxis. Transpl Infect Dis 2008;10(5):369–71.
232. EBPG Expert Group on Renal Transplantation. European best practice guidelines for renal transplantation. Section IV: long-term management of the transplant recipient. IV.7.1. Late infections. *Pneumocystis carinii* pneumonia. Nephrol Dial Transplant 2002;17(S4):36–9.
233. Godeau B, Mainardi JL, Roudot-Thoraval F, et al. Factors associated with *Pneumocystis carinii* pneumonia in Wegener's granulomatosis. Ann Rheum Dis 1995; 54(12):991–4.
234. Bozzette SA, Finkelstein DM, Spector SA, et al. A randomized trial of three anti-*Pneumocystis* agents in patients with advanced human immunodeficiency virus infection. Niaid AIDS clinical trials group. N Engl J Med 1995;332(11):693–9.
235. Bucher HC, Griffith L, Guyatt GH, et al. Meta-analysis of prophylactic treatments against *Pneumocystis carinii* pneumonia and toxoplasma encephalitis in HIV-infected patients. J Acquir Immune Defic Syndr Hum Retrovirol 1997;15(2): 104–14.
236. Stein DS, Stevens RC, Terry D, et al. Use of low-dose trimethoprim-sulfamethoxazole thrice weekly for primary and secondary prophylaxis of *Pneumocystis*

carinii pneumonia in human immunodeficiency virus-infected patients. Antimicrob Agents Chemother 1991;35(9):1705–9.

237. Schneider MM, Hoepelman AI, Eeftinck Schattenkerk JK, et al. A controlled trial of aerosolized pentamidine or trimethoprim-sulfamethoxazole as primary prophylaxis against *Pneumocystis carinii* pneumonia in patients with human immunodeficiency virus infection. The Dutch AIDS treatment group. N Engl J Med 1992;327(26):1836–41.
238. Antinori A, Murri R, Ammassari A, et al. Aerosolized pentamidine, cotrimoxazole and dapsone-pyrimethamine for primary prophylaxis of *Pneumocystis carinii* pneumonia and toxoplasmic encephalitis. AIDS 1995;9(12):1343–50.
239. Hirschel B, Lazzarin A, Chopard P, et al. A controlled study of inhaled pentamidine for primary prevention of *Pneumocystis carinii* pneumonia. N Engl J Med 1991;324(16):1079–83.
240. Casale L, Gold H, Schechter C, et al. Decreased efficacy of inhaled pentamidine in the prevention of *Pneumocystis carinii* pneumonia among HIV-infected patients with severe immunodeficiency. Chest 1993;103(2):342–4.
241. Kazanjian PH, Fisk D, Armstrong W, et al. Increase in prevalence of *Pneumocystis carinii* mutations in patients with AIDS and *P. carinii* pneumonia, in the United States and china. J Infect Dis 2004;189(9):1684–7.
242. Kazanjian P, Locke AB, Hossler PA, et al. *Pneumocystis carinii* mutations associated with sulfa and sulfone prophylaxis failures in AIDS patients. AIDS 1998; 12(8):873–8.
243. Takahashi T, Hosoya N, Endo T, et al. Relationship between mutations in dihydropteroate synthase of *Pneumocystis carinii* f. sp. hominis isolates in Japan and resistance to sulfonamide therapy. J Clin Microbiol 2000;38(9):3161–4.
244. Mei Q, Gurunathan S, Masur H, et al. Failure of co-trimoxazole in *Pneumocystis carinii* infection and mutations in dihydropteroate synthase gene. Lancet 1998; 351(9116):1631–2.
245. Ma L, Borio L, Masur H, et al. *Pneumocystis carinii* dihydropteroate synthase but not dihydrofolate reductase gene mutations correlate with prior trimethoprim-sulfamethoxazole or dapsone use. J Infect Dis 1999;180(6):1969–78.
246. Nahimana A, Rabodonirina M, Bille J, et al. Mutations of *Pneumocystis jirovecii* dihydrofolate reductase associated with failure of prophylaxis. Antimicrob Agents Chemother 2004;48(11):4301–5.

Acute Tuberculosis

David Schlossberg, MD, FACP[a,b,c,*]

KEYWORDS

• Tuberculosis • TB • Pneumonia • Pneumonitis • CAP

Tuberculosis (TB) can present as an acute process and should be included in the differential diagnosis of community-acquired pneumonia (CAP). It may mimic classic bacterial pneumonia or masquerade as an atypical pneumonia, with nonproductive cough and systemic symptomatology. This review summarizes the clinical and radiologic manifestations of acute forms of TB, emphasizing risk factors and diagnostic clues.

The various presentations of TB reflect its pathogenesis and pathophysiology.

Mycobacterium tuberculosis is inhaled from droplet nuclei that are suspended in air. These nuclei contain from one to three organisms, which are then distributed in the well-ventilated areas of the lung, especially the periphery of the midlung fields, most commonly in the right middle lobe, superior segments of the lower lobes and anterior segments of the upper lobes. Right-sided infection is more common than left. Infection is typically unifocal, although it may be bilateral. Clinical manifestations of the initial infection are characteristically minimal; in fact, most patients are asymptomatic. When symptoms are present, cough and dyspnea are most common, with occasional chest pain, sore throat and systemic complaints of fever and malaise. The most common chest X-ray (CXR) is normal; when present, abnormalities include either peripheral infiltrates or adenopathy or both. The infiltrates are seen in anterior as well as posterior segments, and lower lobes as well as upper. They may be rounded, ill-defined, or dense, and may be segmental or lobar. Hilar or mediastinal adenopathy are characteristic and reflect the lymphatic circulation, in that left-sided infiltrates may result in bilateral adenopathy, whereas a focus in the right lung causes adenopathy only on the right. As with various etiologies of atypical pneumonia, the CXR findings are frequently more dramatic than symptoms would predict. Pleural effusions are common in primary TB and may exist without corresponding parenchymal infiltrates or adenopathy.

Lymph nodes draining the parenchymal focus of primary infection may enlarge and obstruct bronchi either by direct compression or by caseation and rupture through the

[a] Temple University School of Medicine, Philadelphia, PA, USA
[b] University of Pennsylvania School of Medicine, Philadelphia, PA, USA
[c] Tuberculosis Control Program, Philadelphia Department of Public Health, 500 South Broad Street, Philadelphia, PA 19146, USA
* Tuberculosis Control Program, Philadelphia Department of Public Health, 500 South Broad Street, Philadelphia, PA 19146.
E-mail address: dschloss@ix.netcom.com

Infect Dis Clin N Am 24 (2010) 139–146
doi:10.1016/j.idc.2009.10.009
0891-5520/10/$ – see front matter

bronchial wall; in such cases, obstructive emphysema or atelectasis my complicate or even dominate the clinical presentation, sometimes referred to as epituberculosis. Erythema nodosum has also been described.

This primary focus usually heals, with scarring and calcification of the peripheral parenchymal focus and the draining lymph nodes; together, these two remnants of the primary infection are called the Gohn complex or Ranke complex. If, instead of healing, the initial infection progresses (progressive primary), cavitation and bronchogenic spread may occur as part of the initial infection; infants younger than 5 are at particular risk for local progression as well as miliary dissemination. From age 5 to puberty there is a period of relative resistance to such progression, with a return of increased susceptibility in adolescents and young adults. Thus, in adolescents and young adults, primary TB spans a spectrum that includes asymptomatic infection, typical childhood pattern of lower lung field infiltrate with regional adenopathy, or progressive disease with caseation and cavity formation.

During the primary infection, drainage to hilar and mediastinal lymph nodes and subsequent lymphohematogenous spread disseminate the organism throughout the body. In immunologically healthy individuals, there is a 10% risk of reactivation of these distant foci for the remainder of the patient's life; half of that risk (5%) is in the first 2 years after infection.

Signs of reactivation, or post–primary TB, are well known: a subacute to chronic illness with cough, fever, night sweats, and weight loss, with infiltrates and cavitation in the apical or posterior segments of upper lobes and superior segments of the lower lobes—areas of highest oxygen tension. The anterior segment of the upper lobes may also be involved, but never as the exclusive area of involvement. Cavities that form within the area of infiltration are thick or thin walled, with smooth inner contours and no air-fluid levels. This presentation contrasts with the classic aerobic-anaerobic lung abscess, which often has an air-fluid level and typically lacks the infiltrative process surrounding the abscess cavities—often multiple—of reactivation TB. At times, infected secretions from cavities may spread endobronchially to dependent areas of the lungs. Such bronchogenic spread results in acute inflammation with nodular infiltrates in segmental or lobar distribution; such areas of inflammation represent an actual TB pneumonitis and are indistinguishable clinically and radiologically from acute pneumonitis of other etiologies, especially if the cavitary source for the bronchogenic spread is not evident on the CXR. Rarely, an endobronchial lesion may initiate the infection, with a transiently normal CXR; diagnosis in such cases is made by bronchoscopy.

In the United States, TB is often not suspected, particularly by a generation of physicians who have seen relatively little of it. Compounding this phenomenon is a problem of progress: the control of TB in the United States has resulted in an increasingly susceptible adult population. The result has been increased cases of primary TB in adults, including the elderly. In addition, it is now recognized that reinfection, producing a primary complex, is possible, especially but not exclusively in HIV-positive patients.

Both primary and reactivation TB can cause acute manifestations, listed in **Box 1**. The acute forms of primary TB result from the initial infection in susceptible children or adults, reinfection in susceptible hosts, progressive primary TB, and atelectasis from compression of lymph nodes. Atelectasis may result from extrinsic node compression or rupture into a bronchus, as described previously; less commonly, it results from endobronchial spread of disease. Most common in the right middle or lower lobe in children, atelectasis is occasionally seen in adults, typically in the anterior segments of the upper lobes.

Box 1
Acute manifestations of primary and reactivation TB

Primary

1. Classic primary TB in susceptibles (particularly older)
2. Reinfection—especially in HIV-positive patients
3. Progressive primary
4. Atelectasis from lymphadenopathy

Reactivation

1. Advanced HIV with atypical presentation
2. TB pneumonitis from bronchogenic spread

The acute manifestations of TB resulting from reactivation include atypical presentations in HIV-positive patients, in whom a typical primary presentation with peripheral infiltrate and adenopathy is seen in both primary and reactivation disease when there is severe CD4 depletion. CT with contrast may demonstrate low attenuation in the center of the lymph nodes with peripheral rim enhancement; the low attenuation is because of necrosis. This CT pattern is suggestive but not diagnostic, as it is also seen in infection owing to fungi and nontuberculous mycobacteria.[1,2] An additional acute form of reactivation disease is TB pneumonitis from bronchogenic spread, which may present clinically and radiographically as bronchopneumonia. This may affect both upper and lobes of the lungs.

It can be seen from the foregoing that acute forms of TB may present as lower lobe disease in adults; this presentation, which is apt to delay consideration of TB as a diagnosis, may occur under multiple circumstances (**Box 2**).

As a result of the impressive mimicry of TB, the diagnosis must be considered, at least initially, in all cases of acute pneumonitis. There are many clinical and epidemiologic clues that should raise red flags for the clinician; these clues are listed in **Box 3**.

TB is often overlooked as a cause of CAP, particularly when it presents as an acute illness. Rigid adherence to treatment guidelines tends to quickly categorize patients as CAP, after which a treatment algorithm is followed that covers common bacterial and nonbacterial organisms. Frequently there is pressure on physicians to institute appropriate therapy within a certain number of hours. All these factors contribute to a delayed suspicion and diagnosis of TB as a cause of CAP. Thus, in one review of unsuspected tuberculosis in a community hospital, 60% of cases were reported after the patient's death; 92% of the patients were elderly.[3]

Epidemiologic clues that should alert the clinician to the possibility of TB include intravenous drug abuse, immigration from countries of high prevalence, contact

Box 2
Lower lobe TB in the adult

1. Classic reactivation TB in superior segments of the lower lobes
2. Progressive primaries—often in older patients—suspect for slowly resolving pneumonitis
3. Endobronchial spread via infected secretions or rupture of a node into a bronchus
4. Advanced AIDS with atypical reactivation TB

Box 3
Clues to TB etiology of CAP

1. Epidemiologic clues: intravenous drug abuse, immigrants, inner-city residence, contacts with TB
2. Clinical clues

   Chronic symptoms (>2–3 weeks)

   Failure to respond to routine therapy

   Relapse following fluoroquinolone (FQN) administration

   Relapse following corticosteroid administration

   Gram stain with weakly gram-positive or gram-neutral rods (ghosts)

   Signs of healed TB, eg, fibrocalcific changes, apical capping, Ghon complex

   Pneumothorax

   Pleural effusion
3. Immunocompromised patients

   HIV

   Tumor necrosis factor-alpha inhibitor therapy

   Posttransplantation

   Postpartum state
4. Underlying diseases with increased risk for TB

   Renal failure

   Diabetes

   Silicosis

   Gastrectomy

   Jejunoileal bypass

   Carcinoma of the head or neck

with TB cases, and residence in inner cities and underserved areas. In addition to epidemiologic clues, there are many clinical clues that should prompt consideration of a tuberculous etiology.

First, symptoms for 2 to 3 weeks or more should suggest TB. Failure to respond to traditional therapy for CAP is also suggestive.[4] If patients do respond but then relapse after treatment with fluoroquinolones (FQNs), TB should be suspected, because *Mycobacterium tuberculosis* (MTB) may respond, transiently, to fluoroquinolone therapy. In one retrospective review, 48% of 33 adults with TB had received FQNs before the diagnosis of TB was made, and the group that received FQNs had a significant delay in initiation of anti-TB therapy. It has been suggested that alternatives to FQNs be used to treat CAP in patients at increased risk for TB, not just because the FQN may mask and delay a tuberculous etiology, but also because of the threat of FQN resistance on the part of MTB, which may develop within 2 weeks on monotherapy.[5–7]

Relapse after corticosteroid administration should also suggest a tuberculous etiology of pneumonia. Corticosteroids can produce rapid (although transient) radiologic and clinical improvement in patients with TB. However, clinical deterioration may ensue, particularly following corticosteroid withdrawal, which is known to occur in AIDS when presumptive therapy for *Pneumocystis jiroveci* (*carinii*) pneumonia (PCP) is augmented with corticosteroids. Such patients may have had TB misdiagnosed as PCP or have been co-infected with both PCP and TB.[8,9] Anti-PCP therapy should not be augmented with corticosteroids unless a definitive diagnosis of PCP is established or at least pending; TB can mimic any radiologic manifestation of PCP, including diffuse interstitial infiltrates.

Additional clues to a possible tuberculous etiology of CAP are a history of hemoptysis, night sweats, and weight loss; sputum Gram stain showing weakly gram-positive or gram-neutral rods; and radiologic findings of upper lobe infiltrates, pleural effusion, cavitation, pneumothorax, and signs of prior tuberculous infection such as fibrocalcific apical changes, apical pleural capping, and a calcified Gohn or Ranke complex. Often the CXR looks worse than the patient's symptoms would suggest, in both primary and reactivation TB.[10–12]

Several types of immune compromise increase the risk of reactivation of TB. HIV infection is a well-known risk, approximating 10% per year (compared with the 10% lifetime risk of HIV-negative patients). With relatively intact immunity, HIV-positive patients have characteristic radiologic manifestations of TB. As HIV infection advances and immunocompromise becomes more profound, reactivation TB atypically resembles primary TB, with infiltrates in any area of the lung, pleural effusions, and hilar or mediastinal lymphadenopathy. HIV-positive patients are also susceptible to reinfection with MTB. TB is a constant challenge in HIV-positive patients, as occasional HIV-positive patients may have dual infection, with MTB plus an additional opportunist. HIV-positive patients may have active, culture-positive TB with symptoms but a normal CXR, and a small number of patients have been described who had TB with clear CXR and no symptoms. Thus, hospitalized HIV-positive patients with any pulmonary symptoms should be isolated initially, until TB is considered unlikely or the patient is placed on presumptive therapy or an alternative diagnosis is reached.[13,14]

Antagonists of tumor necrosis factor (TNF)-alpha include infliximab, etanercept, and adalimumab. They increase the risk for multiple infectious diseases, including TB. The risk may be greater with infliximab than etanercept, possibly because infliximab is an anti-TNF monoclonal antibody, whereas etanercept is a TNF-neutralizing TNF receptor fusion molecule. Unlike etanercept, infliximab and adalimumab reduce TB-responsive CD4 cells and suppress antigen-induced interferon-gamma production. As a result, mice given a receptor fusion molecule were able to control TB, whereas mice given anti-TNF antibody were not.[15] In addition to increasing the risk of TB reactivation, these agents may also increase the likelihood of immune reconstitution syndromes following their use. Physicians should treat for latent infection before using TNF-alpha antagonists, and probably should use two-step testing if the initial tuberculin skin test (PPD) is negative.

The related agent rituximab depletes peripheral CD20 B lymphocytes and may also be associated with mycobacterial infection.[16]

Organ transplantation is a recognized risk for TB. Depending on the specific organ transplanted, the incidence is as high as 74 times (for cardiac transplantation) that of the general population,[17] usually by activation of latent TB infection in the recipient when immunosuppressive medications are administered. In the United States, no standard evaluation is required to assess the risk of a donor having latent tuberculosis infection. However, when TB develops in organ recipients, it is severe and often atypical, reflecting the immunosuppressed state of the recipient. Thus, half of such patients have disseminated or extrapulmonary TB, with a mortality of approximately one-third. As a result, the index of suspicion for TB must be high, not just for suggestive febrile or infectious syndromes, but also for graft rejection or bone marrow suppression. The situation is made more difficult by false-negative pretransplantation PPDs, seen in as many as 75% to 80% of patients; this phenomenon is attributed to anergy in patients with end-stage organ failure. Patients who are screened should have two-step testing when possible, and 5 mm should be used as the cutoff size of the PPD induration.[17,18]

Because pregnancy is a state of mild immunosuppression, postpartum women may manifest a variety of immune reconstitution syndromes, including exacerbation or unmasking of TB. Most of these cases are extrapulmonary, and they occur within the first month after delivery, corresponding to the return of lymphocyte reactivity to PPD antigen.[19]

A final category of clues comprises specific clinical conditions that place the patient at increased risk for TB. **Table 1** lists selected clinical states with their relative risk for reactivation of TB. Renal failure is a known risk for reactivation of tuberculosis. Recent concern has focused on the effect of immigrants with renal failure from countries with a high prevalence of TB; such patients by necessity attend medical facilities where nosocomial spread from undiagnosed TB would be a constant threat.[20] Diabetes mellitus also increases the risk of TB. This is of particular interest given the rising incidence of diabetes in both the developed and the developing world. The World Health Organization and the International Diabetes Federation consider diabetes to be a global pandemic; as one-third of the world is infected with MTB, the implications for the incidence of tuberculosis are significant.[21] Additional risks for reactivation of TB are gastrectomy, jejunoileal bypass, carcinoma of the head or neck, and silicosis.[22] Such points in a patient's history may be overlooked in a busy emergency department, but they are crucial considerations in a patient in whom TB is a possibility.

Current investigations to increase the diagnostic yield in TB presenting as CAP include assays of procalcitonin[23] and quantiferon.[24,25] Although promising, both modalities should presently be considered experimental for this indication.

In conclusion, TB should always be considered, at least initially, in the differential diagnosis of CAP. Epidemiologic and clinical clues may suggest a possible tuberculous etiology, as should various forms of immune compromise and multiple underlying clinical states. TB remains a formidable foe and a resourceful mimic, and the consequences of missing the diagnosis can be disastrous. The clinician should err on the side of caution and expand the initial differential diagnosis.

Table 1
Relative risk for tuberculosis (compared with the general population, independent of PPD status)

Clinical Condition	Relative Risk
Chronic renal failure/hemodialysis	10.0–25.3
Diabetes mellitus	2.0–4.1
Gastrectomy	2–5
Jejunoileal bypass	27–63
Carcinoma of head or neck	16
Silicosis	30

Adapted from Centers for Disease Control and Prevention. Targeted tuberculin testing and treatment of latent tuberculosis infection. MMWR Recomm Rep 2000;49:9.

REFERENCES

1. Gharib AM, Stern EJ. Radiology of pneumonia. Med Clin North Am 2001;85:1461–91.
2. Ketai L, Jordan K, Marom EM. Imaging infection. Clin Chest Med 2008;29:77–105.
3. Counsell SR, Tan JS, Dittus RS. Unsuspected pulmonary tuberculosis in a community teaching hospital. Arch Intern Med 1989;149:1274–8.
4. Weyers CM. Nonresolving pneumonia. Clin Chest Med 2005;26(1):143–58.
5. Dooley KE, Golub J, Goes FS, et al. Empiric treatment of community-acquired pneumonia with fluoroquinolones, and delays in the treatment of tuberculosis. Clin Infect Dis 2002;34:1607–12.
6. Grupper M, Potasman I. Fluoroquinolones in CAP when tuberculosis is around: an instructive case. Am J Med Sci 2008;335:141–4.
7. Ginsburg AS, Woolwine SC, Hooper N, et al. Rapid development of fluoroquinolone resistance in *M. tuberculosis* [letter]. N Engl J Med 2003;349:1977–8.
8. Lui G, Lee N, Wong B, et al. Incidental administration of corticosteroid can mask the diagnosis of tuberculosis. Am J Med 2007;120:e7–10.
9. Castro JG, Manzi G, Espinoza L, et al. Concurrent PCP and TB pneumonia in HIV infected patients. Scand J Infect Dis 2007;39:1054–8.
10. Kunimoto D, Long R. Tuberculosis: still overlooked as a cause of community-acquired pneumonia—how not to miss it. Respir Care Clin N Am 2005;11:25–34.
11. Liam CK, Pang YK, Poosparajah S. Pulmonary tuberculosis presenting as CAP. Respirology 2006;11:786–92.
12. Nyamande K, Lalloo UG, John M. TB presenting as community-acquired pneumonia in a setting of high TB incidence and high HIV prevalence. Int J Tuberc Lung Dis 2007;11:1308–13.
13. Mtei L, Matee M, Herfort O, et al. High rates of clinical and subclinical tuberculosis among HIV-infected ambulatory subjects in Tanzania. Clin Infect Dis 2005;40:1500–7.
14. Kato-Maeda M, Small PM. HIV and tuberculosis. In: Schlossberg D, editor. Tuberculosis and nontuberculous mycobacterial infections. 5th edition. New York: McGraw-Hill; 2006. p. 388–400.
15. Plessner HL, Lin PL, Kohlo T, et al. Neutralization of TNF by antibody but not TNF receptor fusion molecule exacerbates chronic murine tuberculosis. J Invest Dermatol 2007;195:1643–50.
16. Winthrop KL, Yamashita S, Beekman SE, et al. Mycobacterial and other serious infections in patients receiving anti-tumor necrosis factor and other newly-approved biologic therapies: case finding through the emerging infections network. Clin Infect Dis 2008;46:1738–40.
17. Transplantation-transmitted tuberculosis. MMWR Morb Mortal Wkly Rep 2008;57:333.
18. Mycobacterium tuberculosis [editorial]. Am J Transplant 2004;4(Suppl 10):37–41.
19. Singh N, Perfect JR. Immune reconstitution syndrome and exacerbation of infections after pregnancy. Clin Infect Dis 2007;45:1192–9.
20. Moore David AJ, Lightstone Liz, Javid Babak, et al. High rates of tuberculosis in end-stage renal failure: the impact of international migration. Emerg Infect Dis 2002;8:77–8.
21. Diabetes mellitus increases the risk of active tuberculosis: a systematic review of 13 observational studies. PLoS Med 2008;5(7):e152. DOI: 10.1371/journal.pmed.0050152.

22. Centers for Disease Control and Prevention. Targeted tuberculin testing and treatment of latent tuberculosis infection. MMWR Recomm Rep 2000;49:8–9.
23. Nyamande K, Lalloo UG. Serum procalcitonin distinguishes CAP due to bacteria, mycobacteria and PJP. Int J Tuberc Lung Dis 2006;10:510–5.
24. Kobashi Y, Mouri K, Yagi S, et al. Clinical utility of the QuantiFERON TB-2G test for elderly patients with active TB. Chest 2008;133:1196–202.
25. Kobashi Y, Mouri K, Obase Y, et al. Usefulness of the Quantiferon TB-2G test for the differential diagnosis of pulmonary tuberculosis. Intern Med 2008;47:237–43.

Cytomegalovirus Pneumonia: Community-Acquired Pneumonia in Immunocompetent Hosts

Burke A. Cunha, MD, MACP[a,b,*]

KEYWORDS

- Leukopenia • Relative lymphopenia • Atypical lymphocytes
- Thrombocytopenia • CMV cytopathic effects

HISTORY

In 1881, Ribbert noted large cells in kidney cells of a stillborn, which he later described as "protozoan-like" in 1904. These large cells had eccentric nuclei surrounded by a clear halo. Ribbert did not appreciate the significance of his findings until he read the report by Gesionek and Kiolemenoglou published in the same year, describing similar structures in the lungs, liver, and kidney of an 8-month-old fetus. In Ribbert's laboratory in 1907, Lowenstein found these protozoan-like large cells in the parotid glands of infants. Lowenstein was the first to appreciate that these large inclusions were in the nucleus. In 1911, Pettavel described similar inclusions in the thyroid gland of a premature infant. Later, in 1921, Goode, Pasteur, and Talbot reported a case of a 6-week-old infant with intranuclear eosinophilic inclusions similar to those previously described and were the first to use the term "cytomegalia." They did not believe that the large inclusion bodies in the nucleus represented protozoa. In 1925, von Glahn and Pappenheimer described the first adult case of cytomegalovirus (CMV) infection in a male who had an amebic liver abscess; inclusion bodies were found in the lungs and in the intestines. They concluded that the inclusions in this case were similar to those seen in other herpes virus infections. In 1934, Chaudry was the first to definitively link intracellular inclusion bodies with specific viral infections. In 1950, Wyatt

[a] Infectious Disease Division, Winthrop-University Hospital, 259 First Street, Mineola, Long Island, NY 11501, USA
[b] State University of New York School of Medicine, Stony Brook, NY, USA
* Infectious Disease Division, Winthrop-University Hospital, 259 First Street, Mineola, Long Island, NY 11501.

Infect Dis Clin N Am 24 (2010) 147–158
doi:10.1016/j.idc.2009.10.008
id.theclinics.com

and colleagues reported that inclusions (CMV) were always present in renal tubules and reasoned that inclusions might be present in urine specimens. They also coined the term, "generalized cytomegalic inclusion disease," which was first described by Wolbach in 1932. Wyatt was the first to diagnose cytomegalic inclusion disease (CID) antemortem in an infant. In the early 1950s, Mercer and Margileth also showed that CID could be diagnosed by demonstrating inclusion cells in voided urine. Electron microscopy was first used by Minder in 1953 to visualize intracellular inclusions of CMV in the pancreas.[1–5]

In the history of CMV, 1905 to 1954 represented the "period of cytopathology," later followed by the "virological period." Until Enders was able to culture human cells, isolation of human CMV was not possible because human CMV cannot be cultured in nonhuman cell lines. In the late 1950s, Enders and his colleagues developed tissue culture techniques to isolate poliovirus. In 1954, Smith isolated mouse CMV in cell culture and human CMV was cultured in human cell lines Boston and Bethesda. In 1965, Clemola and Kariainen first described CMV (heterophile-negative) infectious mononucleosis in adults. The isolation and identification of CMV led the way to more sophisticated diagnostic methods. Widespread organ transplantation increased interest in CMV because it was the most important pathogen isolated in these immunosuppressed patients. In cases of human immunodeficiency virus (HIV) infection, retinitis, acalculous cholecystitis, esophagitis, colitis, or encephalitis, CMV is an important infection most commonly presenting as a prolonged febrile response, which is a hallmark of CMV infection. Not unexpectedly, CMV has been reported as a cause of fever of unknown origin in children and adults. CMV continues to be an important infection in immunocompetent hosts, for example, CMV infectious mononucleosis and postperfusion syndrome. In other compromised hosts (eg, patients with systemic lupus erythematosus [SLE]) and those on immunosuppressive drugs (eg, patients with Crohn's disease), CMV not uncommonly presents as CMV infectious mononucleosis, fever of unknown origin (FUO), or severe community-acquired pneumonia (CAP).[1,4,5]

In 1968, Carlstrom and colleagues[6] first reported a case of CMV CAPin their series of CMV infection of immunocompetent hosts. One of the patients was a 26-year-old woman who developed CMV CAP. In 1970, Sterner and colleagues[7] reported the case of a 27-year-old woman with CMV postperfusion syndrome who later developed CMV CAP. In 1972, Klemola and colleagues[8] reported 2 more cases of CMV CAP in immunocompetent adults. Klemola's report was the first to describe in detail the features of CMV CAP in immunocompetent adults. He reported that prolonged fever was the predominant presenting sign of CMV CAP. His 2 patients with CMV CAP, a 35-year-old woman and a 60-year-old woman, had no cough or respiratory symptoms but did have prolonged fevers and bilateral basilar patchy/interstitial infiltrates on chest radiograph (CXR). The CMV infiltrates resolved slowly over 6 weeks. He noted that the diagnostic clues to CMV CAP were relative lymphopenia, atypical lymphocytes, and mildly elevated serum transaminases. Typically, initial CMV IgM titers were negative in his patients, but later they developed elevated CMV IgM/IgG titers. CMV viruria was present in both of his cases.

MICROBIOLOGY

CMV DNA viruses are of the murine and human variety. CMVs are DNA viruses with an icosahedral capsid with 162 capsomers, and the viral particles have a diameter of 120 to 200 nm. The capsid is surrounded by a phospholipid-rich envelope.

CMVs are members of the Herpesviridae family, which consists of 8 human herpes viruses (HHVs). The family Herpesviridae includes herpes simplex virus type 1 (HSV-1 or HHV-1) and type 2 (HSV-2 or HHV-2), varicella-zoster virus (HHV-3), Epstein-Barr virus (EBV, HHV-4), and CMV (formerly known as HHV-5). Also there are human herpes viruses HHV-6, HHV-7, and HHV-8. The family of Herpesviridae is divided into 3 subfamilies, representing the HSVs (Alphaherpesvirinae), CMVs (Betaherpesvirinae), and the lymphocryptoviruses (Gammaherpesvirinae). Human CMV (HHV-5), one of the Betaherpesvirinae CMVs, has distinctive characteristics; it (1) has DNA molecular weight of 150×10^6; (2) grows only in human cells and has a narrow host range, that is, humans; (3) grows best in human fibroblasts; (4) has a relatively slow reproductive cycle (>24 hours); and (5) has distinctive inclusion bodies contained in the nuclei and cytoplasm. Infected host cells are enlarged cytomegalia with nuclear and cytoplasmic inclusions. CMV has a predilection for salivary glands but is not present in parotid or submandibular glands or sublingual glands. After the kidneys, the lungs are the most common sites of infection in acquired-CMV infection.[1,4,5]

Morphologically, CMV resembles other herpes viruses, particularly HSV, with important cytopathic differences. Although cellular penetration of HSV and CMV takes place rapidly, the intracellular replication of CMV is much slower (approximately 4 days) compared with that of HSV (approximately 8 hours). The reason for the slow intracellular replication of CMV is not well understood. Although both HSV and CMV produce intranuclear inclusions, only CMV produces cytoplasmic inclusions (dense bodies). Because only CMV produces perinuclear cytoplasmic inclusions, cytopathologic diagnosis is possible. Cytopathologic changes in host tissue indicates active infection, not inactive or latent infection.[1,4,5,9,10]

EPIDEMIOLOGY

Typical bacterial causes of CAP may be differentiated from the atypical CAPs by the presence or absence of extrapulmonary findings. Patients presenting with CAP without extrapulmonary findings have infection caused by typical bacterial CAP pathogens (ie, *Streptococcus pneumoniae*, *Haemophilus influenzae*, or *Moraxella catarrhalis*). Patients presenting with CAP with extrapulmonary findings have atypical CAP that may be caused by zoonotic or nonzoonotic atypical pathogens. The most common causes of nonzoonotic atypical CAP are legionnaires disease, *Mycoplasma pneumoniae*, or *Chlamydophila (Chlamydia) pneumoniae.* Aside from the usual zoonotic and nonzoonotic atypical pathogens causing CAP, there are other viral pathogens that not infrequently present in atypical CAP, such as CMV, adenovirus, influenza (human, avian, swine), and *Pneumocystis (carinii) jiroveci* (PCP). PCP and CMVs are recognized pathogens in compromised hosts, for example, those who undergo transplants and those on immunosuppressive drugs or steroids. However, CMV, influenza (human, avian, swine), and adenovirus are the 3 most common causes of severe viral CAP in immunocompetent adults.

CLINICAL PRESENTATION

In immunocompromised hosts and in those who are on immunosuppressive drugs, the clinical presentation of CMV CAP has been well described. CMV is present in the lungs in approximately 75% of patients with HIV and PCP. The presence of CMV in lung biopsy specimens of HIV-infected patients with PCP does not indicate a causal role in the patients' clinical presentation of severe CAP. In such patients, if PCP is treated, CAP resolves without specific anti-CMV therapy.

CMV CAP in immunocompetent hosts is an uncommon but is being recognized more frequently, particularly when presenting as severe viral CAP. As with other CAP pathogens, the severity of presentation of CMV CAP in normal hosts varies.

Certainly, many mild and moderately severe cases of CMV CAP go undetected because they are easily missed as "mild flu" or are ascribed to "a respiratory virus." CMV in normal hosts is most likely to be recognized when presenting as severe viral CAP.[1,6–8,11–13]

Severe CAP implies that the patient is sufficiently ill with CAP to require hospitalization and, often, ventilatory support. Patients presenting with severe CAP may be approached clinically by the degree of hypoxemia and the appearance and distribution of infiltrates on the CXR. Severe CAP may also be mimicked by noninfectious disorders presenting with severe hypoxemia, hypotension, and infiltrates on the CXR. The most common noninfectious disorders mimicking severe CAP are pulmonary embolus, congestive heart failure, pulmonary drug reactions, pulmonary hemorrhage, collagen vascular diseases (eg, SLE pneumonitis, sarcoidosis), and clinical decompensation in patients with preexisting severe interstitial lung disease. These mimics of severe CAP can usually be eliminated from further clinical consideration on the basis of history, physical examination, and routine nonspecific laboratory features, which point to the diagnosis. If the noninfectious mimics of severe CAP are eliminated, the clinician should then consider patients with focal/segmental pulmonary infiltrates (ie, bacterial CAPs) versus patients with either minimal/no infiltrates or bilateral symmetric interstitial infiltrates (ie, PCP/viral CAPs).[14–17]

The 2 most common bacterial pathogens that cause severe CAP are *S pneumoniae* and *Legionella* (legionnaires disease), which present with focal segmental or lobar infiltrates on CXR. The differential diagnosis of patients who present without focal/lobar infiltrates on CXR with hypoxemia with either minimal or no infiltrates or bilateral symmetric interstitial infiltrates on CXR includes HIV-infected patients with PCP, immunosuppressed patients, or patients with viral pneumonias, such as, influenza (human, avian, swine); severe acute respiratory syndrome (SARS); hantavirus pulmonary syndrome (HPS); or CMV. The viral CAPs, presenting as severe CMV infection, initially present with minimal or no pulmonary infiltrates on CXR but are accompanied by various degrees of hypoxemia. The degree of hypoxemia is related to the degree of oxygen diffusion defect caused by interstitial pathogens. The severity of viral CAP in normal hosts is directly related to the degree and duration of hypoxemia. The magnitude of the oxygen diffusion defect caused by viral involvement of the lung interstitium in severe viral CAPs is best assessed by the alveolar-arterial (A-a) gradient. Patients presenting with severe viral CAP typically have increased A-a gradients of more than 35. The CXR appearance of CMV CAP is not distinctive (**Fig. 1**).[11,12,14] The CXR is most helpful in excluding other pathogens or disorders in the differential diagnosis, that is, either focal infiltrates due to typical/atypical bacterial CAP pathogens or disorders that may mimic severe CAP. Typically, severe CMV CAP presents with no infiltrates, rapidly followed by bilateral patchy interstitial infiltrates most prominent in both lung bases. In immunocompetent patients presenting with otherwise unexplained severe CAP, with minimal or no infiltrates or bilateral symmetric interstitial infiltrates and hypoxemia with an increased A-a gradient. CMV should be included in the differential diagnosis when there are other clinical features of CMV that suggest CMV versus other causes of severe viral CAP. The associated features obtained from history, physical examination, and nonspecific laboratory tests can limit differential diagnostic possibilities and should prompt specific CMV diagnostic testing (**Table 1**).[1,3,8,14]

DIFFERENTIAL DIAGNOSIS

CMV is an immunomodulatory virus that may cause or perturbate immune disorders, such as SLE.[1,13,18] Not uncommonly, in patients with SLE, CMV presents with flare and CAP. SLE pneumonitis, per se, does not usually present as CAP with severe

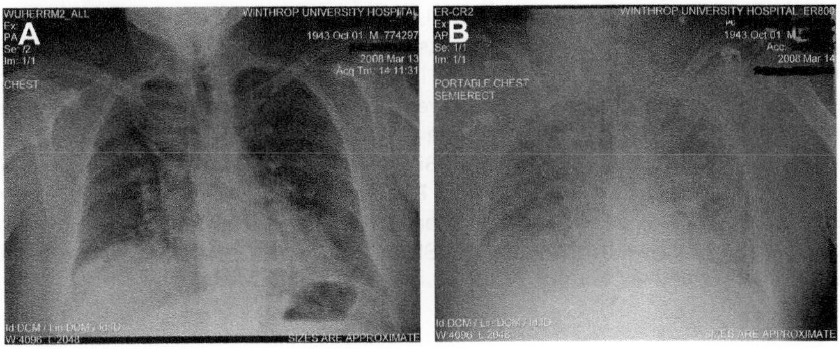

Fig. 1. CMV CAP on chest X-rays (*A, B*).

hypoxemia.[13] The clinical problem is to recognize that pulmonary infiltrates in a patient with SLE during flare may represent CAP, not SLE pneumonitis. Pneumonitis is characterized by migratory pulmonary infiltrates with or without pleural effusions.[11] SLE is a multisystem disorder that affects nearly all organs except the liver. If a patient with SLE flare has increased serum transaminases, CMV should be suspected as the cause of the SLE flare.[13,14,17,19] CMV characteristically involves the liver, which is manifested by mild elevations of the serum transaminases. SLE patients with flare and increased serum transaminases do not have lupoid hepatitis (autoimmune hepatitis) and should be viewed as having CMV-precipitated SLE flare until proved

Table 1
CMV spectrum of infection: preferred organ involvement in immunocompetent patients

Common Sites of CMV Involvement	Clinical Features	Uncommon Sites of CMV Involvement	Clinical Features
Lung	Severe CAP	Kidney	CMV viruria
Liver	Increased serum transaminases (AST/ALT)	Adrenals	Adrenalitis
Spleen	Splenomegaly	Salivary glands	Sialitis
Gastrointestinal tract	Segmental/pancolitis Colitis	Pancreas	Pancreatitis
Central nervous system	Encephalitis[a]	Esophagus	Esophageal ulcers Esophagitis
Hematologic	Leukopenia Relative lymphopenia Atypical lymphocytes Thrombocytopenia Aplastic anemia Increased procoagulant activity	—	—
Multisystem involvement	FUO	—	—

Abbreviations: AST/ALT, aspartate aminotransferase/alanine aminotransferase; FUO, fever of unknown origin.

[a] May present as the sole manifestation of CMV infection.

otherwise. CMV not only can induce the SLE flare but also may infect lung interstitium and present as severe viral CAP in patients with SLE. SLE pneumonitis, per se, is not accompanied by severe hypoxemia or a high A-a gradient.[13,14] With SLE flare, the presence of severe hypoxemia and increased A-a gradient and mildly increased serum transaminases (aspartate aminotransferase/alanine aminotransferase) should suggest superimposed CMV. Untreated SLE patients have impaired humoral immunity with impaired B lymphocyte function. Patients with SLE who are on immunosuppressive therapy, in addition, have impaired cell-mediated immunity (CMI) and T-lymphocyte function. In patients with SLE, CMV further intensifies the degree of immunosuppression, ie, impaired CMI.

DIAGNOSIS

Clinical

Clinically in normal hosts, the differential diagnosis of severe viral CAP may be due to a wide variety of viruses. It is usually possible, based on epidemiologic and clinical features, to eliminate some viral causes presenting as severe CAP, such as avian influenza (H5N1), SARS, and HPS. Other viral causes of severe CAP include human influenza, swine influenza (H1N1), adenovirus, and CMV. The most common differential diagnostic problem with severe viral CAP is to clinically differentiate influenza, adenovirus, and CMV. Severe human influenza A infection has characteristic clinical presentation in adults. Unlike CMV and adenovirus, human influenza has a seasonal distribution. Swine influenza (H1N1) should also be considered as a cause of severe viral CAP.[14,18,20–22]

Adenovirus is a great masquerader and may mimic viral and bacterial infections. It is usually relatively straightforward to differentiate influenza from adenoviral CAP. It is not the CXR appearance or degree of hypoxemia that permits clinical differentiation between influenza and adenoviral CAP. Rather, the associated clinical features may suggest the correct diagnosis. The clinical features that suggest adenoviral CAP include lobar infiltrates, conjunctival suffusion, leukopenia, relative lymphopenia, and thrombocytopenia. CMV CAP has, in common with seasonal human influenza and swine influenza (H1N1), otherwise unexplained relative lymphopenia or thrombocytopenia.[14] However, increased serum transaminases, nearly always a feature of CMV, may also occur in influenza, swine influenza (H1N1), or adenoviral infection.[23–25] The presence of atypical lymphocytes argues against the diagnosis of influenza (human, avian, swine) and, to a lesser extent, adenoviral infection, in a patient with viral CAP should suggest CMV CAP (**Table 2**).[14,25]

Patients presenting with severe viral CAP and a negative recent travel or zoonotic contact history with otherwise unexplained leukopenia, relative lymphopenia, thrombocytopenia, atypical lymphocytes with mildly increased serum transaminases should suggest CMV CAP and prompt specific diagnostic testing to confirm or rule out CMV.[1,3,14,25,26]

Although CMV is an uncommon but important cause of severe viral CAP, it is not a cause of late ventilator-associated pneumonia (VAP). In late-onset VAP, unlike in HSV-1, CMV does not present as otherwise unexplained hypoxemia after 1 to 2 weeks in ventilated patients. HSV-1 late-onset VAP often presents as “failure to wean.” HSV-1 reactivation occurs secondary to reactivation of HSV-1 from the trauma of intubation/ventilation. Whereas CMV reactivation in blood lymphocytes is detected by CMV antigen, a positive CMV polymerase chain reaction (PCR) is common in septic/ventilated patients without clinical CMV infection.[27–35] Late-onset VAP caused by CMV occurs very rarely.[31,36–38]

Table 2
Differential diagnosis of severe viral CAP in adults

	Influenza	Adenovirus	CMV
Symptoms			
Onset	Acute	Acute	Subacute/acute
Myalgias	+	±	±
Neck/back myalgias	+	–	–
Signs			
Fever	+	+	+
Dry cough	+	±	±
Conjunctival suffusion	±	±	–
Blood-tinged sputum	±	–	–
Laboratory tests			
Leukocytosis	±	–	±
Leukopenia	±	+	±
Relative lymphopenia	+	+	±
Atypical lymphocytes	–	±	+
Thrombocytopenia	+	+	±
Mildly elevated cold agglutinin titers	±	±	±
Mildly elevated serum transaminases (AST/ALT)	±	±	+
Severe hypoxemia (A-a gradient >35)	±	±	±
Chest radiograph			
No/minimal infiltrates (early, <48 h)	+	+	+
Bilateral/patchy infiltrates (later, >48 h)	+	±	±
Focal segmental/lobar infiltrates	–[a]	+	–
Diagnostic tests			
DFA for respiratory viruses	+	+	–
↑ Adenoviral IgM titers	–	+	–
↑ CMV IgM titers	–	–	+[b]
Positive CMV PCR	–	–	±
Diagnostic cytopathology			
BAL	–	–	+
TBB	–	+	+

Abbreviations: AST/ALT, aspartate aminotransferase/alanine aminotransferase; BAL, bronchoalveolar lavage; DFA, direct fluorescent antibody; IgM, immunoglobulin M; PCR, polymerase chain reaction; TBB, transbronchial biopsy; ↑, increase.

[a] Only with simultaneous bacterial CAP (*S aureus*).

[b] May be falsely positive with rheumatoid factors (RFs) in acute Epstein-Barr virus infectious mononucleosis.

Adapted from Cunha BA. Pneumonia essentials. 3rd edition. Sudbury (MA): Jones and Bartlett; 2010; with permission.

Laboratory Tests

CMV may be diagnosed by isolating the virus from body fluids, such as respiratory secretions and urine; multiple specimens may be needed to demonstrate CMV viruria. CMV cultured from body fluids or biopsy specimens suggests infection, but after primary CMV infection, some patients become long-term shedders of the virus into the urine. Care must be taken in interpreting the clinical significance of CMV viruria. However, if a patient has an infection compatible with CMV and other pathogens are not isolated, CMV cultured from the urine may have a diagnostic significance. In immunocompetent older children and sometimes adults, CMV viruria may occur after CMV infection. CMV viruria indicates infection in immunocompetent individuals but is uncommon in nonimmunosuppressed hosts. In contrast, viremia is associated with immunocompetent and immunosuppressed adults. CMV viremia may be demonstrated in buffy coat specimens by CMV culture.[1,4,5,9,10]

Viral isolation

Human fibroblast cultures should be observed twice a week for CMV cytopathic effect (CPE). CMV CPEs resemble that of HSV in the first 1 to 2 days. Because CMV CPE changes occur slowly, CMV cultures should be maintained for 3 weeks before being reported as negative. CMV monoclonal antibodies are used to detect CMV in cell cultures approximately 2 days before CPE changes become apparent.[5,9,10,14]

Serologic tests

Serologic testing is the most common method used to demonstrate current or past CMV infection. The diagnosis of recent CMV infection depends on demonstrating either a single elevated CMV IgM titer or a 4-fold increase in CMV IgG titers. Care must be taken in interpreting a single elevated CMV IgM titer because there may be falsely elevated IgM titers in patients with elevated rheumatoid factors (RFs), EBV, or HHV-6 infection. False-positive CMV IgM test results may occur in patients with EBV or HHV-6 infectious mononucleosis because such individuals may produce heterotypic IgM antibodies. RF is an IgM antibody that reacts with IgG. IgM RF forms a complex with CMV IgG. The CMV IgG binds to CMV antigen together with nonviral RF IgM, resulting in false-positive results. False-negative results may occur if there is competitive inhibition of the binding of RF IgM to CMV antigen. For this reason, separate IgM and IgG titers should be ordered to minimize the incidence of false-positive and false-negative CMV IgM results. If there is any discrepancy between CMV IgM titers and the clinical presentation (ie, false-positive/negative tests), RF, EBV VCA IgM, and HHV-6 IgM titers should be obtained.[1,4,5]

CMV antigen assays

CMV semiquantitative antigenemia assay is a sensitive/specific and rapid method to detect CMV activation in lymphocytes. More important than an isolated elevated level are serial increases in CMV antigen titers. In general, a low-titer positive antigenemia indicates asymptomatic infection. Usually with CMV reactivation infection, CMV antigen titers are higher or increase over time. However, in immunosuppressed patients, such as transplant patients, even low or modest CMV antigenemia may indicate reactivation/infection.[5,9,10,18,22]

CMV PCR

CMV PCR is very sensitive and indicates reactivation of CMV in lymphocytes. The main difficulty in using CMV PCR is that it does not distinguish between asymptomatic or latent infection and active infection. Because PCR is so sensitive, serial qualitative PCR, as with semiquantitative CMV antigen levels, may be more clinically useful. As with CMV antigenemia, very high levels or increasing levels suggest active/impending CMV infection. Particularly in immunocompromised hosts, eg, transplants a negative CMV PCR argues strongly against reactivation but not CMV infection. Importantly, in immunocompetent hosts with primary CMV CAP, CMV PCR is usually negative.[4,5,10,18]

CMV cytopathology

Because CMV produces characteristic large cells (cytomegalic cells) with intranuclear basophilic inclusions and cytoplasmic eosinophilic inclusions, active CMV infection can be diagnosed by demonstrating characteristic CMV intracellular inclusions with hematoxylin-eosin, Giemsa, Wright, or Papanicolaou stains in tissue specimens. CMV intranuclear inclusions are surrounded by a clear halo giving them the typical appearance of an "owl's eye," but dense granular cytoplasmic inclusions, although not present in all cells, are diagnostic of CMV active infection (**Table 3**).[1,4,5,14]

THERAPY

CMV, like other herpes viruses, is characterized by its latency, ability to evade host defenses/survive indefinitely, and by its ability to be reactivated resulting in subclinical or clinical infection. CMV reactivation is a function of the host's CMI. CMV is a major problem in compromised hosts with impaired CMI and in those on steroids or immunosuppressive therapy that facilitates the reactivation of CMV. In immunocompetent hosts, most CMV infections are mild-to-moderately severe. However, in some cases, CMV infection in normal hosts may be severe. Excluding HIV with PCP, CMV CAP in compromised hosts, particularly in organ transplants, is usually severe and may be fatal. Anti-CMV therapy may be lifesaving in such cases. CMV is an uncommon cause of severe viral CAP in immunocompetent adults. Severe CMV CAP is treated with CMV antivirals. Often, in normal hosts, CMV CAP resolves during CMV therapy (induction).[18,22]

Table 3
Cytopathologic effects of CMV, HSV, and adenoviral pneumonias

Cytopathologic Findings	CMV[a]	HSV[b]	Adenovirus
Cytopathic effects	+	+	+
Intranuclear inclusions	Early	Late	
Intracytoplasmic inclusions	Late	–	Early (multiple, small) Late (large dense)
Cytomegalia (enlarged infected cell size)	+++	++	+
Intranuclear Inclusions			
Ground glass appearance	–	+	–
Prominent perinuclear halo	+	–	+ (Late)
Kidney bean–shaped nucleus (nuclear molding)	–[e,f]	+[e]	–
Multinucleated giant cells (syncytia)	–	+	–
Eosinophilic intranuclear inclusions	–[c]	+	+[d] (Early)
Nucleolus (basophilic) accessory body	+	–	–
Smudged nucleus	–	–	+
Intracytoplasmic Inclusions			
Dense (basophilic) granular inclusions	+[f]	–	–

[a] CAP.
[b] CAP or Late-onset VAP.
[c] May be eosinophilic early.
[d] Small.
[e] Gomori methenamine silver stain (GMS).
[f] GMS positive and periodic acid-Schiff stain positive.

Adapted from Cunha BA. Pneumonia essentials. 3rd edition. Sudbury (MA): Jones and Bartlett; 2010; with permission.

Although acyclovir is active against other herpes viruses, it is ineffective against CMV. The mainstay of anti-CMV therapy is ganciclovir 5 mg/kg (intravenous) every 12 hours for the duration of infection. The oral equivalent of parenteral ganciclovir is valganciclovir. Valganciclovir is metabolized to ganciclovir in vivo and is as effective as parenteral ganciclovir. Oral valganciclovir may be used to complete therapy after the initial ganciclovir therapy or may be used for the entire duration of therapy. The dosage of oral valganciclovir for induction therapy is 900 mg (by mouth) every 12 hours for 21 days. In immunocompetent hosts, a complete course of therapy with ganciclovir/valganciclovir is usually not necessary because patients usually improve after 1 to 2 weeks of therapy. In such patients, anti-CMV therapy is often continued for an additional week to prevent potential relapse. Foscarnet is alternative CMV therapy, but is administered intravenously and is nephrotoxic.[1,2,4,5,14,18,22]

The decision to treat CMV CAP is based on severity, that is, the degree of hypoxemia. Treatment of CMV CAP in organ transplants is obligatory but not so in patients with HIV. In patients with HIV, CAP may be caused by the usual typical CAP pathogens or *Mycobacterium tuberculosis*. CAP in patients with HIV may also be caused by an atypical CAP pathogen, for example, legionnaires disease. However, the most common CAP in patients with HIV with mild/moderately decreased CD4 cell counts is PCP. Even though patients with HIV are, by definition, immunosuppressed with various degrees of impaired CMI, CMV is an "innocent bystander" and not a pathogen in such patients. In patients with HIV with PCP CAP, CMV is present in lung tissue in 75% of such patients as an "innocent bystander" and is not responsible for the hypoxemia due to PCP. As PCP is treated in patients with HIV, hypoxemia gradually resolves and CMV does not reactivate but remains an "innocent bystander". For this reason, in HIV patients with PCP CAP, CMV is not treated.[14,25]

COMPLICATIONS AND PROGNOSIS

In patients with organ transplants, CMV CAP may be fatal. The severity of CMV CAP in such patients is related to the degree of impaired CMI. In immunocompetent hosts, even with severe CMV CAP, the prognosis is good. Most mild or moderately severe cases resolve before the diagnosis of CMV CAP is confirmed. In organ transplants with severe CMV CAP, CMV therapy with ganciclovir/valacyclovir is essential.[14,32] CMV CAP in immunocompetent hosts, even if severe, rarely requires a full course of anti-CMV therapy.

REFERENCES

1. Ho M. Cytomegalovirus biology and infection. 2nd edition. New York: Plenum Publishing Corp; 1991.
2. Cohen JL, Corey GR. Cytomegalovirus infection in the normal host. Medicine 1985;64:100–14.
3. Klotman ME, Hamilton JD. Cytomegalovirus pneumonia. Semin Respir Infect 1987;2:95–103.
4. Pass RF. Cytomegalovirus. In: Knipe DM, Howley PM, editors. Fields virology, vol. 2. 4th edition. Philadelphia: Lippincott Williams & Wilkins; 2001. p. 2675–705.
5. Sanghavi SK, Rowe DT, Rinaldo CR. Cytomegalovirus, varicella-zoster virus, and Epstein-barr virus. In: Specter S, Hodinka RL, Young SA, et al, editors. Clinical virology manual. Washington, DC: ASM Press; 2009. p. 454–61.
6. Carlstrom G, Alden J, Belfrage S, et al. Acquired cytomegalovirus infection. Br Med J 1968;2:521–5.

7. Sterner G, Agell BO, Wahren B, et al. Acquired cytomegalovirus infection in older children and adults. Scand J Infect Dis 1970;2:95–103.
8. Klemola E, Stenstrom R, von Essen R. Pneumonia as a clinical manifestation of cytomegalovirus infection in previously healthy adults. Scand J Infect Dis 1972; 4:7–10.
9. Treanor JJ. Respiratory infections. In: Richman DD, Whitley RJ, Hayden FG, editors. Clinical virology. 3rd edition. Washington, DC: ASM Press; 2009. p. 7–28.
10. Griffiths PD, Emery VC, Milne R. Cytomegalovirus. In: Richman DD, Whitley RJ, Hayden FG, editors. Clinical virology. 3rd edition. Washington, DC: ASM Press; 2009. p. 475–506.
11. Cunha BA, Pherez F, Walls N. Severe cytomegalovirus (CMV) community-acquired pneumonia (CAP) in an immunocompetent host. Heart Lung 2009;38:243–8.
12. Rafailidis PI, Mourtzoukou E, Varbobitis IC, et al. Severe cytomegalovirus infection in apparently immunocompetent patients: a systematic review. Virol J 2008;5:47.
13. Vasquez V, Barzaga RA, Cunha BA. Cytomegalovirus-induced flare of systemic lupus erythematosus. Heart Lung 1992;21:407–8.
14. Cunha BA. Pneumonia essentials. 3rd edition. Sudbury (MA): Jones and Bartlett; 2010.
15. Cunha BA. The atypical pneumonias. Clinical diagnosis and importance. Clin Microbiol Infect 2006;12:12–24.
16. Cunha BA. Ambulatory community-acquired pneumonia: the predominance of atypical pathogens. Eur J Clin Microbiol Infect Dis 2003;22:579–83.
17. Ramos-Casals M, Cuadrado MJ, Alba P, et al. Acute viral infections in patients with systemic lupus erythematosus. Description of 23 cases and review of the literature. Medicine 2008;87:311–8.
18. Kotton CN, Fishman JA. Viral infection in the renal transplant recipient. J Am Soc Nephrol 2009;16:1758–74.
19. Cunha BA, Gouzhva O, Nausheen S. Severe cytomegalovirus (CMV) community-acquired pneumonia (CAP) precipitating a systemic lupus erythematosis (SLE) flare. Heart Lung 2009;38:249–52.
20. Falsey AR, Walsh EE. Viral pneumonia in older adults. Clin Infect Dis 2006;42: 518–24.
21. Mera JR, Whimbey E, Elting L. Cytomegalovirus pneumonia in adult nontransplantation patients with cancer: review of 20 cases occurring from 1964 through 1990. Clin Infect Dis 1996;22:1046–50.
22. Akhter J, Al-Johani S, Ali MA, et al. Post-renal transplantation viral infections. Infectious Disease Practice 2008;32:657–61.
23. Cunha BA. Severe adenovirus community-acquired pneumonia mimicking *Legionella*. Eur J Clin Microbiol Infect Dis 2009;28:313–5.
24. Cunha BA. Atypical pneumonias: current clinical concepts focusing on Legionnaires' disease. Curr Opin Pulm Med 2008;14:183–94.
25. Forward K. Community acquired pneumonia due to cytomegalovirus HSV-1 and HHV-6. In: Marrie TJ, editor. Community acquired pneumonia. New York: Plenum Publishers; 2001. p. 665–77.
26. Eddleston M, Peacock S, Juniper M, et al. Severe cytomegalovirus infection in immunocompetent patients. Clin Infect Dis 1997;24:52–6.
27. Jaber S, Chanques G, Borry J, et al. Cytomegalovirus infection in critically ill patients: associated factors and consequences. Chest 2005;127:233–41.
28. von Muller L, Klemm A, Weiss M, et al. Active cytomegalovirus in infection in patients with septic shock. Emerg Infect Dis 2006;12:1517–22.

29. Chiche L, Forel JM, Roch A, et al. Active cytomegalovirus infection is common in mechanically ventilated medical intensive care unit patients. Crit Care Med 2009; 37:1850–7.
30. Cohen JI. Cytomegalovirus in the intensive care unit: pathogen or passenger? Crit Care Med 2009;37:2095–6.
31. Cunha BA. Cytomegalovirus (CMV) reactivation is not a cause of late ventilator associated pneumonia (VAP) in the ICU. Crit Care Med 2010;38:341–2.
32. Laing RB, Dykhuizen RS, Smith CC, et al. Parenteral ganciclovir treatment of acute CMV infection in the immunocompetent host. Infection 1997;25:44–6.
33. Robinson CC. Respiratory viruses. In: Specter S, Hodinka RL, Young SA, et al, editors. Clinical virology manual. Washington, DC: ASM Press; 2009. p. 203–48.
34. French CA. Respiratory tract. In: Cibas ES, Ducatman BS, editors. Cytology: diagnostic principles and clinical correlates. Philadelphia: Saunders Elsevier; 2009.
35. Eisenberg MJ, Kaplan B. Cytomegalovirus-induced thrombocytopenia in an immunocompetent adult. West J Med 1993;158:525–6.
36. Limaye AP, Kirby KA, Rubenfeld GD, et al. Cytomegalovirus reactivation in critically ill immnocompetent patients. JAMA 2008;300:413–22.
37. Heininger A, Jahn G, Engel C, et al. Human cytomegalovirus infections in nonimmunosuppressed critically ill patients. Crit Care Med 2001;29:541–7.
38. Kutza AS, Muhl E, Hackstein H, et al. High incidence of active cytomegalovirus infection among septic patients. Clin Infect Dis 1998;25:1076–82.

Hantavirus Pulmonary Syndrome

Steven Q. Simpson, MD*, Leslie Spikes, MD, Saurin Patel, MD, Ibrahim Faruqi, MD, MPH

KEYWORDS

• Hantavirus • Pneumonia • Viral pneumonia
• Acute respiratory failure • Hemorrhagic fever

Hantavirus pulmonary syndrome (HPS), a disease now known to have been present for centuries, if not millennia, in the Americas was discovered only 16 years ago in the southwestern United States.[1] Two young long-distance runners who lived together in the New Mexican desert fell victim in early May, 1993, to what seemed to be a rapidly progressive pulmonary infection, and both of them died within days. The unusual circumstance of two highly fit individuals succumbing in this manner, especially in the spring, led health officials to investigate the cause and initiate surveillance for other, similar cases. It soon became evident that they were in the midst of an outbreak of a seriously deadly infectious agent and that the syndrome was one that had not been previously described by the medical community.

The causative agent for the illness was soon (<6 weeks after the index cases were identified) determined to be an unidentified North American member of the *Hantavirus* genus. The clinical syndrome caused by this agent, ultimately named *Sin Nombre virus* (SNV), came to be called the *hantavirus pulmonary syndrome*. This designation distinguished it from previously described hantaviral illnesses, which were characterized as hemorrhagic fever with renal syndrome (HFRS). Early in the course of events it became evident that cardiac function, and respiratory function, are markedly impaired by infection with this virus. For that reason, some authors have adopted the moniker *Hantavirus cardiopulmonary syndrome*. Although that name certainly has logic, the Centers for Disease Control and Prevention (CDC) continue to refer to the illness as HPS, as does this article.

HANTAVIRUSES

The hantaviruses are an enveloped genus of the family Bunyaviridae. Virions are spherical and encapsulated by a bilayered phospholipid membrane. The composition of each virion is greater than 50% protein, 20% to 30% lipid, and 2% to 7% carbohydrate,

Division of Pulmonary and Critical Care Medicine, University of Kansas, 3901 Rainbow Boulevard, Mail Stop 3007, Kansas City, KS 66160-7381, USA
* Corresponding author.
E-mail address: ssimpson3@kumc.edu (S.Q. Simpson).

Infect Dis Clin N Am 24 (2010) 159–173
doi:10.1016/j.idc.2009.10.011 **id.theclinics.com**

making them easily disrupted with heat, detergents, organic solvents, and hypochlorite solutions.[2] Diameters range from 71 to 200 nm, with an average of approximately 100 nm.[3] The genome consists of three single-stranded, negative-sense RNA segments: long (L), medium (M), and short (S). Each of the segments encodes only one protein. The S segment codes for the nucleocapsid protein (N protein), the M segment codes for the viral envelope glycoproteins (two proteins, G1 and G2), and the L segment codes for viral transcriptase.[4] The 3′ terminal and 5′ terminal end are complementary sequences, resulting in the RNA strand forming "pan-handle" structures that seem to be important in viral transcription and replication.[5] Each segment also has short noncoding regions, the function of which is yet to be elucidated. **Fig. 1** shows a schematic of SNV based on CDC electron micrographs.[6]

Hantaviruses principally target vascular endothelial cells, but also infect alveolar macrophages and follicular dendritic cells. Renal tubular epithelium can also be a site for infection. Cell entry of hantaviruses is mediated by binding to β3 integrins.[7] Sin Nombre and New York viruses enter human cells by way of αvβ3 and αIIbβ3

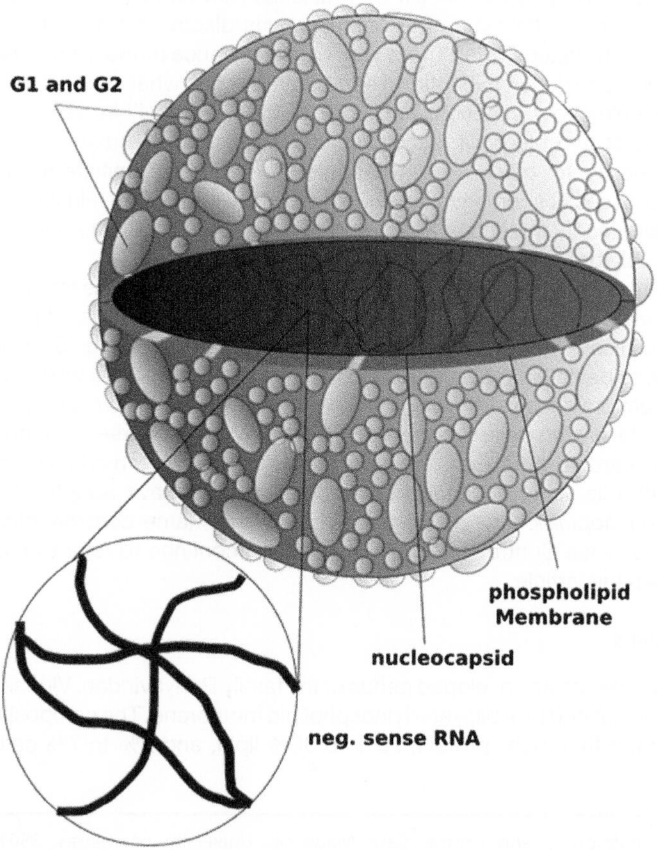

Fig. 1. Schematic diagram of Sin Nombre virus, based on Centers for Disease Control and Prevention electron micrographs. Structures are not drawn to scale. *G1* and *G2* represent glycoproteins that mediate attachment of virions to human cells by way of β3 integrins. The virus consists of a phospholipid bilayer envelope surrounding a nucleocapsid protein. Three strands of negative sense RNA constitute the viral genome. (*Courtesy of* N. Simpson, Fairway, KS.)

integrins, whereas Prospect Hill, a nonpathogenic hantavirus, does not, suggesting a role for these particular molecules in human pathogenesis. Uptake of these viruses is inhibited by various competitive ligands. SNV glycoprotein is processed through the Golgi apparatus, where virions likely are packaged, but later in the course of in vitro infection glycoprotein antigens can be found at the cell surface of human pulmonary endothelial cells.[8] Likewise, SNV and Black Creek Canal viruses localize to the apical membrane of polarized Vero cells.[3,9]

EPIDEMIOLOGY AND ECOLOGY

Reservoirs

Like other members of the Bunyavirus family, each hantavirus is closely associated with a specific rodent reservoir. The hantaviruses chronically infect rodents that are members of subfamilies of the family Muridae without causing illness in the rodents. **Table 1** shows known pathogenic hantaviruses, their rodent hosts, and their geographic locations. The Murinae subfamily hosts the Old World hantaviruses Hantaan and Dobrava, and other nonpathogenic strains.

The Arvicolinae, or voles, are hosts to Puumala virus, which causes HFRS in Scandinavia, and to Prospect Hill virus which is found in the Ohio River valley but does not cause disease. The pathogenic New World hantaviruses chronically infect rodents of the Sigmodontinae subfamily. The single interloper in this relationship between the Muridae and the hantaviruses is Seoul virus, whose host is *Rattus norvegicus*. In keeping with the travel habits of that host, Seoul virus–induced HFRS has been diagnosed throughout Asia and the Americas, mostly in coastal areas, and infected rodents have been identified on every continent, except Antarctica. Indigenous hantaviruses had not been identified in Africa until 2006, when the Sangassou virus was detected in the wood mouse *Hylomyscus simus*, a member of the Murinae subfamily; no human infections with this virus have yet been detected.[10]

In the United States, the principal virus causing HPS is SNV, which chronically infects the deer mouse, *Peromyscus maniculatis*. The deer mouse habitat occupies a huge swath of the North American continent, sparing only areas nearing the Arctic Circle, a few states in the southeastern United States, and southern Mexico. Approximately 10% of tested deer mice in this range are infected with SNV.[11] Additionally, closely related hantaviruses are hosted by other sigmodontine rodents in areas where deer mice are sparse, including Black Creek Canal virus, hosted by the cotton rat *Sigmodon hispidus* in Florida, and the Bayou virus, hosted by the swamp rat *Oligoryzomus palustris* in Louisiana and Texas.

In November of 1996, an outbreak of HPS was detected in the Neuquen region of southern Patagonia, and the source was traced to yet another sigmodontine rodent, the "coli largo" or long-tailed rice rat, *Oligoryzomus longicaudatus*. The hantavirus detected in both patients and rats was named the *Andes virus*.[12] Heightened awareness of the disease, its causative agents, and its presenting features led to the identification of HPS cases, along with new strains of hantaviruses and newly identified hosts, in multiple South American countries, including Bolivia, Brazil, Chile, Paraguay, and Uruguay. By 1999, HPS caused by Choclo virus was identified in Central America (Panama), carried by the pygmy rice rat *Oligoryzomus fulvescens*.[13] Based on the broad distribution of sigmodontine rodents throughout the Americas, the CDC estimates that it is only a matter of time before HPS is detected in every American country.[14]

Mode of Transmission

In contrast to other Bunyaviridae, transmission of hantaviruses does not involve an arthropod intermediate. Transmission largely occurs through inhalation of aerosolized

Table 1
Pathogenic hantaviruses

Hantaviruses	Host	Geographic Range	Syndrome	Yearly Incidence/ Mortality Rate
Eurasian				
Dobrava-belgrade (DOB)	*Apodemus flavicollis* (yellow-necked field mouse)	Balkans	HFRS	100/15%
Hantaan (HTN)	*Apodemus agrarius* (striped-field mouse)	China, Korea, Russia	HFRS	100,000/1%–5%
Puumala (PUU)	*Clethrionomys glareolus* (red bank vole)	Europe	NE	30,000/1%
Saaremaa (SAA)	*Apodemus agrarius* (Striped field mouse) *Microtus arvalis* (European common vole)	Northern Europe	HFRS	Unknown/0%
Seoul (SEO)	*Rattus norvegicus* (Norway [brown] rat); *Rattus rattus* (black rat)	Worldwide	HFRS	Unknown/1%–2%
Tula (TUU)	*Microtus arvalis* (European common vole)	Europe	HFRS	Unknown/0%
North American				
Bayou (BAY	*Oryzomys palustris* (rice rat)	Southeastern United States	HPS	5 cases/1 fatality
Black creek canal (BCC)	*Sigmodon hispidus* (cotton rat)	Florida	HPS	1 case/0 fatality
New York (NY)	*Peromyscus leucopus* (white-footed mouse)	Eastern United States	HPS	3 cases/ 1 fatality

Sin Nombre (SN)	*Peromyscus maniculatus* (deer mouse)	Western United States	HPS	20–80/35%–40%
Central and South American				
Andes (AND)	*Oligoryzomys longicaudatus* (long-tailed pygmy rice rat)	Argentina and Chile	HPS	50–200/35%–40%
Araraquara (ARA)	*Bolomys lasiurus* (hairy-tailed bolo mouse)	Central Brazil	HPS	20–50/25%
Bermejo (BMJ)	*Oligoryzomys chacoensis* (Chacoan pygmy rice rat)	Northern Argentina	HPS	Unknown/20%
Castelo dos sonhos (CAS)	Unknown	Central Brazil	HPS	Unknown/25%
Choclo (CHO)	*Oligoryzomys fulvescens* (pygmy rice rat)	Western Panama	HPS	2–30/10%
Juquitiba (JUQ)	*Oligoryzomys nigripos* (black-footed pygmy rice rat)	Southern Brazil	HPS	Unknown/25%
Laguna Negra (LN)	*Calomys laucha* (vesper mouse)	Northwestern Argentina, Bolivia, and Paraguay	HPS	2–30/9%
Lechiguanas (LEC)	*Oligoryzomys flavescens* (yellow pygmy rat)	Central Argentina	HPS	Unknown/30%
Oran (ORN)	*Oligoryzomylongicaudatus* (long-tailed rice rat)	Northwestern Argentina and Bolivia	HPS	Unknown/35%

Abbreviations: HFRS, hemorrhagic fever with renal syndrome; HPS, hantavirus pulmonary syndrome; NE, Nephropathia epidemica (a form of HFRS).

urine, feces, or saliva of the rodent host. Within species, the viruses are also commonly transmitted through aggressive behavior, such as biting, especially among males, and males have a higher prevalence of infection than females.[15,16] Both HFRS and HPS are predominantly rural diseases, with associated risk factors of farming, land development, hunting, and camping, because each of these activities brings humans into closer contact with the natural rodent reservoirs, which are all sylvan or agrarian in their choice of habitat. However, HPS is nearly always acquired indoors or within closed spaces, such as peridomestic buildings on farms or ranches, livestock feed containers, or the cabs of abandoned pickup trucks.[17]

Several factors contribute to the propensity for indoor acquisition by humans. Animals captured in the peridomestic environment have a higher prevalence of active infection than those captured in a sylvan environment (25% vs. 10%), likely because of greater supplies of foodstuffs and higher murine population densities.[18] Higher population densities lead to more interaction among mice and higher rates of intraspecies transmission. Likewise, humans are more likely to encounter rodent excreta when population densities are higher.

Although SNV and other hantaviruses are capable of withstanding desiccation for days, they are inactivated by ultraviolet light, which is less plentiful in the indoor environment. Humans are prone to cleaning and other activities that stir up virus-carrying dust particles, and without the diluting effect of outdoor air they are subject to inhaling higher concentrations of virus.

Incidence and Prevalence

Since 1993, approximately 465 cases of HPS have been documented in the United States, a few of which were retrospectively identified.[14] The overwhelming majority (>90%) of these infections are isolated, not in clusters. Although SNV-induced HPS has occurred throughout the range of the deer mouse, the incidence is highest in the western United States, and SNV accounts for the vast majority of North American disease. Canada reports approximately 10% to 15% of the North American cases each year. In the United States, approximately two thirds of HPS cases have been among men. The average age of patients who have HPS is 38 years, with a range of 10 to 83 years. There has been a striking absence of severe HPS among prepubertal individuals in the United States, although disease in 11 children aged 10 to 16 years had clinical courses similar to those described in adults.[19] The United States mortality rate is 35%.[14]

The incidence of HPS in Latin America is largely unknown but cases have been reported from Central America to southern Patagonia. The Andes virus was responsible for outbreaks in Argentina and Chile and is closely related to the Bayou virus. Although most North American cases have been sporadic and isolated, most South American cases have occurred in clusters. The Patagonian outbreak in 1996 was unique in that it occurred in an area with a relatively low rodent population density, and human-to-human transmission was suspected when physicians treating infected patients became ill themselves.[20] Gene sequencing of virus recovered from cases with rodent exposure and from their contacts who had no possibility of rodent exposure confirmed human-to-human transmission.[21,22] As of this writing, human-to-human transmission of hantaviruses has been shown only for the Andes virus.

The seroprevalence of IgG antibodies to hantaviruses differs between North and South American populations. In the United States, the Four Corners area has the highest incidence of infection; however, presence of antibodies among tested individuals in that region is less than 1%.[23,24] Childhood infection in North America is also rare. In contrast, some endemic areas in South America have a much higher rate of infection, including in children, with seroprevalence as high as 42.7% in areas of Paraguay.[25] In all areas studied, the seroprevalence is higher in South America than in North America, suggesting the occurrence of mild and asymptomatic infections.[26]

CLINICAL FEATURES

Although the dramatic and well-publicized feature of HPS is its effect on cardiopulmonary function, the disease actually comprises four clinical phases: prodrome, pulmonary edema and shock, diuresis, and convalescence.[27] During the initial prodromal phase, symptoms are virtually identical to the febrile phase of HFRS.[1] This phase typically lasts 3 to 6 days, at which time the onset of respiratory symptoms and shock is abrupt. Mortality most commonly occurs in the first 24 hours of the pulmonary edema and shock phase of the illness, which also tends to last from 3 to 6 days. Patients who survive the shock phase enter the diuretic phase of the illness. In this phase, patients may have urine flow rates ranging from 300 to 500 mL/hr, simultaneous with rapid (24–48 hours) resolution of respiratory and hemodynamic abnormalities.[28] After diuresis and extubation, patients enter the convalescent phase of the illness, which typically lasts for a few months, but some patients have taken up to 2 years for full recovery.

Presentation

The most common signs and symptoms in the prodromal phase are identical to those of other, less-severe viral illnesses. Nearly all patients complain of subjective fever or chills on presentation, and most have myalgias or headache. Many patients initially have nausea/vomiting, diarrhea, or abdominal pain. In fact, several patients have been admitted to the hospital for treatment of gastroenteritis before HPS is diagnosed.

Cough is present in nearly two thirds of patients on presentation. The cough is most often nonproductive, but occasionally a patient produces amber-colored pulmonary secretions that are confused with purulent sputum. This sputum is actually alveolar edema fluid and manifests at the onset of the shock phase of illness. Despite the central role that pulmonary problems play in HPS, dyspnea is not a common early complaint. Dyspnea is associated with advanced disease and often is a sign of impending respiratory failure. **Box 1** shows presenting symptoms of HPS, and symptoms that are uncommon in the syndrome. These latter symptoms have been helpful in distinguishing HPS from other acute febrile illnesses.

The most frequent initial physical findings in HPS are tachypnea, fever, and tachycardia.[1,28] The pulmonary examination is unrevealing early in the illness, but with the onset of pulmonary edema, fine rales are present, which become more pronounced with progression of disease. Severe abdominal tenderness is present in approximately 10% of patients and may mimic appendicitis. Hypotension is unusual on presentation, but when it is present indicates advanced disease and requires aggressive resuscitation. Although many patients are thrombocytopenic, petechiae are rare in North American HPS. Several findings that are common in HFRS, such as conjunctival hemorrhage, flushing, and peripheral edema, are virtually never present in people who have North American HPS but are relatively more prevalent among people who have Andes virus infection.[29,30]

Laboratory Findings

A trio of hematologic findings, including thrombocytopenia, leukocytosis with a left shift, and circulating immunoblastoid lymphocytes, is unique to HPS in the Americas, although these findings are reported in HFRS in Asia.[31] Thrombocytopenia is present in 79% of patients at presentation and is the most common initial laboratory

Box 1
Presenting sign and symptoms in hantavirus pulmonary syndrome

Common (>40% of cases)
Fever
Myalgia
Nausea/vomiting/diarrhea
Conjunctival injection[a]
Cough
Headache
Facial flushing[a]
Uncommon (<5% of cases)
Odynophagia
Rhinorrhea
Sinusitis
Otalgia
Meningismus
Petechiae
Pleuritic pain
[a] In Andes virus infection but not Sin Nombre.

abnormality; it develops in all patients during their hospital course. The white blood cell count is increased, and immature neutrophils such as myelocytes and promyelocytes are frequently present. All patients have a lymphocyte population that includes at least 10% immunoblasts and plasma cells, a finding not seen in similar disorders such as acute respiratory distress syndrome (ARDS). These immunoblasts may often be reported as atypical lymphocytes by laboratory personnel. Hemoconcentration is common, with hematocrits as high as 77%; this finding is believed to result from massive capillary leaking of plasma but not cells.[32]

Liver enzymes, including aspartate aminotransferase and alanine aminotransferase, tend to be increased, but not dramatically so. Hypoalbuminemia is a common finding, possibly caused by resuscitation with crystalloid solutions, but bilirubin and alkaline phosphatase are typically normal.[33] Serum lactate dehydrogenase level is frequently increased with an electrophoretic pattern consistent with lung and liver injury. Creatinine rises mildly in most North American cases, but only 20% of patients achieve creatinine levels greater than 2.0 mg/dL in North America, and only a couple of renal failure cases have been reported.[34–36] Case series from South America indicate a 48% prevalence of renal insufficiency.[37–39]

Serum lactate levels help establish disease severity. An increased serum lactate level identifies patients who have poor tissue perfusion and those who require immediate resuscitative efforts. In early series, all patients who had a serum lactate level of 4.0 mmol/L or higher died despite aggressive treatment, except some patients who were treated with extracorporeal membrane oxygenation (ECMO).[28,40,41]

Radiographic Findings

Chest radiographic abnormalities are noted on admission in most patients, even in the absence of dyspnea. Major findings are interstitial edema, and include Kerley's B lines, hilar indistinctness, and peribronchial cuffing.[42,43] Many patients develop severe airspace disease and progressive hypoxemia. Airspace flooding typically begins in dependent areas of the lung and progresses to involve all lung fields. This progression may be as rapid as 4 to 6 hours from presentation. Cardiac silhouettes are not enlarged, and pleural effusions develop in all patients as the disease progresses. Lobar infiltrates are not seen in HPS, and their presence should strongly suggest another diagnosis.

Respiratory Function

Disease often progresses abruptly from prodrome to full-blown HPS, and patients presenting with dyspnea typically require intubation and mechanical ventilation within 1 to 6 hours.[28,41] All patients who have HPS develop pulmonary edema, with severity ranging from mild interstitial edema to diffuse alveolar flooding with profound hypoxemia. PaO_2 to fraction of inspired oxygen (FIO_2) ratios may be as low as 28 during mechanical ventilation with high levels of positive end-expiratory pressure (normal PaO_2/FIO_2 range is 350–500, dependent on elevation), which would equate to a PaO_2 of 28 mm Hg while breathing 100% oxygen. Chest radiography demonstrates diffuse interstitial or alveolar infiltrates, and low respiratory system compliance is evident. Alveolar flooding seems to result from a very low reflection coefficient in the alveolar capillaries; in other words, the barrier between capillary blood and alveolar gas is porous.[27] The result is that relatively low intracapillary hydrostatic pressures can cause massive fluid flux across the membrane. In this disease, pulmonary artery occlusive pressures (wedge pressures) exceeding 10 to 12 mm Hg result in profound alveolar edema,[28] (S.Q. Simpson, unpublished data, 1997). Pleural effusions develop in most patients and can be massive; the mechanisms for accumulation of pleural fluid are believed to be similar to those for alveolar fluid formation.[44]

In patients who survive an initial crisis period of 24 to 72 hours, recovery is often nearly as rapid as the decline, and these patients are most frequently extubated in less than a week. After hospital discharge, pulmonary function testing may show air trapping or diminished carbon monoxide diffusing capacity for up to 6 months, during which most patients have returned to their pre-HPS activities. However, patients who remain dyspneic for more than a year after recovering from the acute illness have been reported.

Hemodynamics

Nearly all patients who have HPS fit accepted criteria for the diagnosis of severe sepsis, having serologic evidence of infection, fever, tachypnea, tachycardia, and evidence of organ dysfunction.[45] However, the hemodynamic parameters in HPS are unique compared with other forms of septic shock and are closely associated with mortality. Shock caused by other viruses, bacteria, and fungi has been associated with an increased cardiac index and low systemic vascular resistance.[46–48] Patients who have HPS nearly uniformly have a diminished cardiac index and normal or increased systemic vascular resistance.[28] At presentation, many patients who have HPS have intravascular volume depletion, as evidenced by increased hematocrit and decreased pulmonary artery occlusive pressures. Patients who have hypotension have a low cardiac stroke volume and low cardiac output because of inadequate left ventricular preload. However, intravascular volume repletion does not improve cardiac output, suggesting the presence of myocardial depression. Echocardiography also shows poor left ventricular systolic function. Death, when it occurs, is caused by progressive myocardial insufficiency, and the terminal event is almost uniformly progressive hypotension, which evolves to pulseless electrical activity.

Pathology

At autopsy, the lungs of patients who have HPS are grossly edematous and have an average combined weight nearly twice normal.[33] Pleural effusions are uniformly present, with volume ranging from 200 to 8400 mL. Histologically, variable amounts of alveolar and septal edema are found.[32,33] Hyaline membranes with little cellular debris are usually present, the respiratory epithelium is intact, and type II pneumocytes appear nonactivated. An interstitial infiltration of mononuclear cells is present and many of the mononuclear cells are enlarged and have the characteristics of immunoblasts. Intravascular neutrophils are common, but only rarely in the interstitium, alveoli, and bronchioles. No vasculitis has been identified in pulmonary vessels, and no viral inclusions or cytopathic effects are seen on light microscopy, although immunologic staining shows viral antigens in the pulmonary endothelium. Electron microscopy shows rare endothelial inclusions of 90 to 110 nm particles consistent in appearance with hantavirus virions. These histopathologic findings distinguish HPS from diffuse alveolar damage or ARDS, in which the infiltrate is predominantly neutrophilic, type II pneumocytes are activated, and extensive cellular debris is present. Immunohistochemistry shows abundant staining of pulmonary endothelial cells.[32] A fine, granular-appearing stain localizes in the pulmonary microvascular endothelium and is rarely seen in the endothelium of larger veins and arteries. When sections of multiple lung segments are available, the microvascular staining appears uniform throughout the lungs.

The heart of patients who have fatal SNV infection is grossly and histologically normal, with no evidence of significant coronary artery disease or recent myocardial infarction.[33] Neither myocarditis nor cardiomyopathy are found. However, myocarditis was present in fatal cases of HPS in both Argentina and Brazil.[49,50] A small pericardial effusion was seen in one patient. Myocardial capillaries contain SNV antigens in most specimens, with antigen loads ranging from focal involvement to extensive, diffuse staining. In the Brazilian series myocytes stain for hantaviral antigens, a finding that has not been seen in North American HPS.[50]

Examination of the liver shows a portal triaditis in approximately half of the cases, with expanded pools of lymphocytes, including large immunoblasts, but without necrosis.[32,33] The spleen and lymph nodes typically contain an infiltrate of immunoblasts. Lymphocytes within splenic lymphoid follicles typically contain SNV antigens, and macrophages in several tissues, including the lungs, also stain positively. The brain, kidneys, adrenals, pancreas, skeletal muscle, and skin are normal both macroscopically and histologically. SNV antigens are seen in multiple other tissues, including skeletal muscle, adrenal glands, intestine, and brain, although these tissues stain less intensely and less consistently than the lungs.

DIAGNOSIS AND TREATMENT

The key to treatment of HPS lies in recognition of the illness, but that can be a challenge for clinicians, because the prodromal phase of the illness is nondistinguishing.[1] One must have a high index of suspicion, especially in rural locales, and it would be wise to query all patients who have fever, chills, myalgias, and gastrointestinal symptoms for recent history of dust exposure in enclosed spaces or exposure to rodents. Such recent activities as cleaning closets, garages, feed bins, or other outbuildings in rural locations must raise the index of suspicion and should prompt further investigation. In Patagonia it is clearly wise to obtain any history of HPS in close contacts, because of the prospect of human-to-human transmission. However, family members are frequently exposed to common risk factors in their home environment, and therefore this bit of history-taking can also be useful in other regions of the Americas.

If the patient's history is compatible with appropriate rodent exposure, a complete blood cell count should be obtained to evaluate for thrombocytopenia, which is the earliest laboratory abnormality in HPS.[31] The combination of a compatible history and thrombocytopenia should prompt hospitalization, especially if atypical lymphocytes are present. Commercial laboratories can serologically confirm or rule out the diagnosis of HPS within 24 hours; IgM antibodies to nucleocapsid antigen are universally present in symptomatic patients, and IgG antibodies are present in most.[51] The state health department should also be contacted and a blood specimen submitted for in-state testing or testing at the CDC. If the patient has cough, dyspnea, or other respiratory symptoms, a chest radiograph should be obtained. If there is evidence of pulmonary interstitial edema, the patient should be moved to an intensive care unit. Careful consideration must be given to transferring any patient who has HPS or suspected HPS to a facility with expertise in the management of shock and severe acute respiratory failure. Patients can and do deteriorate extremely rapidly, and waiting for the onset of shock to initiate transfer is often futile.[28,40,41]

Patients transitioning into the shock/respiratory failure stage of illness should have a flow-directed pulmonary artery catheter placed, and an arterial catheter for continuous blood pressure monitoring. Pulmonary artery occlusive pressure should be optimized between 8 and 12 mm Hg, but no higher. If the patient is hypotensive with these cardiac filling pressures, then a cardiac inotrope, preferably dobutamine, should be initiated. Vasopressor agents should be avoided, if possible, because they increase cardiac afterload. If pulse oximetry or serial arterial blood gases show a downward trend in arterial oxygenation, patients should be intubated early in their course.

The University of New Mexico (UNM) has extensive experience with ECMO in the treatment of patients who have HPS.[41] Because ECMO replaces or augments the function of both heart and lungs, it may offer the best hope of survival for patients for whom more conventional intensive are unit therapies fail. UNM reported on a series of 38 patients treated in this manner, with a mortality rate of 40%. Unfortunately, the descriptive nature of this study makes it difficult to draw conclusions regarding the efficacy of ECMO. The mortality rate in the study is roughly equivalent to the 35% overall mortality rate in the United States. However, patients in the study were chosen because they met criteria that in 1994 were believed to be associated with 100% mortality.[40] A randomized trial of ECMO probably will not be undertaken. Instituting ECMO at a moment's notice, especially among adults, is not possible even in most tertiary hospitals, and therefore more conventional therapies will remain the mainstay of HPS treatment.

As of this writing, no specific therapy exists for hantaviral diseases in the Americas. A multicenter randomized trial of intravenous ribavirin was closed because of a low rate of enrollment.[52] No clear effect of ribavirin was detected, in either direction. Although the possibility of passive immunization has been discussed for 15 years, and neutralizing antibodies remain present for years in survivors, no cases of administering immune human sera have been reported.[53] For now, cautious supportive care remains preferred treatment.

PREVENTION

With a case fatality rate of 35% to 40% and no proven effectiveness of antiviral therapy, preventing viral transmission and augmenting viral immunity in appropriate individuals are critical.[54] Satellite imagery allows evaluation of ecologic conditions and prospective prediction of areas of high rodent population, thereby enabling measurement of rodent infection rates to predict times of extraordinary risk.[55]

Less predictable is human to rodent contact; hence the need for measures aimed at decreasing rodent-to-human transmission, including those that decrease the risk for inhalation of aerosolized rodent excreta. To this effect, CDC recommends the "Seal Up! Trap Up! Clean Up!" approach: seal up holes inside and outside the home to prevent entry by rodents, trap rodents, and take precautions before and while cleaning rodent-infested areas. Before cleaning a space or an unused building, ventilate the area by opening doors and windows for at least 30 minutes to diffuse potentially infectious aerosolized material. Do not stir up dust by sweeping or vacuuming up droppings, urine, or nesting materials. Wear rubber, latex, vinyl, or nitrile gloves when cleaning excreta and handling dead rodents or rodent nests.[54]

Although evidence for human-to-human transmission of HPS in Argentina led the CDC to conduct a comprehensive review of the HPS registry, it found that SNV infection rarely, if ever, transmits from person-to-person, and that existing guidelines for preventing HPS remain appropriate for North America.[21,22,56,57] However, exercising contact and airborne precautions in the hospital and clinic is appropriate if infection with the Andes strain is suspected, as is remaining vigilant for new evidence of human-to-human transmission of other hantaviruses.[58]

Effective, though expensive, recombinant vaccines against Hantaan (HTNV), Puumala (PUUV), Dobrava (DOBV), and Seoul (SEOV) strains, causative agents of HFRS, have been tested in clinical trials and are selectively used in Asia.[58,59] An inactivated bivalent HTNV/PUUV vaccine protected hamsters against subsequent infection by HTNV, SEOV, DOBV, and PUUV, but not SNV or New York Virus.[58] In a recent study, Rhesus macaques vaccinated with nucleic acid vaccine (Gene Gun method) containing M genome segment of Andes virus developed neutralizing antibodies that also cross-neutralized other HPS-associated hantaviruses, including SNV. Sera from the vaccinated monkeys delayed the onset of HPS and death when injected into hamsters 1 day before challenge. Injection on day 4 or 5 after challenge provided 100% protection.[60] No human vaccination trials for the New World hantaviruses are currently in progress.

REFERENCES

1. Duchin JS, Koster FT, Peters CJ, et al. Hantavirus pulmonary syndrome: a clinical description of 17 patients with a newly recognized disease. The Hantavirus Study Group. N Engl J Med 1994;330(14):949–55.
2. Gonzalez-Scarano F, Nathanson N. Bunyaviridae. In: Fields BN, Knipe DM, Howley PM, editors. Fields virology. 3rd edition. Philadelphia: Lippincott-Raven Publishers; 1996. p. 1473–504.
3. Goldsmith CS, Elliott LH, Peters CJ, et al. Ultrastructural characteristics of Sin Nombre virus, causative agent of hantavirus pulmonary syndrome. Arch Virol 1995;140(12):2107–22.
4. Schmaljohn CS, Dalrymple JM. Hantaviruses. In: Webster GW, Granoff A, editors, Encylopedia of virology, vol. 2. London: Academic Press; 1994. p. 538–45.
5. Elliott RM, Schmaljohn CS, Collett MS. Bunyaviridae genome structure and gene expression. Curr Top Microbiol Immunol 1991;169:91–141.
6. National Center for Infectious Diseases. Special Pathogens Branch. All About Hantaviruses. Available at: http://cdc.gov/ncidod/diseases/hanta/hps/index.htm. Accessed February 25, 2009.

7. Gavrilovskaya IN, Shepley M, Shaw R, et al. beta3 Integrins mediate the cellular entry of hantaviruses that cause respiratory failure. Proc Natl Acad Sci U S A 1998;95(12):7074–9.
8. Spiropoulou CF, Goldsmith CS, Shoemaker TR, et al. Sin Nombre virus glycoprotein trafficking. Virology 2003;308(1):48–63.
9. Ravkov EV, Rollin PE, Ksiazek TG, et al. Genetic and serologic analysis of Black Creek Canal virus and its association with human disease and Sigmodon hispidus infection. Virology 1995;210(2):482–9.
10. Klempa B, Fichet-Calvet E, Lecompte E, et al. Hantavirus in African wood mouse, Guinea. Emerg Infect Dis 2006;12(5):838–40.
11. Lonner BN, Douglass RJ, Kuenzi AJ, et al. Seroprevalence against Sin Nombre virus in resident and dispersing deer mice. Vector Borne Zoonotic Dis 2008; 8(4):433–41.
12. Lopez N, Padula P, Rossi C, et al. Genetic identification of a new hantavirus causing severe pulmonary syndrome in Argentina. Virology 1996;220(1):223–6.
13. Bayard V, Kitsutani PT, Barria EO, et al. Outbreak of hantavirus pulmonary syndrome, Los Santos, Panama, 1999–2000. Emerg Infect Dis 2004;10(9): 1635–42.
14. Addressing emerging infectious disease threats: a prevention strategy for the United States. Executive summary. MMWR Recomm Rep 1994;43(RR-5): 1–18.
15. Douglass RJ, Semmens WJ, Matlock-Cooley SJ, et al. Deer mouse movements in peridomestic and sylvan settings in relation to Sin Nombre virus antibody prevalence. J Wildl Dis 2006;42(4):813–8.
16. Calisher CH, Mills JN, Sweeney WP, et al. Do unusual site-specific population dynamics of rodent reservoirs provide clues to the natural history of hantaviruses? J Wildl Dis 2001;37(2):280–8.
17. Armstrong LR, Zaki SR, Goldoft MJ, et al. Hantavirus pulmonary syndrome associated with entering or cleaning rarely used, rodent-infested structures. J Infect Dis 1995;172(4):1166.
18. Kuenzi AJ, Douglass RJ, White D Jr, et al. Antibody to sin nombre virus in rodents associated with peridomestic habitats in west central Montana. Am J Trop Med Hyg 2001;64(3–4):137–46.
19. Ramos MM, Overturf GD, Crowley MR, et al. Infection with Sin Nombre hantavirus: clinical presentation and outcome in children and adolescents. Pediatrics 2001;108(2):E27.
20. Enria D, Padula P, Segura EL, et al. Hantavirus pulmonary syndrome in Argentina. Possibility of person to person transmission. Medicina (B Aires) 1996;56(6): 709–11.
21. Padula PJ, Edelstein A, Miguel SD, et al. Hantavirus pulmonary syndrome outbreak in Argentina: molecular evidence for person-to-person transmission of Andes virus. Virology 1998;241(2):323–30.
22. Martinez VP, Bellomo C, San Juan J, et al. Person-to-person transmission of Andes virus. Emerg Infect Dis 2005;11(12):1848–53.
23. Auwaerter PG, Oldach D, Mundy LM, et al. Hantavirus serologies in patients hospitalized with community-acquired pneumonia. J Infect Dis 1996;173(1):237–9.
24. Vitek CR, Breiman RF, Ksiazek TG, et al. Evidence against person-to-person transmission of hantavirus to health care workers. Clin Infect Dis 1996;22(5): 824–6.
25. Ferrer JF, Galligan D, Esteban E, et al. Hantavirus infection in people inhabiting a highly endemic region of the Gran Chaco territory, Paraguay: association with

Trypanosoma cruzi infection, epidemiological features and haematological characteristics. Ann Trop Med Parasitol 2003;97(3):269–80.
26. Pini N. Hantavirus pulmonary syndrome in Latin America. Curr Opin Infect Dis 2004;17(5):427–31.
27. Levy H, Simpson SQ. Hantavirus pulmonary syndrome. Am J Respir Crit Care Med 1994;49(6):1710–3.
28. Hallin GW, Simpson SQ, Crowell RE, et al. Cardiopulmonary manifestations of hantavirus pulmonary syndrome. Crit Care Med 1996;24(2):252–8.
29. Baro M, Vergara J, Navarrete M. [Hantavirus in Chile: review and cases analysis since 1975]. Rev Med Chil 1999;127(12):1513–23 [in Spanish].
30. Cantoni G, Lazaro M, Resa A, et al. Hantavirus pulmonary syndrome in the Province of Rio Negro, Argentina, 1993–1996. Rev Inst Med Trop Sao Paulo 1997; 39(4):191–6.
31. Koster F, Foucar K, Hjelle B, et al. Rapid presumptive diagnosis of hantavirus cardiopulmonary syndrome by peripheral blood smear review. Am J Clin Pathol 2001;116(5):665–72.
32. Zaki SR, Greer PW, Coffield LM, et al. Hantavirus pulmonary syndrome. Pathogenesis of an emerging infectious disease. Am J Pathol 1995;146(3):552–79.
33. Nolte KB, Feddersen RM, Foucar K, et al. Hantavirus pulmonary syndrome in the United States: a pathological description of a disease caused by a new agent. Hum Pathol 1995;26(1):110–20.
34. Hjelle B, Goade D, Torrez-Martinez N, et al. Hantavirus pulmonary syndrome, renal insufficiency, and myositis associated with infection by Bayou hantavirus. Clin Infect Dis 1996;23(3):495–500.
35. Dara SI, Albright RC, Peters SG. Acute sin nombre hantavirus infection complicated by renal failure requiring hemodialysis. Mayo Clin Proc 2005;80(5): 703–4.
36. Peters CJ, Simpson GL, Levy H. Spectrum of hantavirus infection: hemorrhagic fever with renal syndrome and hantavirus pulmonary syndrome. Annu Rev Med 1999;50:531–45.
37. Centers for Disease Control and Prevention (CDC). Hantavirus pulmonary syndrome – Chile, 1997. MMWR Morb Mortal Wkly Rep 1997;46(40):949–51.
38. Castillo C, Naranjo J, Sepulveda A, et al. Hantavirus pulmonary syndrome due to Andes virus in Temuco, Chile: clinical experience with 16 adults. Chest 2001; 120(2):548–54.
39. Riquelme R, Riquelme M, Torres A, et al. Hantavirus pulmonary syndrome, southern Chile. Emerg Infect Dis 2003;9(11):1438–43.
40. Crowley MR, Katz RW, Kessler R, et al. Successful treatment of adults with severe Hantavirus pulmonary syndrome with extracorporeal membrane oxygenation. Crit Care Med 1998;26(2):409–14.
41. Dietl CA, Wernly JA, Pett SB, et al. Extracorporeal membrane oxygenation support improves survival of patients with severe Hantavirus cardiopulmonary syndrome. J Thorac Cardiovasc Surg 2008;135(3):579–84.
42. Ketai LH, Williamson MR, Telepak RJ, et al. Hantavirus pulmonary syndrome: radiographic findings in 16 patients. Radiology 1994;191(3):665–8.
43. Ketai LH, Kelsey CA, Jordan K, et al. Distinguishing hantavirus pulmonary syndrome from acute respiratory distress syndrome by chest radiography: are there different radiographic manifestations of increased alveolar permeability? J Thorac Imaging 1998;13(3):172–7.
44. Bustamante EA, Levy H, Simpson SQ. Pleural fluid characteristics in hantavirus pulmonary syndrome. Chest 1997;112(4):1133–6.

45. Bone RC, Fisher CJ Jr, Clemmer TP, et al. Sepsis syndrome: a valid clinical entity. Methylprednisolone Severe Sepsis Study Group. Crit Care Med 1989;17(5): 389–93.
46. Parker MM, Parrillo JE. Septic shock. Hemodynamics and pathogenesis. JAMA 1983;250(24):3324–7.
47. Parrillo JE. Pathogenetic mechanisms of septic shock. N Engl J Med 1993; 328(20):1471–7.
48. Parrillo JE, Burch C, Shelhamer JH, et al. A circulating myocardial depressant substance in humans with septic shock. Septic shock patients with a reduced ejection fraction have a circulating factor that depresses in vitro myocardial cell performance. J Clin Invest 1985;76(4):1539–53.
49. Lazaro ME, Resa AJ, Barclay CM, et al. [Hantavirus pulmonary syndrome in southern Argentina]. Medicina (B Aires) 2000;60(3):289–301 [in Spanish].
50. Saggioro FP, Rossi MA, Duarte MI, et al. Hantavirus infection induces a typical myocarditis that may be responsible for myocardial depression and shock in hantavirus pulmonary syndrome. J Infect Dis 2007;195(10):1541–9.
51. Hjelle B, Jenison S, Torrez-Martinez N, et al. Rapid and specific detection of Sin Nombre virus antibodies in patients with hantavirus pulmonary syndrome by a strip immunoblot assay suitable for field diagnosis. J Clin Microbiol 1997; 35(3):600–8.
52. Mertz GJ, Miedzinski L, Goade D, et al. Placebo-controlled, double-blind trial of intravenous ribavirin for the treatment of hantavirus cardiopulmonary syndrome in North America. Clin Infect Dis 2004;39(9):1307–13.
53. Ye C, Prescott J, Nofchissey R, et al. Neutralizing antibodies and Sin Nombre virus RNA after recovery from hantavirus cardiopulmonary syndrome. Emerg Infect Dis 2004;10(3):478–82.
54. Mills JN, Corneli A, Young JC, et al. Hantavirus pulmonary syndrome—United States: updated recommendations for risk reduction. Centers for disease control and prevention. MMWR Recomm Rep 2002;51(RR-9):1–12.
55. Peters CJ, Khan AS. Hantavirus pulmonary syndrome: the new American hemorrhagic fever. Clin Infect Dis 2002;34(9):1224–31.
56. Padula PJ, Edelstein A, Miguel SD, et al. [Epidemic outbreak of Hantavirus pulmonary syndrome in Argentina. Molecular evidence of person to person transmission of Andes virus]. Medicina (B Aires) 1998;58(Suppl 1):27–36 [in Spanish].
57. Toro J, Vega JD, Khan AS, et al. An outbreak of hantavirus pulmonary syndrome, Chile, 1997. Emerg Infect Dis 1998;4(4):687–94.
58. Kruger DH, Ulrich R, Lundkvist AA. Hantavirus infections and their prevention. Microbes Infect 2001;3(13):1129–44.
59. McClain DJ, Summers PL, Harrison SA, et al. Clinical evaluation of a vaccinia-vectored Hantaan virus vaccine. J Med Virol 2000;60(1):77–85.
60. Custer DM, Thompson E, Schmaljohn CS, et al. Active and passive vaccination against hantavirus pulmonary syndrome with Andes virus M genome segment-based DNA vaccine. J Virol 2003;77(18):9894–905.

Severe Acute Respiratory Syndrome (SARS)

Dennis J. Cleri, MD, FACP, FAAM, FIDSA[a,b,c,*],
Anthony J. Ricketti, MD, FCCP[a,b,c,d], John R. Vernaleo, MD, FACP[e]

KEYWORDS

- Acute respiratory distress syndrome (ARDS)
- Angiotensin-converting enzyme 2 (ACE-2)
- Chinese horseshoe bats (genus *Rhinolophus*)
- Himalayan (masked) palm civets (*Paguma larvata*)
- Severe acute respiratory syndrome coronavirus
- Superspreading events

To-morrow, and to-morrow, and to-morrow,
Creeps in this petty pace from day to day,
To the last syllable of recorded time;
And all our yesterdays have lighted fools
The way to dusty death. Out, out, brief candle!
Life's but a walking shadow
William Shakespeare, Macbeth

Disclaimer: The authors have indicated there is no funding in support of this document. Additionally, there are no other relationships that might pose a conflict of interest by any of the authors. None of the authors has any professional or financial relationships relevant to the subject matter in this paper. This manuscript and any tables or figures therein, have not been submitted to or are under consideration by any other publisher or publication.

[a] Internal Medicine Residency Program, St Francis Medical Center, 601 Hamilton Avenue, Trenton, NJ 08629, USA
[b] Seton Hall University School of Health and Medical Sciences, 400 South Orange Avenue, South Orange, NJ 07079, USA
[c] Department of Medicine, St Francis Medical Center, Room B-158, 601 Hamilton Avenue, Trenton, NJ 08629-1986, USA
[d] Section of Allergy and Immunology, St Francis Medical Center, 601 Hamilton Avenue, Trenton, NJ 08629, USA
[e] Division of Infectious Diseases, Wyckoff Heights Medical Center, 374 Stockholm Street, Brooklyn, New York 11237, USA
* Corresponding author. Department of Medicine, St Francis Medical Center, Room B-158, 601 Hamilton Avenue, Trenton, NJ 08629-1986.
E-mail address: dcleri@StFrancisMedical.org (D.J. Cleri).

Infect Dis Clin N Am 24 (2010) 175–202
doi:10.1016/j.idc.2009.10.005
id.theclinics.com

INTRODUCTION AND VIROLOGY

From November 2002 to July 2003, severe respiratory distress syndrome (SARS) quickly spread from Foshan (Shunde district), Guangdong Province in the People's Republic of China to 33 other countries or regions on 5 continents.[1–3] The details of the rapidity of the early epidemic are given by Lam and colleagues.[4] There were 8447 cases, 21% occurring in health care workers (HCWs), and 813 deaths (9.6% overall mortality) by the time SARS was contained in July 2003.[1,5–7] In the Hong Kong and Hanoi outbreaks, 46% and 63% of cases occurred in HCWs, respectively.[7] The case-fatality rate in 2003 was estimated at 13.2% for patients younger than 60 years and 50% for patients more than 60 years of age. Fifty percent of patients with acute respiratory distress syndrome (ARDS) died.[2,3,8] Laboratory-acquired cases resulted in transmission to family contacts.[2] A few patients were "superspreaders" of the virus.[3] In 1 hospital, exposure to a single patient resulted in infection in 138 patients and HCWs.[9] Two hundred fifty-two cases were reported in Canada (February 23 to June 12, 2003) and 29 cases were reported in the United States (February 24 to July 13, 2003).[1,3]

The pathogen, the human coronavirus (CoV) group 2b, SARS-CoV, is of animal origin.[10–12] The SARS-like-CoV (SL-CoV) virus from animal hosts has a nucleotide homology greater than 99% with SARS-CoV.[13] From virus sequence data, it seems that the masked (Himalayan) palm civet (*Paguma larvata*) acted as an amplification host. The epidemic strains (including SARS-Urbani) evolved because of civet-human interaction in Chinese animal markets.[14] Serologic evidence of natural SL-CoV infection is also found in the Chinese ferret-badger (*Melogale moschata*). SARS-CoV strains from the 2002 to 2003 outbreak (referred to as the "late human SARS-CoV" strains based on presumed evolutionary characteristics) differ from the strains from the 2003 to 2004 epidemic ("early human SARS-CoV" strains) in (1) spike protein genetic homogeneity, rate of nonsynonymous mutation, and binding affinity to angiotensin-converting enzyme 2 (ACE-2); (2) severity of disease; (3) epidemic potential; (4) transmission (animal/human-to-human, early strains (2003–2004 isolates); human-to-human, late strains (2002–2003 isolates)); and (5) the presence of a 415 nucleotide deletion in some of the late strains.[13]

There are 26 known species of CoV infecting 36 animal species.[10,15,16] In addition to SARS-CoV, 4 other human CoVs (HCoV-229E, HCoV-OC43, HCoV-NL63, HCoV-HKU1) cause illness. SL-CoV does not cause disease in humans. HCoV-NL63 and HCoV-HKU1 have a worldwide distribution, and cause respiratory tract infections, especially in the winter months.[17] A survey of nasopharyngeal swabs from patients with acute respiratory tract infections (Hong Kong, n = 4181), found 2.1% to be infected with 1 of these other (non-SARS-CoV) viruses.[11] In children (in France), these pathogens were isolated from 9.8% of respiratory specimens from hospitalized children and immunocompromised adults.[18,19]

Evidence that SARS-CoV is a new virus of animal origin is based on: (1) genetic sequencing; (2) retrospective human serologic studies finding no evidence of SARS-CoV or related viral infections; (3) during the 2002 to 2003 SARS epidemic, serologic surveys among market traders found a higher seroprevalence for antibodies against SARS-CoV or related viruses amongst animal traders than controls; (4) the earliest SARS cases lived near produce markets but not near farms, and almost half were food handlers with likely animal contact; and, (5) SARS-CoVs isolated from animals in markets were almost identical to human isolates.[20]

CoVs, named for their crownlike morphology, are 80 to 160 nm, positive-sense single stranded RNA viruses with helical nucleocapsids. They belong to the

Coronaviridae family of the Nidovirales order, and have the largest known RNA genome, increasing the likelihood of genetic variation.[10,21] In wild and domestic animals, CoVs cause mild to severe enteritis, respiratory, neurologic, and systemic disease.[21] In humans, they cause the common cold in addition to SARS (SARS-CoV).[10] Necrotizing enterocolitis in newborns has been associated with a CoV-like agent.[22] Animals and humans are infected by group 1 and 2 CoVs, and birds are infected by group 3.[10] Rodents and bats are also infected by CoVs. Group 2 CoVs include human CoVs (HCoV-OC43 and HCoV-HkU1), mouse hepatitis virus, rat CoV, bovine CoV, porcine hemaglutinating encephalomyelitis virus, equine CoV, and canine respiratory CoV.[10] Interspecies transmission of CoVs is well documented. Animals and birds may act as natural reservoirs for CoV-related diseases in domestic animals and humans. A study conducted by the US Centers for Disease Control and Prevention (CDC) found no evidence of SARS-CoV transmission from bats to humans among bat biologists who were "always" or "most of the time" (66%–68% of test subjects) exposed to bat blood, saliva, tissue, bites, or scratches.[23] The virology and pathogenesis of SARS-CoV are discussed by Weiss and Navas-Martin.[21]

SARS-CoV has been isolated from Himalayan (masked) palm civets (*Paguma larvata*), raccoon dogs (*Nyctereutes procyonides*), and Chinese ferret-badgers (*Melogale moschata*) in wild live markets in (Shenzhen) China.[6,12,20,24] More than 10 mammalian species are susceptible to SARS-CoV, including cynomolgus macaque (*Macaca facicularis*), rhesus macaque (*Macaca mulatta*), African green monkey (*Cercopithecus aethiops*), ferret (*Mustela furo*), golden hamster (*Mesocricetus auratus*), guinea pig (*Cavia porcellus*), mouse (*Mus musculus*), rat (*Rattus rattus*), domestic cat (*Felis domesticus*), and pig (*Sus scrofa*).[21]

The common marmoset is susceptible to SARS-CoV. It develops disease similar to human illness (pneumonia, hepatitis, mild colitis with watery diarrhea).[2]

SL-CoV has been isolated from Chinese horseshoe bat species (*Rhinolophus pearsoni*, *R macrotis*, *R pussilus*, and *R ferrumequinum*) and the cave-dwelling fruit bat (*Rousettus leschenault*).[5,7,12] Serologic or polymerase chain reaction (PCR) evidence of infection by closely related SARS-CoV viruses in bats found in Chinese provinces 1000 to 2000 km apart and in Hong Kong strongly suggest that bats are the natural reservoir. Other CoVs have been isolated from bat species from the People's Republic of China: *R sinicus*, *R pearsoni*, *R ferrumequinum*, *R macrotis*, *R ferrumequinum*, *Myotis ricketti*, *Miniopterus magnater*, *M pusillus*, *M schreibersii*, *Scolophlus kuhlii*, *Tylonycteris pachypus*, *Pipistrelius abramus*, *and P pipistrellus*.[20,25] In the United States (in wild and zoo-kept animals), CoVs have been isolated from bats (*Myotis occultus*, *Eptesicus fuscus*), sambar deer (*Cevus unicolor*), white-tailed deer (*Odocoileus virginianus*), waterbuck (*Kobus ellipsipyrmnus*), elk (*Cervus elephus*), caribou (*Rangifer tarandus*), sitatunga (*Tragelaphus spekei*), giraffe (*Giraffa camelopardalis*), and musk oxen (*Ovibus moschatus*).[10,23]

Bats are sold in the live markets in southern China for consumption and use in traditional medicine. No one has observed civets becoming ill from naturally occurring infection. However, when injected with SARS-CoV, they develop fever, lethargy, loss of aggressiveness, and decreased appetite. This result and there being no evidence of infection in wild and farmed civets make them an unlikely animal reservoir.[12,20]

The SL-CoV has greater genetic variation than SARS-CoV. Pteropid bats (flying foxes or fruit bats) are reservoirs for Hendra and Nipah viruses, which are emerging infections in Australia and Southeast Asia. In the henipaviruses, the bat-derived viruses have greater genetic diversity than the viruses isolated in the Nipah virus outbreaks in Malaysia and Bangladesh in 1999 and 2004.[12]

Bats tolerate these and other viral infections without any outward signs,[12,20] which suggests that civets became infected in the markets while captive in proximity to the bats.[26] The civet (a "naive" species) in turn infects man.[12]

Hamsters, guinea pigs, young mice (4–6 weeks old), rats, cats, and pigs remain asymptomatic when experimentally infected with SARS-CoV. Rats are a particular problem as they are ubiquitous. The only animal contact of the first human case in 2004 in Guangdong was rats. Birds are not susceptible to SARS-CoV infection.[20,21]

Of the 3 structural membrane proteins of SARS-CoV, the spike (S) protein has a 76% similarity with bat SL-CoV, and 78% similarity with civet CoV. The membrane (M) and envelope (E) proteins have 96% and 100% similarity, respectively. Variation in the S protein is believed to be responsible for host range, interspecies transmission, and adaptation.[21,24]

HISTORY

There are more things in heaven and earth, Horatio,
Than are dreamt of in your philosophy.
William Shakespeare, Hamlet

Dr Carlo Urbani of the World Health Organization (WHO) and President of the Italian branch of Médecins Sans Frontières first identified the disease in an American businessman hospitalized in Hanoi, Vietnam, in February 2003. WHO designated the new disease "SARS" on March 15, 2003. Dr Urbani died of SARS on March 29 that same year.[1,4] Most of the cases were reported from China (5327) and the Far East (Hong Kong: 1755; Taiwan: 678; and Singapore: 206).[1,3]

The pathogen, a novel CoV, was isolated in Vero-cell culture and detected by reverse transcriptase PCR (RT-PCR) from patients' respiratory secretions. The disease was reproduced by inoculation into cynomolgus macaques, and identified in these animals by negative-contrast electron microscopy and RT-PCR. The genome has been completely sequenced, and that analysis indicates that SARS-CoV is not closely related to any of the other 3 CoV groups.[1]

PATHOLOGY

At post mortem, the highest concentration of virus is found in the lungs and small bowel. This is probably related to the density of SARS-CoV receptors.[27] The alveolar epithelium has the highest intensity of infection followed by alveolar macrophages. There is little involvement of the bronchiolar epithelium, and no involvement of the bronchial epithelium or regional lymph nodes.[28] Other autopsy studies reveal little pathology in the upper respiratory tract, and no peribronchial or hilar adenopathy. There are limited serous pleural effusions, and pronounced pulmonary edema and consolidation.[28]

Histologically, there is diffuse alveolar damage, pulmonary edema, and hyaline membranes. Some areas reveal interstitial thickening. Some patients display intraalveolar organization of exudates and granulation tissue in the small airways, especially in the subpleural areas. Atypical pneumocytes, either multinucleated giant cells or cells with large atypical nuclei, are present in most patients. Vascular fibrin thrombi are common and often accompanied by pulmonary infarcts.[29] Some patients have evidence of bacterial (including methicillin-resistant *Staphylococcus aureus* and *Stenotrophomonas maltophilia*), fungal (*Aspergillus* and *Candida* species) or viral (cytomegalovirus) superinfections. Viral-like particles that represent viral nucleocapsids are seen in scanty pneumocytes.[9,29–31]

Spleen and lymph node histology reveals lymphocyte depletion, and white pulp atrophy in the spleen.[30]

Pathologic changes from biopsy or autopsy specimens from the gastrointestinal tract are minimal (mucosal lymphoid depletion), but evidence of viral replication is found in the small and large intestine.[30,32]

In patients who died with acute renal failure (ARF), pathology reveals acute tubular necrosis without glomerular disease.[33]

In the central nervous system, there was edema, and degeneration of neurons with evidence of viral infection. Bone marrow abnormalities, in some but not all patients, included hemophagocytosis. Necrosis and infiltration of the adrenal gland with monocytes and lymphocytes, destruction of follicular epithelial cells in the thyroid, germ cell destruction, and apoptotic spermatogenetic cells in the testes, and edema and atrophy of myocardial fibers were seen.[30] Myofiber degeneration with myofiber necrosis, macrophage infiltration, myofiber atrophy, and rare regenerative fibers were present. Necrotic fibers accumulated IgG, IgM, C3, and fibrinogen, but without other chronic inflammatory or lymphocytic infiltration.[34]

In animal models (cats and ferrets), ACE-2 and CD209L (also known as L-SIGN, a SARS-CoV binding receptor that mediates proteasome-dependent viral degradation and is expressed in cytokeratin$^+$ respiratory epithelia) are the SARS-CoV receptors in the respiratory tract, although ACE-2 is the most efficient.[2,35] SARS-CoV antigen expression and lesions developed in the respiratory tract of animals 4 days post inoculation. Diffuse alveolar damage associated with SARS-CoV antigen expression evolved in all infected animals. Cats developed a unique tracheobronchoadenitis. Antigen expression was seen in type I and II pneumocytes and serous cells of the tracheobronchial submucosal glands in cats, and serous epithelial cells and type II pneumocytes in ferrets. The difference between these animal models and humans is that humans develop syncytial and hyaline membranes.[35]

The renin-angiotensin system plays an important role in the pathogenesis of pulmonary hypertension and pulmonary fibrosis.[36] ACE cleaves angiotensin I, producing the peptide, angiotensin II. ACE-2 reduces angiotensin II levels. ACE-2 knockout mouse studies demonstrate that ACE-2 protects the animals from ARDS. SARS-CoV injections, and injections of SARS-CoV S protein reduces ACE-2 expression and worsens ARDS.[37,38]

ACE-2 is highly expressed in the enterocytes of the small intestine, and this organ becomes infected with SARS-CoV. In other organs, cell types without ACE-2 expression may become infected. Some endothelial cells, which express ACE-2 to a high level, do not become infected.[39]

Another postulated pathologic mechanism is that human long interspersed nuclear element 1 endonuclease domain protein seems to be the target of SARS-associated autoantibodies. These antibodies were found in 40.9% of patients with SARS.[40]

On presentation, virus may be detected in patients by RT-PCR in nasopharyngeal aspirates (80%), stool (84.4%), and urine (33.3%). All 3 sites were positive in 28.9% of patients, and 40% of patients remained positive (at least at 1 site) on discharge.[41] Shedding peaks 10 days after the onset of symptoms.[42] Patients do not stop shedding for another 13 days (range 2–60 days). The median time to becoming RT-PCR negative was 30 days (range 2–81 days).[41]

The virus survives drying on inanimate surfaces for as long as 6 days.[43] It is inactivated by 500 ppm hypochlorite (laundry bleach), exposure for 5 minutes or less to 75% ethanol, and household detergents. Disinfection of waste systems, elimination of rodents and cockroaches, and care in garbage disposal are all considered important in preventing infection.[5,43–47] Standard disinfectants or detergent disinfectants approved by the Environmental Protection Agency are recommended for decontamination (see Centers for Disease Control and Prevention – public health guidance for community-level preparedness and response to severe acute respiratory syndrome [SARS]. Version 2. Available at: http://www.cdc.gov/ncidod/sars/guidance/I/pdf/healthcare.pdf).[46]

Disease containment is problematic. Virus was found in 97% of fecal samples from the Amoy Gardens outbreak, yet no rectal swabs were positive in hospital-acquired SARS cases in a Taiwan hospital. This was attributed to nosocomial respiratory spread.[48]

Preventing spread of SARS-CoV is made difficult by: (1) the potential spread by fomites, and conversion from droplet to airborne transmission[49]; (2) an incubation period averaging 6.4 days (usually 2–10 days; Hong Kong and Toronto 4.7 days,[50] but it may be as long as 16 days); (3) 3 to 5 days between disease onset and hospitalization; (4) the absence of specific symptoms; (5) often presenting as atypical (community-acquired) pneumonia[51]; (6) the lack of a reliable diagnostic test for early disease, putting HCWs at particular risk; (7) atypical presentations including diarrhea and bloody diarrhea without respiratory symptoms; and (8) early diagnosis depending solely on exposure to SARS or travel through epidemic or endemic areas.[3,5,52–55] This makes SARS-CoV an ideal agent for terrorists.

HUMAN EPIDEMIOLOGY

There were 2 major SARS outbreaks: (1) the early outbreak originating in Guangdong province in late 2002 (to early 2003); (2) isolated clusters in Taiwan, Singapore, and mainland China from the accidental release of the virus in 2003; and (3) a second outbreak beginning in late 2003 to early 2004, again reported from Guangdong province, in individuals with animal contacts with different SARS-CoV strains.[13] Molecular studies separated the human SARS-CoV isolated into early, middle, and late phase outbreak viruses. Human SARS-CoV isolates from 2003 to 2004 (sporadic cases from the same area of China) were more closely related to animal isolates than human isolates from 2002 to 2003 (the "pandemic" outbreak). This finding suggested "an independent species-crossing" event.[13]

Excluding "superspreading events" (SSEs), SARS-CoV has a calculated base-case reproduction number (R_0) of 2 to 4.[5] Attack rates range from 10.3% to 60%, with a risk of 2.4 to 31.3 cases/1000 exposure-hours.[3] SSEs include patients excreting high titers of virus, aerosol generation, contamination of the environment (fomites), and close contact in health care settings. These instances have resulted in as many as 300 infections from a single patient. SSEs have occurred in a hotel in Hong Kong, health care facilities in Hong Kong, Beijing, Singapore, and Toronto, and an air flight from Hong Kong to Beijing.[5,52]

In the Amoy Gardens high-rise apartments (Hong Kong), more than 300 residents developed SARS-CoV infections.[56] High concentrations of SARS-CoV were found in indoor aerosols originating from the plumbing in the building. Virus can survive 14 days in sewage at 4°C, and 2 days at 20°C.[57] The aerosols entered the apartments through bathroom drains, infecting the inhabitants, and were subsequently blown by prevailing winds and contaminated other buildings.[56,58] Meteorologic factors (ambient winds, low mixing heights preventing dispersion of aerosols, and a decrease in temperature enabling the virus to survive for longer periods) are believed to have played a crucial role in the outbreak.[1,59] A positive association (although not cause and effect) between air pollution and SARS case-fatality rates exists.[60,61]

Nasopharyngeal swab SARS-CoV concentrations were directly related to the distance from the index case. Individuals (45% of patients) in adjacent units on the same block (Amoy Gardens Block E) as the index case had higher viral concentrations than those living further away (55% of patients living within 6 blocks), suggesting airborne spread.[56,62] The possibility of rodents and fomites playing a role could not be excluded.[62]

Other factors that contribute to nosocomial contagion include: (1) 1 m or less between beds; (2) lack of hand-washing facilities; (3) lack of changing facilities for the staff; (4) resuscitation performed on the ward; (5) HCWs working while symptomatic; (6) patients requiring oxygen therapy; and (7) patients requiring positive airway pressure ventilation. Viral loads might be high and shedding prolonged in immunocompromised patients. In addition, airflows around oxygen masks disseminate potentially infectious particles up to 0.4 m.[5,63] Use of a closed oxygen delivery mask with a respiratory filter can prevent droplet dispersal without increased positive pressure or end-tidal CO_2.[64]

Recommendations for containing the spread of disease include: (1) hand washing; (2) appropriate well-fitted facemasks; (3) isolation (airborne precautions); and (4) quarantine of asymptomatic contacts, thus significantly decreasing the time from onset of disease to isolation.[5] The application of infection control procedures in Singapore resulted in a significant drop in the R_0 (week 1, $R_0 = 7$; week 2, $R_0 = 1.6$; after week 2, $R_0<1$).[5]

HCWs remained at significant risk after initiation of infection control precautions. In Toronto, risk factors included performance of high-risk patient care procedures, inconsistent use of personal protective equipment, fatigue, and lack of adequate training. In this group of HCWs, 47% wore jewelry, 27% ate meals on the unit where they worked, and only 60% received any formal training. All HCWs interviewed indicated that they visited at least once the room of a patient with SARS who was not wearing a mask. Masks were not fit-tested until late in the outbreak. Forty percent reused items (stethoscopes, goggles, and cleaning equipment) elsewhere on the ward, and about one-third of HCWs assisted in endotracheal intubation of a patient with SARS.[65] There is evidence that SARS-CoV was transmitted to HCWs during cardiopulmonary resuscitation.[66]

Simulations based on stochastic susceptible-infected-recovered dynamics of hospital social networks predict that HCWs, particularly physicians, are the principle vector of disease. This model suggests that control of outbreaks could be achieved more effectively by (1) restricting physician visits to different hospital units (wards) and (2) vaccinating physicians and individuals with widespread contacts as a priority (when a vaccine becomes available).[67]

Another study screened asymptomatic HCWs' nasopharyngeal swabs with a more sensitive second-nested RT-PCR. This test can detect less than 800 copies of RNA/mm^3. These individuals were considered "first line...well protected" HCWs caring for patients infected with SARS-CoV. They all employed gloves, gowns, goggles, and N-95 masks. Second-nested RT-PCR assays (for SARS-CoV) were positive in 11.5% of these HCWs. No asymptomatic HCW became seropositive despite being RT-PCR positive. Those HCWs with positive second-nested RT-PCR were either required to stay at home or in central accommodation for 3 days before follow-up testing. Second and third tests were always negative. These investigators additionally recommended addition of regular nasopharyngeal swab screening to daily recording of temperature for all first-line HCWs.[7]

In Toronto, there were 358 cases, 2132 investigations, and 23,103 contacts that required health department attention. Only 13,291 of the contacts complied with quarantine recommendations, 8058 were not contacted until after the quarantine period, and 1754 could not be contacted. SARS-CoV transmission was limited to nosocomial and household spread. Health departments should expect to quarantine 100 contacts and investigate 8 possible cases for each case of SARS that meets the epidemiologic criteria.[50]

CLINICAL PRESENTATIONS

The WHO case definition for probable SARS includes: (1) fever greater than 38°C or history of fever in the preceding 48 hours; (2) new infiltrates on chest radiograph consistent with pneumonia; (3) chills or cough or malaise or myalgia or history of exposure; and (4) 1 or more positive tests for SARS-CoV.[4] Statistical analysis using "frequentistic" and Bayesian approaches when applied to SARS show that border (ie, airport) entry screening with a diagnostic test is rarely an efficacious method for preventing importation of a disease into a country.[68] Resources should be placed at entry points into the health care system and not international borders.[53]

Most patients present with flulike symptoms (fever, chills, cough, and malaise). Most patients (70%) develop dyspnea, and recurrent or persistent fever. Thirty percent significantly improve within 1 week. Mortality is 6.8% in patients less than 60 years old, and 43% in older patients. Male sex and comorbid conditions (eg, diabetes, hyperglycemia independent of diabetes, chronic hepatitis) increase mortality.[30,54,69] Overall, patients with and without comorbid conditions have 46% and 10% mortality, respectively.[30] Advanced age, high admission neutrophil count, and initial elevated lactic dehydrogenase (LDH) are independent correlates of an adverse outcome.[54]

During the first week (March 6–16th) of the 2003 Hong Kong SARS epidemic, there was an outbreak of human metapneumovirus (hMPV). hMPV RNA was detected in 20% of nasopharyngeal aspirates of SARS patients. HCWs and epidemiologic association with the SARS unit were risk factors for the hMPV infection. Coinfected patients had more cough (22.6%) and coryza (15.9%), but this was not statistically significant. Severity of illness and outcomes did not differ among those solely infected with SARS-CoV and those infected with both viruses.[70]

Table 1 enumerates clinical presentations.[3,4,7,32,48,51,52,71–75]

Table 2 describes the laboratory findings.[4,51,74,76,77]

Watery diarrhea is part of the initial presentation in approximately 20% of patients. In the outbreak at Amoy Gardens, Hong Kong, 73% of patients developed diarrhea with positive RT-PCR for SARS-CoV in 97% of their stool samples.[48,71] Cumulatively, 38.4% of patients develop a self-limited watery diarrhea (mean: 3.7 ± 2.7 days' duration) some time during their illness.[32,71] In HCWs who were believed to have acquired SARS by the respiratory route, 18.8% to 19.6% developed diarrhea. In 1 study, none of the HCWs had positive rectal swabs for SARS-CoV (by RT-PCR).[48]

Some contacts of SARS patients have been asymptomatically infected.[78] The most frequent symptom is fever higher than 38°C for more than 24 hours. Other symptoms vary and are nonspecific. They include sore throat, myalgia, and nausea. In up to 21% of patients, the initial chest radiographs may be normal.[77]

Pregnancy

Infants born to pregnant women with SARS did not seem to acquire the infection by vertical transmission.[79] In 1 study, there were 3 deaths among 12 pregnant women (25% mortality). In another study, 4 of 10 patients required intubation compared

Table 1
SARS-CoV infection signs and symptoms in patients at presentation

Signs and Symptoms	Frequency (Results Reported from Multiple Centers) — Adult Cases	Pediatric Cases (5.5 Months to 18 Years)
Asymptomatic viral colonization	11.5% of "well protected" first-line HCWs who did not seroconvert or later develop disease	
Fever	99%–100%	98%–100%
Chills or rigors	55%–90%	14.5% (rigor: 8.1%)
Cough (productive/ nonproductive)	43%–100%	60%–62.9%
Shortness of breath	10%–80%	
Myalgia	20–60.9%	17.7%
Malaise/lethargy	35%–70%	6.5%
Headache	11%–70%	11.3%
Sputum production	10%–29%	
Sore throat	23.2%–30%	9.7% (independent predictor of severe disease)
Coryza	22.5% (not reported in all studies)	22.6%
Nausea or vomiting	10%–19.6%	41%
Diarrhea	11%–15% Fever and diarrhea, sometimes bloody diarrhea without respiratory symptoms at presentation.[46] Other studies have found 20.3% have watery diarrhea on presentation and 38.4% develop a self-limited diarrhea (most frequently in the first week) some time during the illness.[30] In the community outbreak in Amoy Gardens, Hong Kong, 73% of 75 patients had watery diarrhea and 97% had positive stools.[65,73] Hospital-acquired SARS less frequently presents with diarrhea (18.8%)[73]	

Data from Refs.[3,4,7,32,48,51,52,71–75]

with 12.5% of nonpregnant patients.[80] Four of 7 patients (57%) in the first trimester had spontaneous miscarriages, and 4 or 5 patients who became ill after 24 weeks' gestation delivered prematurely. Two pregnant women recovered and carried their babies to term, but the pregnancies were complicated by intrauterine growth restriction. No newborn presented with clinical SARS or had evidence of SARS-CoV infection (examining cord blood, placenta, and follow-up neonatal serology).[81]

Table 2
SARS-CoV infection: radiologic and laboratory findings in adult patients at presentation

Radiologic and Laboratory Findings	Frequency
Abnormal chest radiograph	78.3%–100% (One report: 35.5% of children have normal chest radiographs at presentation. Another report indicates 97% of children had abnormal chest radiographs)
Of those with abnormal chest radiographs	
Unilateral focal disease	56.4%
Progressive disease	90%
Detection of infiltrates by CT scan of:	
87% positive chest radiograph:	13% detected by chest CT scan
96% positive chest radiographs:	4% detected by chest CT scan
Anemia	Decrease in hemoglobin by 2 g/dL: 49% Hemolysis: 76%
Lymphopenia	69.6%–90% Wong et al[71] reported 98% developed lymphopenia (absolute counts <1000/mm^3)
CD4 and CD8 lymphocyte counts	Decreases during the early course of disease. Low CD4 and CD8 counts at presentation a poor prognostic sign (associated with admission to the ICU or death)
Leukopenia	22–34.1% Wong et al[71] documented transient leukopenia in 64% of patients during the first week (WBC <4.0 × 10^6/dL). 2.5% developed transient neutropenia (absolute count <0.5 × 10^6/dL)
Leukocytosis	61% of patients in second and third week of illness (WBC >11.0 × 10^6/dL).[30] Elevated absolute neutrophil count an independent predictor of an adverse outcome.
Thrombocytopenia	33%–44% (1 study reported thrombocytopenia to be mild and self-limited: platelet counts <40,000/mm^3). 2.5% with platelet counts <50,000/mm^3[71]
Hyponatremia	20.3%–60%
Hypokalemia	25.2%–47%
Hypocalcemia	60%
Increased ALT	23.4%–56%
Increased LDH	47%–87% High peak LDH independent predictor of an adverse outcome
Increased CPK	19%–56%
Prolonged activated partial thromboplastin time	18%–42.8%
Increased D-dimer	45% (reported from 1 center)

Data from Refs.[4,51,74,76,77]

Neonatal Disease

Of the 5 infants born to mothers with SARS, no infant had laboratory or clinical evidence of infection. Four of the 5 infants were born prematurely (28 weeks, 26 weeks, 32 weeks, 33 weeks, and 37 weeks). One infant developed necrotizing enterocolitis and ileal perforation, and another developed a perforation of the jejunum. The mother of the infant with necrotizing enterocolitis died 14 days after delivery.[82]

Pediatric Disease

Between February and June 2003, an outbreak of SARS occurred in Toronto, Canada. Children with potential exposure to SARS were classified as suspect SARS if they developed symptoms within 10 days of exposure, and probable SARS if the chest radiograph revealed lower respiratory tract disease.

Clinical disease manifestations included the following: fever higher than 38°C (70% of probable and 100% of suspect); respiratory symptoms (80% of probable and 60% of suspect); and headache, lethargy, vomiting, and diarrhea in a minority of patients. No children exhibited irritability or myalgia. Focal minor alveolar infiltrates were seen in 8 of 10 probable cases, and single cases of progressive lower lobe infiltrates, and perihilar peribronchial thickening. The patient with the bilateral infiltrates, a 17-year-old girl, developed respiratory distress and required supplemental oxygen. Nine children received intravenous ribavirin and 1 child received intravenous and aerosolized ribavirin. The clinical course for most children was described as "mild and brief."[1] There is only 1 published report of transmission of SARS-CoV from a pediatric patient with SARS.[73] In some children, exercise impairment and radiologic abnormalities persisted 6 months after diagnosis.[83] Thin-section computed tomography (CT) abnormalities have persisted in 32% of children up to 12 months after diagnosis, but were most often minor.[84]

The most common laboratory finding was lymphopenia. Some, but not all children exhibited neutropenia, mild thrombocytopenia, elevated liver enzymes (aspartate transaminase, alanine transaminase [ALT], and LDH), and elevated creatine phosphokinase (CPK) (1 case).[1]

Two to 3 months after the onset of illness, ~40% of children reported a self-limited thinning and shedding of hair (telogen effluvium).[75]

Patients on Dialysis

Patients on dialysis have a higher risk for acquiring SARS. They display the same typical symptoms (fever, myalgia, chills, rigors, gastrointestinal symptoms), but these are less severe. Although these patients sought medical attention at later stages of disease, the changes in their chest radiographs tended to be less severe than in patients not on dialysis (17% vs 45% with bilateral or multifocal changes). Patients on dialysis shed virus for longer periods, have greater transfusion requirements, require longer hospitalization, but have similar mortality compared with the control group.[85]

Mild or Subclinical Disease

In 1 study, 6 of 910 patients suspected of SARS-CoV infection and managed as outpatients had serologic evidence of infection. Five patients had normal chest radiographs and 2 patients had no symptoms. Those with symptoms complained of myalgia, fever, cough, and chills. However, more than half of these patients did not have follow-up serology.

Serologic testing of asymptomatic close contacts (1068 individuals) found 2 (0.19%) with IgG SARS-CoV antibodies. None of 29 household contacts of 13 SARS patients showed serologic evidence of infection. In another study, 1 symptomatic household contact was identified, but that individual had traveled to a SARS-"endemic" area. The investigators conclude that few individuals have mild or subclinical disease.[86–89]

COMPLICATIONS

HLA-B* 4601 haplotype (Taiwanese patients), HLA-B*0703 and HLA-DRB1*0301 (Hong Kong Chinese patients) alleles, low or deficient mannose binding lectin serum levels, and increased expression of the IP-10 gene (increased IP-10 concentrations) seem to be risk factors for SARS.[30,90] Liver/lymph node specific intercellular adhesion molecule 3 (ICAM3)-grabbing nonintegrin homozygotic individuals (L-SIGN or *CLEC4M*) have a lower risk.[30,91] In Hong Kong Chinese patients, interferon gamma (IFN-γ) +874 AA and IFN-$_{\gamma}$ AT genotypes were associated with a 5.19- and 2.57-fold increased risk of developing SARS.[91] Excessive induction of proinflammatory cytokines and chemokines, and recruitment of immune cells are postulated as the mechanisms for the most serious lung injury.[30,90]

Respiratory Complications

Patients discharged after SARS-CoV infection frequently have abnormal chest radiographs (15 of 24 patients). These abnormalities include patchy opacification, and volume loss. Abnormalities persisted in 15 of 25 patients 18 days after discharge. Opacifications and volume loss remained unchanged in 5 patients. CT studies of these patients revealed that 62% developed pulmonary fibrosis. Those who developed CT evidence of pulmonary fibrosis were older (mean age 45 vs 30.3 years), men (8:7 male/female ratio), were more often admitted to the intensive care unit (ICU) (26.6% vs 11.1%), had higher peak LDH levels (438.9 U/L vs 355.6 U/L), more often required pulsed steroid therapy, had more radiographic opacification, and more abnormal segments on thin-section CT.[92]

CT findings (at $\sim$52 $\pm$ 20 days) revealed air trapping (92%), ground glass opacities (90%), reticulation (70%), parenchymal bands (55%), bronchiectasis (18%), consolidation (10%), and honeycombing (8%). A second CT (at $\sim$141 $\pm$ 27 days) demonstrated resolution of ground glass and interstitial opacities, but air trapping persisted.[93]

The incidence of spontaneous pneumothorax (in nonventilated patients) is 1.7%. In half of these patients, the pneumothorax was bilateral. In 1 study, all patients had higher LDH levels, and all had received steroids.[94] In patients receiving mechanical ventilation, 14% developed pneumomediastinum with subcutaneous emphysema, and 24% developed a pneumothorax.[9]

Cardiovascular Complications

Cardiovascular complications were seen in most patients. Overall, 50.4% of the patients became hypotensive (28.1% in week 1; 21.5% in week 2; and, 14.8% in week 3). Tachycardia that could not be explained because of either fever or hypotension was present in 71.9% of patients (62.8% in week 1; 45.4% in week 2; and, 35.5% in week 3). Tachycardia was weakly associated with steroid therapy during the second and third weeks of illness, and persisted at follow-up in 38.8% of patients. Transient bradycardia was seen in 14.9% of patients. Reversible cardiomegaly without heart failure occurred in 10.7% of patients. Transient atrial fibrillation was seen in 1 patient.[95]

ARF

ARF occurred in 17% of patients admitted with probable SARS.[96] Most of the patients were men (77%), older, and more often had underlying illnesses (diabetes: 38% vs 6%, $P<.01$; and, heart failure: 38% vs 2%, $P<.001$). There was an increased incidence of respiratory failure (85% vs 26%, $P<.001$) and death (77% vs 8%, $P<.001$).[96]

In patients who initially had normal serum creatinines, the incidence of ARF was 6.7%, occurring 5 to 48 days into their illness (median 20 days). In this study, 91.7% of the patients died (vs 8.8% of patients without ARF: $P<.0001$).[33]

Complicating the ARF were hypotension (77%) from sepsis, gastrointestinal bleed, ARDS, and rhabdomyolysis (10%–43%).[96,97] In 1 study, 2 of the 3 patients with rhabdomyolysis died with multiple organ failure.[97]

Osteonecrosis

Joint pain is a common complaint after SARS-CoV infection. Osteonecrosis of the hip and knee is a risk for patients receiving steroid therapy. The risk for this complication for low total dose steroid therapy was 0.6%. For higher total dose steroid therapy and for therapy for more than 18 days, the risk is 9.9% to 13%.[98,99] Tumor necrosis factor α polymorphisms of promoter region (1031CT/CC and -863 AC genotypes) are not associated with susceptibility to SARS-CoV infection or the risk of interstitial lung fibrosis, but do represent risk factors for femoral head necrosis.[100] Bone density is reduced in patients receiving steroid therapy.[101] Bone resorption and formation biochemical tests cannot predict the development of this complication.[99]

Bacterial and Fungal Superinfection

Bacterial and fungal superinfection, related to prolonged duration of illness, prolonged ventilator support, and high-dose steroid therapy have been reported. These infections include *Aspergillus* species, *Mucor* species, *Pseudomonas aeruginosa*, *Klebsiella* species, methicillin-resistant *Staphylococcus aureus*, α-hemolytic *Streptococcus* species, and cytomegalovirus.[30]

Endocrine

Hypocortisolism is found in 39.3% of survivors of SARS-CoV infection. A few patients (3.3%) with hypocortisolism had transient subclinical thyrotoxicosis. Almost 7% were biochemically either centrally or primarily hypothyroid. Most hypothalamic-pituitary-adrenal axis abnormalities returned to normal within 1 year.[102]

Hepatitis

Reactive hepatitis is a common finding in 24% of patients having elevated ALT on admission, and up to 69% developing ALT elevation during the course of their illness. Concomitant hepatitis B was not associated with an adverse clinical outcome, but severe hepatitis was.[103] Liver damage seems to be directly caused by SARS-CoV rather than hypoxia.[104]

Psychiatric Complications

Psychiatric complications that significantly and negatively affected the quality of life have been seen in other survivors of ARDS. After intensive care treatment, 17% to 43% of patients suffered at least once from clinically significant psychiatric symptoms (point prevalence). Posttraumatic stress disorder (PTSD) was diagnosed in 21% to 35% of patients, and nonspecific anxiety in 23% to 48% of patients. Prevalence of PTSD at hospital discharge, and 5 and 8 years later, were 44%, 25%, and 24%, respectively. PTSD and depression were associated with longer length of stay in the ICU and longer duration of mechanical ventilation and sedation.[105]

PTSD was diagnosed in Toronto residents who were quarantined in 28.9% of respondents to a voluntary survey. The presence of PTSD correlated with depressive symptoms (31.2%) and duration of quarantine.[106]

HCWs were more likely to suffer from PTSD if there was: (1) a perception of risk to themselves; (2) a significant impact on their work routines; (3) a depressive affect; and (4) assignment to a high-risk unit. HCWs caring for more than 1 patient with SARS experienced less PTSD.[107]

RADIOLOGY

Approximately one-fifth of patients presented with a normal chest radiograph, but developed infiltrates within 7 days (median 3 days) of onset of fever.[77] Of the 78.3% who presented with opacities on the chest radiographs, 54.6% were unilateral and the remainder were bilateral. The mean parenchymal involvement was 5% (range 1%–63% opacification). Radiographic changes appeared to peak at 8.6 days, which corresponded approximately to the initial treatment with steroids.[77]

The involvement of more than 1 lung zone and bilateral versus unilateral disease were associated with a higher risk of ICU admission and death.[77] Patients who died were older (56.9 ± 17.2 years vs 40.4 ± 16.6 years, P = .002), and had a higher frequency of comorbid conditions.[108] Abnormalities on thin-section CT in adults improved with time. Extent and persistence of the findings correlated with advanced age, severity of the disease, and diffusion capacity adjusted for hemoglobin.[109]

In children, SARS cannot be distinguished from other forms of viral pneumonia.[110] One report indicates that 35% of children present with normal chest radiographs. The most common chest radiograph finding was consolidation (45.2%), sometimes with peripheral multifocal disease (22.6%), peribronchial thickening (14.5%), and rarely pleural effusion. Interstitial disease was not observed. In another report, 97% of cases had abnormal chest radiographs.[72,73]

LABORATORY TESTING

Sensitivity of RT-PCR collected in the first 3 days of the illness is inadequate. The 6-item clinical score for emergency room triage during a SARS outbreak of febrile patients, most of whom were otherwise healthy, seems to be 92.6% sensitive and 71.2% specific. These figures were generated in a noninfluenza season.[5] A promising RT-PCR is under development to detect viremic blood donor samples early in the symptomatic disease.[111]

Confirmation of infection is made by identifying the SARS-CoV nucleocapsid (N) protein in the serum by N antigen-capture enzyme-linked immunosorbent assay (ELISA) and N antigen-capture chemiluminescent immunoassay. Serology can be accomplished by commercially available indirect ELISA kit, and indirect immunofluorescent assay (IFA).[78] ELISA and IFA results nearly always tend to be in agreement. Serology is positive in 8.3% of patients in the first 2 weeks. Paired serology was positive in 96.2% of patients in whom RT-PCR was positive in 64% of the same patients.[112] SARS-CoV patients' serums falsely cross-react by ELISA and Western blot for human T-lymphotropic virus (HTLV-1 and HTLV-II).[113]

Viral cultures are performed in African green monkey Vero E6 cell monolayers. Confirmation is by RT-PCR.[114] RNA amplification by real-time nucleic acid sequence-based amplification seems to be at least as sensitive as RT-PCR.[115]

During the first 2 weeks of illness, RT-PCR has a diagnostic yield for tracheal aspirates of 66.7%, and 56.5% for stool.[114] Pooled throat and nasal swabs, rectal swab, nasal swab, throat swab, and nasopharyngeal aspirate had yields from 29.7% to 40% for the first 2 weeks of illness. Throat washing and urine had lower yields (17.3% and 4.5%, respectively). Viral cultures had lower yields, and no specimens were positive by culture that were negative by RT-PCR.[114]

In the first 4 to 5 days of illness, it seems that nasopharyngeal aspirates and throat swabs are more useful in detecting virus, whereas stool specimens are more valuable after 5 days of illness (20% sensitivity). Urine samples are of little or no use. Clinical specimens remain stable at 4°C or −70°C for weeks and may be stored for later testing.[116]

RT-PCR can detect SARS-CoV after 30 days in respiratory secretions, stool, and urine in some patients, but virus cannot be isolated by culture after 3 weeks.[116] Quantitative RT-PCR (RTq-PCR) used to measure the viral load in nasopharyngeal aspirates (obtained from day 10–15 after the onset of symptoms) correlated with oxygen desaturation, the need for mechanical ventilation, diarrhea, abnormal liver function studies, and death. Serum RTq-PCR is predictive of oxygen desaturation, the need for mechanical ventilation, and death. Stool viral load is associated with diarrhea, and urine viral load correlates with abnormal urine analysis.[117]

Nasopharyngeal viral loads tend to peak at day 10 and decrease to less than initial levels by day 15. It seems, however, that the worsening of the clinical condition in week 2 is not directly related to viral replication but more to the immunopathology of the infection.[71] The applications of surface-enhanced laser desorption/ionization (SELDI) ProteinChip technology producing proteomic fingerprints examined more than 800 common proteomic features. SELDI found that 95% of SARS patients had similar serum proteomic profiles. For specific proteomic features, sensitivity and specificity ranged from 95% to 97% and 97% to 100%, respectively. Combining all the biomarkers produced a SARS-specific fingerprint. Immunoglobulin κ light chain presence correlated with SARS-CoV viral load and seems to be helpful in diagnosing the infection.[118] Serum amyloid protein levels detected by SELDI, peptide mapping, and tandem mass spectrometric analysis correlated with the extent of pneumonia on serial chest radiographs.[119]

Monoclonal antibody has been used to identify viral infection by immunofluorescence staining, Western blot, or immunohistology.[120]

Immune Response

Antibodies develop late in the first week after the onset of symptoms. Specific IgG antibodies (seroconversion) are found in more than 95% of patients by day 25. $CD4^+$ and $CD8^+$ cells are stimulated to produce antibody and kill infected cells, respectively. Proinflammatory cytokines released by activated macrophages are believed to contribute to local inflammation and contribute to SARS pathology.[121]

Laboratory and Autopsy

All specimens from suspected SARS patients must be handled using biosafety laboratory level 3 (BSL-3) practices in a BSL-2 facility. These specimens should be stored in a secure place using BSL-3 precautions with strict access control, inventorying of specimens, and the inventory audited at frequent intervals. Unneeded specimens should be sterilized and discarded according to BSL-3 protocols. All personnel should be appropriately trained for BSL-3 precautions, retrained at designated intervals, drills conducted, and laboratory procedures audited on a regular basis.[47]

In community hospitals, generally the acid-fast bacilli room, a closed separate negative-pressure room with a biologic safety hood vented through a high efficiency particulate air (HEPA) filter may be adapted for handling these specimens. Viral isolation and cultures must never be attempted in these facilities, and are permitted only in a BSL-3 facility.

Postmortem examinations on SARS patients should be undertaken only in a specially designed BSL-3 laboratory. This facility should be physically separated from the rest of the health care facility; it should be divided into 5 sections (a clean area, a semi-contaminated area, a contaminated area, and 2 buffer zones); it should be 2 ventilation systems separate from the remainder of the building; laminar flow should be from clean areas to progressively contaminated areas; negative pressures should be from clean, semi-contaminated to contaminated areas with pressure gradients; and there should be no tap water or sewage system. Use of personal protective equipment must be strictly adhered to. The mortuary must be adjacent to the buffer zone next to the contaminated (autopsy) room, and a downdraft table ventilation system with HEPA filtration must be employed.[122] Details are described in Ref.[122] and in Refs.[2–5] therein.

DIFFERENTIAL DIAGNOSIS

Bacterial community-acquired pneumonias that may result in ARDS and mistaken for SARS-CoV infection include *Streptococcus pneumonia*, *Haemophilus influenzae*, *Moraxella catarrhalis*, community-associated methicillin-resistant *Staphylococcus aureus*, and atypical pneumonias (eg, *Legionella* species).[55] The differential diagnosis of viruses that commonly cause ARDS with fever includes seasonal influenza (A or B), parainfluenza virus, avian influenza, respiratory syncytial virus, adenovirus, varicella, hMPV, and hantavirus.[55,123] Other organisms likely to require “mass” critical care, have the potential to spread disease to HCWs, and result in an extensive community epidemic with high morbidity and mortality are smallpox, viral hemorrhagic fever, plague, tularemia, and anthrax.[55]

TREATMENT AND PREVENTION

Eye of newt, and toe of frog,
Wool of bat, and tongue of dog,
Adder's fork, and blind-worm's sting,
Lizard's leg, and howlet's wing,–
For a charm of powerful trouble,
Like a hell-broth boil and bubble.
William Shakespeare, Macbeth

Aerosolized SARS-CoV viral droplets are 0.1 to 0.2 μm (as opposed to the 4- to 8-μm droplets produced by coughing, sneezing or talking). SARS-CoV remains viable for several days at normal ambient room temperatures and humidity. Suspect patients must be immediately isolated using contact, droplet, and airborne isolation precautions in a negative-pressure single room.[55,124] In 1 study, no virus was detected in the air from the negative-pressure room of a patient on mechanical ventilation (with a 0.023-μm filter on the exhalation circuit) before and after extubation.[124] Viral inactivating methods and agents are listed in **Table 3**.[43–46]

Immunity to SARS-CoV has been achieved in animal models by the induction of neutralizing antibodies using live-attenuated vaccinia virus Ankara expressing S glycoprotein vaccine, recombinant spike protein polypeptide vaccine (generated in

Table 3
SARS-CoV stability and inactivating agents

Agent or Activity	Comments
Povidone-iodine	2-minute treatment reduced infectivity to less than detectable levels
70% ethanol	Equivalent to povidone-iodine
Formalin Glutaraldehyde Methanol Acetone	Fixation of Vero E6 SARS-CoV for 5 minutes with these agents eliminated all infectivity
Heating at 56°C for 60 minutes in absence of protein	Eliminates infectivity
Solvent/detergents	For virus inactivation: Triton X-100 required 2 hours; Tween 80 required 4 hours; and sodium cholate required up to 24 hours
Octanoic acid	Does not inactivate virus
Heating at 56°C for 60 minutes in the presence of 20% protein	Residual infectivity remains
Heating at 60°C for at least 30 minutes in the presence of protein	Minimal requirement to eliminate infectivity in the presence of protein
Ultraviolet subtype C	Inactivated virus in 40 minutes. The presence of bovine serum albumin limited ability to inactivate virus
Ultraviolet A light	Requires the addition of psoralen to enhance inactivation of virus. The presence of bovine serum albumin limited ability to inactivate virus
Virus in suspension	Maintains infectivity for 9 days
Dried virus	Maintains infectivity for 6 days
Virus in fomites and stool	Maintains infectivity 24–72 hours

Data from Refs.[43–46]

Escherichia coli with spike polypeptide DNA), adenoviral-based (expressing either N or S proteins) virus, recombinant baculovirus, Newcastle disease virus, attenuated vesicular stomatitis virus expressing S protein, attenuated *Salmonella enterica* serovar Typhi and serovar Typhimurium, S protein on *Lactobacillus casei*, rhabdovirus-based vaccines, attenuated parainfluenza virus expressing S protein, and inactivated SARS-CoV vaccine, among others.[6,21,125–137] Comprehensive reviews of vaccine development are referenced.[2,21]

Human monoclonal antibody (hmAbs) 80 R directed against the SARS-CoV S protein, acting as a viral entry inhibitor by blocking its binding to the ACE-2 receptor, protects mice against infection.[138] ACE-2 itself protects murine lungs from acute lung injury, and SARS-spike protein-mediated lung injury.[139]

The SARS-CoV strain from the first outbreak (2002/early 2003) could be neutralized by the hmAbs 80R and S3.1. The SARS-CoV GD03 strain from the second SARS outbreak (2003/2004) was resistant to both these products. Two other hmAbs products (m396 and S230.15) were able to neutralize strain GD03, isolates from the first SARS outbreak (Urbani, Tor2), and isolates from palm civets.[140] The use of 2 noncompeting hmAbs may allow for the use of lower doses as the result of synergy, and prevent the emergence of resistant mutants.[141]

Conversely, antibodies that neutralize most (human) SARS-CoV S glycoproteins enhanced entry mediated by the civet virus S glycoprotein. This result occurs because of the antibody interaction with conformational epitopes in the human ACE-2 binding domain.[142]

Pathogen-free chickens immunized with inactivated SARS-CoV produced eggs from which anti-IgY (egg yolk) anti-SARS-CoV antibody was extracted. The product had a neutralization titer of 1:640. It could be lyophilized, reconstituted without loss of activity, and maintain good thermal stability.[143]

Other theoretic treatments include treatment of SARS ARDS by blocking the pulmonary renin-angiotensin system or treatment with ACE-2.[37,38]

Uncontrolled trials suggest that IFN alfacon-1 (a synthetic interferon) with steroids, protease inhibitors with ribavirin, or convalescent plasma with neutralizing antibody may be useful for treatment. Some investigators suggest considering prophylaxis with IFN or hyperimmune globulin for unprotected exposures.[42] A hybrid IFN (IFN-α B/D) and a mismatched double-stranded (ds) RNA IFN inducer (Ampligen [poly I: poly C124]), also display antiviral activity.[144]

Randomized controlled trials are not available to evaluate treatment regimens. Early positive outcomes using ribavirin and steroids led to widespread use of that combination. In 1 study of 71 cases (97% laboratory confirmed), antibiotics, ribavirin plus a 3-week step-down steroid therapy and pulsed methylprednisolone "rescue" resulted in 3.4% mortality, all in patients older than 65 years. Complications suffered by these patients included hyperglycemia (58%), pneumomediastinum (13%), psychiatric symptoms (7%), and ventilator associated pneumonia (2%).[145] Steroid therapy, including pulsed steroids, has been used in critically ill patients. High-dose and prolonged steroid therapy predisposed patients to multiple adverse outcomes, especially avascular necrosis (in 1 study, 12% of patients).[146]

Some reports demonstrate ribavirin antiviral activity and synergy with type I IFN (IFN-β1a or leukocytic IFN-α).[8] Subsequent reports indicated that ribavirin and mizoribine (both inosine-5′ monophosphate dehydrogenase inhibitors) had poor in vitro antiviral activity and were associated with frequent toxicity.[146,147]

Concern exists about the adverse effects of ribavirin. These effects include dose-dependent anemia with doses 1.2 g/d or greater for more than 10 days (hemolysis or bone marrow suppression), arrhythmia, elevated lactate and pyruvate levels, hypocalcemia, and hypomagnesemia. Patients have complained of chest pain and dizziness. Less frequently, patients develop hyperuricemia, hyperbilirubinemia, interstitial pneumonia, leukopenia, and thrombocytopenia. Ribavirin therapy resulted in anemia in 72.7% of patients, with 50% decreasing more than 2 g/dL of hemoglobin. Hypoxemic and anemic patients receiving ribavirin had a higher mortality (29%).[148]

Indomethacin has significant in vitro anti-SARS-CoV activity.[149] Other antiinflammatory agents (chloroquine, amodiaquine, and pentoxifylline) were inactive in vitro.[144] Niclosamide and several interferons have demonstrated in vitro (in Vero E6 cells) activity.[150,151] Several nucleoside analogues, protease inhibitors, reverse transcriptase inhibitors, neuraminidase inhibitors, amantadine, and foscarnet did not adequately inhibit cytopathic effect.[151]

Ritonavir/lopinavir (Kaletra), the human immunodeficiency virus protease inhibitor combination (400 mg ritonavir and 100 mg lopinavir) has been suggested for the early treatment of SARS. IFN, although not recommended as standard therapy, possesses in vitro antiviral activity. Cases reported suggest that they should be subjected to clinical trial.[146,152] In 1 study, the combination of lopinavir/ritonavir and ribavirin resulted in a lower incidence of intubation with a matched cohort (0% vs 11%, respectively),[153] and ARDS or death (2.4%) versus historical control (28.8%, $P<.001$) at 3 weeks.[152]

Novel CoV-inhibiting agents that seem theoretically promising include carbohydrate-binding agents, nucleoside analogues with 6-chloropurine nucleobase, ranpirnase (onconase, an amphibian oocyte/early embryo ribonuclease), and drugs targeting viral envelope protein.[135,154,155] Safety testing of equine anti-SARS-CoV F(ab′)2 has been undertaken in macaques.[156] Patent applications for cathepsin L inhibitors (inhibitors of SARS-CoV entry into cells), SARS-CoV protease inhibitors, IFN, and short interfering RNAs that inhibit the expression of SARS-CoV genes, have either been made or are under consideration.[21,157] ACE-2 cellular receptor and the SARS-CoV spike protein are likewise therapeutic targets.[158]

A review in 2006 of SARS therapy administered during the epidemic found that finding clear-cut treatment benefits was elusive. There were 26 reports of inconclusive benefits and 4 reports of possible harm related to ribavirin therapy, 25 inconclusive reports and 4 reports of possible harm from steroid therapy, and inconclusive reports for lipinavir/ritonavir therapy (2), IFN-α therapy (3), and convalescent plasma or immunoglobulin therapy (7).[8]

Virus-encoded enzymes (3C-like cysteine protease and papainlike cysteine protease, nucleoside triphosphate hydrolase/helicase and RNA-dependent RNA polymerase) have been considered therapeutic targets. Other compounds exhibiting in vitro activity include valinomycin, glycopeptide antibiotics, plant lectins, hesperetin, glycyrrhizin, aurintricarboxylic acid, niclosamide, nelfinavir, and calpain inhibitors.[159]

SUMMARY

Once more unto the breach, dear friends, once more;
Or close the wall up with our English dead.
In peace there's nothing so becomes a man
As modest stillness and humility;
But when the blast of war blows in our ears,
Then imitate the action of the tiger:
Stiffen the sinews, summon up the blood.
William Shakespeare, Henry V

Identification of a possible SARS patient must be made on admission to the hospital. Symptoms almost if not always overlap common respiratory diseases present in the community, making the epidemiologic history critical. Rapid definitive laboratory testing of patients (and HCWs) must be available. Recognizing the patient as a risk for SARS becomes a difficult task if this is a result of a bioterrorist attack, and the patient is 1 of the first to present to the institution.

Placement of the patient in a negative-pressure room, strict enforcement of infection control measures, and the use of personal protective equipment are essential. The use of a closed oxygen delivery mask with a respiratory filter is mandatory in all patients requiring supplemental oxygen. Regular screening of HCWs for nasopharyngeal carriage may be necessary. In addition, the laboratory needs to be warned of the possibility of a SARS-CoV infection as soon as possible. The danger of nosocomial spread, HCW-, and laboratory-acquired infection is significant, even after implementation of infection control practices.

As shown by the Amoy Gardens outbreak, SARS may represent an environmental hazard through contamination by viral aerosols associated with plumbing.

There are no definitive treatment modalities. Ribavirin and steroid therapy seems to be the most frequent choice of clinicians during the epidemics, yet there is a lack of clear evidence of benefit.

The horseshoe bat is the natural reservoir for the SARS-CoV, with civets as the amplification host, and "wet markets" and farms as the amplification centers.[16] SARS-CoV has significant similarities to avian CoVs and SARS-CoV-like viruses found in mammals (masked palm civets and racoon dogs) from the Chinese live-animal markets. The 5′ polymerase gene is of mammalian origin, whereas the 3′ end structural gene excluding the S glycoprotein is of avian origin. The S glycoprotein is of feline and avian origin. The SARS-CoV rapidly evolved from the group 2 CoVs. It still circulates in animal reservoirs, ready to reemerge and cause a new epidemic.[160,161]

Challenges faced by the health care institution include closure of the ICU beds, loss of staff through quarantine and illness, emergent introduction of new, complex, and restrictive infection control procedures, rapid staff education, system planning, and maintaining morale.[162] Booth and Stewart (Toronto)[162] indicate that coordinated leadership, communication infrastructure, and systems in place to quickly expand and modify critical care services is essential to meeting the demands of a SARS outbreak.

REFERENCES

1. Bitnun A, Allen U, Heurter H, et al. Children hospitalized with severe acute respiratory syndrome-related illness in Toronto. Pediatrics 2003;112:e261.
2. Gillim-Ross L, Subbarao K. Emerging respiratory viruses: challenges and vaccine strategies. Clin Microbiol Rev 2006;19:614–36.
3. Christian MD, Poutanen SM, Loutfy MR, et al. Severe acute respiratory syndrome. Clin Infect Dis 2004;38:1420–7.
4. Lam CW, Chan MH, Wong CK. Severe acute respiratory syndrome: clinical and laboratory manifestations. Clin Biochem Rev 2004;25:121–32.
5. Chen YC, Chang SC, Tsai KS, et al. Certainties and uncertainties facing emerging respiratory infectious diseases: lessons from SARS. J Formos Med Assoc 2008;107:432–42.
6. Liu L, Fang Q, Deng F, et al. Natural mutations in the receptor binding domain of spike glycoprotein determine the reactivity of cross-neutralization between palm civet coronavirus and severe acute respiratory syndrome coronavirus. J Virol 2007;81:4694–700.
7. Ho HT, Chang MS, Wei TY, et al. Colonization of severe acute respiratory syndrome–associated coronavirus among health-care workers screened by nasopharyngeal swab. Chest 2006;129:95–101.
8. Stockman LJ, Bellamy R, Garner P. SARS: systematic review of treatment effects. PLoS Med 2006;3:e343.
9. Sung JJ, Wu A, Joynt GM, et al. Severe acute respiratory syndrome: report of treatment and outcome after a major outbreak. Thorax 2004;59:414–20.
10. Hasoksuz M, Alekseev K, Vlasova A, et al. Biologic, antigenic, and full-length genomic characterization of a bovine-like coronavirus isolated from a giraffe. J Virol 2007;81:4981–90.
11. Lau SK, Woo PC, Yip CC, et al. Coronavirus HKU1 and other coronavirus infections in Hong Kong. J Clin Microbiol 2006;44:2063–71.
12. Li W, Shi Z, Yu M, et al. Bats are natural reservoirs of SARS-like coronaviruses. Science 2005;310:676–9.
13. Jiang S, He Y, Liu S. SARS vaccine development. Emerg Infect Dis 2005;11:1016–20.
14. Sheahan T, Rockx B, Donaldson E, et al. Pathways of cross species transmission of synthetically reconstructed zoonotic severe acute respiratory syndrome cornonavirus. J Virol 2008;82:8721–32.

15. Yang H, Bartlam M, Rao Z. Drug design targeting the main protease, the Achilles' heel of coronaviruses. Curr Pharm Des 2006;12:4573–90.
16. Cheng VC, Lau SK, Woo PC, et al. Severe acute respiratory syndrome coronavirus as an agent of emerging and reemerging infection. Clin Microbiol Rev 2007;20:660–94.
17. van der Hoek L. Human coronaviruses: what do they cause? Antivir Ther 2007; 12:651–8.
18. Pyrc K, Berkhout B, van der Hoek L. Antiviral strategies against human coronaviruses. Infect Disord Drug Targets 2007;7:59–66.
19. Vabret A, Dina J, Gouarin S, et al. Human (non-severe acute respiratory syndrome) coronavirus infections in hospitalized children in France. J Paediatr Child Health 2008;44:176–81.
20. Wang LF, Shi Z, Zhang S, et al. Review of bats and SARS. Emerg Infect Dis 2006;12:1834–40.
21. Weiss SR, Navas-Martin S. Coronavirus pathogenesis and the emerging pathogen severe acute respiratory syndrome coronavirus. Microbiol Mol Biol Rev 2005;69:635–64.
22. Chany C, Moscovici O, Lebon P, et al. Association of coronavirus infection with neonatal necrotizing enterocolitis. Pediatrics 1982;69:209–14.
23. Stockman LJ, Haynes LM, Miao C, et al. Coronavirus antibodies in bat biologists. Emerg Infect Dis 2008;14:999–1000.
24. Bai B, Hu Q, Hu H, et al. Virus-like particles of SARS-like coronavirus formed by membrane proteins from different origins demonstrate stimulating activity in human dendritic cells. PLoS One 2008;3:e2685.
25. Cui J, Han N, Streicker D, et al. Evolutionary relationships between bat coronaviruses and their hosts. Emerg Infect Dis 2007;13:1526–32.
26. Normile D. Virology. Researchers tie deadly SARS virus to bats. Science 2005; 309:2154–5.
27. Tang JW, To KF, Lo AW, et al. Quantitative temporal-spatial distribution of severe acute respiratory syndrome-associated coronavirus (SARS-CoV) in post-mortem tissue. J Med Virol 2007;79:1245–53.
28. Nicholls JM, Butany J, Poon LL, et al. Time course and cellular localization of SARS-CoV nucleoprotein and RNA in lung from fatal cases. PLoS Med 2006;3:e27.
29. Hwang DM, Chamberlain DW, Poutanen SM. Pulmonary pathology of severe acute respiratory syndrome in Toronto. Mod Pathol 2005;18:1–10.
30. Gu J, Korteweg C. Pathology and pathogenesis of severe acute respiratory syndrome. Am J Pathol 2007;170:1136–47.
31. Tse GM, To KF, Chan PK, et al. Pulmonary pathological features in coronavirus associated severe acute respiratory syndrome (SARS). J Clin Pathol 2004;57:260–5.
32. Leung WK, To KF, Chan PK, et al. Enteric involvement of severe acute respiratory syndrome-associated coronavirus infection. Gastroenterology 2003;125: 1011–7.
33. Chu KH, Tsang WK, Tang CS, et al. Acute renal impairment in coronavirus-associated severe acute respiratory syndrome. Kidney Int 2005;67:698–705.
34. Leung TW, Wong KS, Hui AC, et al. Myopathic changes associated with severe acute respiratory syndrome: a postmortem case series. Arch Neurol 2005;62: 1113–7.
35. van den Brand JM, Haagmans BL, Leijten L, et al. Pathology of experimental SARS coronavirus infection in cats and ferrets. Vet Pathol 2008;45:551–62.
36. Kuba K, Imai Y, Penninger JM. Angiotensin-converting enzyme 2 in lung diseases. Curr Opin Pharmacol 2006;6:271–6.

37. Imai Y, Kuba K, Penninger JM. Lessons from SARS: a new potential therapy for acute respiratory distress syndrome (ARDS) with angiotensin converting enzyme 2 (ACE2). Masui 2008;57:302–10.
38. Imai Y, Kuba K, Penninger JM. The discovery of angiotensin-converting enzyme 2 and its role in acute lung injury in mice. Exp Physiol 2008;93:543–8.
39. To KF, Lo AW. Exploring the pathogenesis of severe acute respiratory syndrome (SARS): the tissue distribution of coronavirus (SARS-CoV) and its putative receptor, angiotensin-converting enzyme 2 (ACE2). J Pathol 2004;203:740–3.
40. He WP, Shu CL, Li BA, et al. Human LINE 1 endonuclease domain as a putative target of SARS-associated autoantibodies involved in the pathogenesis of severe acute respiratory syndrome. Chin Med J 2008;5:608–14.
41. Chu CM, Leung WS, Cheng VC, et al. Duration of RT-PCR positivity in severe acute respiratory syndrome. Eur Respir J 2005;25:12–4.
42. Wong SS, Yuen KY. The management of coronavirus infections with particular reference to SARS. J Antimicrob Chemother 2008;62:437–41.
43. Rabenau HF, Cinati J, Morgenstern B, et al. Stability and inactivation of SARS coronavirus. Med Microbiol Immunol 2005;194:1–6.
44. Kariwa H, Fujii N, Takashima I. Inactivation of SARS coronavirus by means of povidone-iodine, physical conditions and chemical reagents. Dermatology 2006; 212(Suppl 1):119–23.
45. Darnell ME, Taylor DR. Evaluation of inactivation methods for severe acute respiratory syndrome coronavirus in noncellular blood products. Transfusion 2006; 46:1770–7.
46. Hota B. Contamination, disinfection, and cross-colonization: are hospital surfaces reservoirs for nosocomial infection? Clin Infect Dis 2004;39:1182–9.
47. Lim W, Ng KC, Tsang DN. Laboratory containment of SARS virus. Ann Acad Med Singapore 2006;35:354–60.
48. Chiu YC, Wu KL, Chou YP, et al. Diarrhea in medical care workers with severe acute respiratory syndrome. J Clin Gastroenterol 2004;38:880–2.
49. Hui DS, Chan PK. Clinical features, pathogenesis and immunobiology of severe acute respiratory syndrome. Curr Opin Pulm Med 2008;14:241–7.
50. Svoboda T, Henry B, Shulman L, et al. Public health measures to control the spread of the severe acute respiratory syndrome during the outbreak in Toronto. N Engl J Med 2004;350:2352–61.
51. Lee N, Hui D, Wu A, et al. A major outbreak of severe acute respiratory syndrome in Hong Kong. N Engl J Med 2003;348:1986–94.
52. Anderson RM, Fraser C, Ghani AC, et al. Epidemiology, transmission dynamics and control of SARS: the 2002-2003 epidemic. Philos Trans R Soc Lond B Biol Sci 2004;359:1091–105.
53. St John RK, King A, de Jong D, et al. Border screening for SARS. Emerg Infect Dis 2005;11:6–10.
54. Tsui PT, Kwok ML, Yuen H, et al. Severe acute respiratory syndrome: clinical outcome and prognostic correlates. Emerg Infect Dis 2003;9:1064–9.
55. Sandrock CE. Severe febrile respiratory illnesses as a cause of mass critical care. Respir Care 2008;53:40–53.
56. Li Y, Duan S, Yu IT, et al. Multi-zone modeling of probable SARS virus transmission by airflow between flats in Block E, Amoy Gardens. Indoor Air 2005;15: 96–111.
57. Wang XW, Li J, Guo T, et al. Concentration and detection of SARS coronavirus in sewage from Xiao Tang Shan Hospital and the 309th Hospital of the Chinese People's Liberation Army. Water Sci Technol 2005;52:213–21.

58. McKinney KR, Gong YY, Lewis TG. Environmental transmission of SARS at Amoy Gardens. J Environ Health 2006;68:26–30.
59. Yip C, Chang WL, Yeung KH, et al. Possible meteorological influence on the severe acute respiratory syndrome (SARS) community outbreak at Amoy Gardens, Hong Kong. J Environ Health 2007;70:39–46.
60. Cui Y, Zhang ZF, Froines J, et al. Air pollution and case fatality of SARs in the People's Republic of China: an ecologic study. Environ Health 2003;2:15.
61. Kan HD, Chen BH, Fu CW, et al. Relationship between ambient air pollution and daily mortality of SARS in Beijing. Biomed Environ Sci 2005;18:1–4.
62. Chu CM, Cheng VC, Hung IF, et al. Viral load distribution in SARS outbreak. Emerg Infect Dis 2005;11:1882–6.
63. Hui DS, Ip M, Tang JW, et al. Airflows around oxygen masks: a potential source of infection? Chest 2006;130:822–6.
64. Somogyi R, Vesely AE, Azami T, et al. Dispersal of respiratory droplets with open vs closed oxygen delivery masks: implications for the transmission of severe acute respiratory syndrome. Chest 2004;125:1155–7.
65. Ofner-Agostini M, Gravel D, McDonald LC, et al. Cluster of cases of severe acute respiratory syndrome among Toronto healthcare workers after implementation of infection control precautions: a case series. Infect Control Hosp Epidemiol 2006;27:473–8.
66. Christian MD, Loutfy M, McDonald LC, et al. Possible SARS coronavirus transmission during cardiopulmonary resuscitation. Emerg Infect Dis 2004;10:287–93.
67. Ueno T, Masuda N. Controlling nosocomial infection based on structure of hospital social networks. J Theor Biol 2008;254:655–66.
68. Dell'Omodarme M, Prati MC. The probability of failing in detecting an infectious disease at entry points into a country. Stat Med 2005;24:2669–79.
69. Yang JK, Feng Y, Yuan MY, et al. Plasma glucose levels and diabetes are independent predictors for mortality and morbidity in patients with SARS. Diabet Med 2006;23:623–8.
70. Lee N, Chan PK, Yu IT, et al. Co-circulation of human metapneumovirus and SARS-associated coronavirus during a major nosocomial SARS outbreak in Hong Kong. J Clin Virol 2007;40:333–7.
71. Peiris JS, Chu CM, Cheng VC, et al. Clinical progression and viral load in a community outbreak of coronavirus-associated SARS pneumonia: a prospective study. Lancet 2003;361:1767–72.
72. Babyn PS, Chu WC, Tsou IY, et al. Severe acute respiratory syndrome (SARS): chest radiographic features in children. Pediatr Radiol 2004;34:47–58.
73. Stockman LJ, Massoudi MS, Helfand R, et al. Severe acute respiratory syndrome in children. Pediatr Infect Dis J 2007;26:68–74.
74. Booth CM, Matukas LM, Tomlinson GA, et al. Clinical features and short-term outcomes of 144 patients with SARS in the greater Toronto area. JAMA 2003;289:2801–9.
75. Leung CW, Kwan YW, Ko PW, et al. Severe acute respiratory syndrome among children. Pediatrics 2004;113:e535–43.
76. Wong RS, Wu A, To KF, et al. Haematological manifestations in patients with severe acute respiratory syndrome: retrospective analysis. BMJ 2003;326:1358–63.
77. Hui DS, Wong KT, Antonio GE, et al. Severe acute respiratory syndrome: correlation between clinical outcome and radiologic features. Radiology 2004;233:579–85.

78. Che XY, Di B, Zhao GP, et al. A patient with asymptomatic severe acute respiratory syndrome (SARS) and antigenemia from the 2003–2004 community outbreak of SARS in Guangzhou, China. Clin Infect Dis 2006;43:e1–5.
79. Ksiezakowska K, Laszczyk M, Wilczynski J, et al. SARS-CoV infection and pregnancy. Ginekol Pol 2008;79:47–50.
80. Lam CM, Wong SF, Leung TN, et al. A case-controlled study comparing clinical course and outcomes of pregnant and non-pregnant women with severe acute respiratory syndrome. BJOG 2004;111:771–4.
81. Wong SF, Chow KM, Leung TN, et al. Pregnancy and perinatal outcomes of women with severe acute respiratory syndrome. Am J Obstet Gynecol 2004; 191:292–7.
82. Shek CC, Ng PC, Fung GP, et al. Infants born to mothers with severe acute respiratory syndrome. Pediatrics 2003;112:e254.
83. Li AM, Chan CH, Chan DF. Long-term sequelae of SARS in children. Paediatr Respir Rev 2004;5:296–9.
84. Chu WC, Li AM, Ng AW, et al. Thin-section CT 12 months after the diagnosis of severe acute respiratory syndrome in pediatric patients. AJR Am J Roentgenol 2006;186:1707–14.
85. Kwan BC, Leung CB, Szeto CC, et al. Severe acute respiratory syndrome in dialysis patients. J Am Soc Nephrol 2004;15:1883–8.
86. Rainer TH, Chan PK, Ip M, et al. The spectrum of severe acute respiratory syndrome-associated coronavirus infection. Ann Intern Med 2004;140:614–9.
87. Leung GM, Chung PH, Tsang T, et al. SARS-CoV antibody prevalence in all Hong Kong patient contacts. Emerg Infect Dis 2004;10:1653–6.
88. Lee CC, Chen SY, Chang IJ, et al. Seroprevalence of SARS coronavirus antibody in household contacts. Epidemiol Infect 2005;133:1119–22.
89. Isakbaeva ET, Khetsuriani N, Beard RS, et al. SARS-associated coronavirus transmission, United States. Emerg Infect Dis 2004;10:225–31.
90. Poutanen SM, Low DE. Severe acute respiratory syndrome: an update. Curr Opin Infect Dis 2004;17:287–94.
91. Chong WP, Ip WK, Tso GH, et al. The interferon gamma gene polymorphism +874 A/T is associated with severe acute respiratory syndrome. BMC Infect Dis 2006;6:82.
92. Antonio GE, Wong KT, Hui DS, et al. Thin-section CT in patients with severe acute respiratory syndrome following hospital discharge: preliminary experience. Radiology 2003;228:810–5.
93. Chang YC, Yu CJ, Chang SC, et al. Pulmonary sequelae in convalescent patients after severe acute respiratory syndrome: evaluation with thin-section CT. Radiology 2005;236:1067–75.
94. Felice GA. SARS, pneumothorax, and our response to epidemics. Chest 2004; 125:1982–4.
95. Yu CM, Wong RS, Wu EB, et al. Cardiovascular complications of severe acute respiratory syndrome. Postgrad Med J 2006;82:140–4.
96. Huang JW, Chen KY, Tsai HB, et al. Acute renal failure in patients with severe acute respiratory syndrome. J Formos Med Assoc 2005;104:891–6.
97. Chen LL, Hsu CW, Tian YC, et al. Rhabdomyolysis associated with acute renal failure in patients with severe acute respiratory syndrome. Int J Clin Pract 2005; 59:1162–6.
98. Griffith JF, Antonio GE, Kumta SM, et al. Osteonecrosis of hip and knee in patients with severe acute respiratory syndrome treated with steroids. Radiology 2005;235:168–75.

99. Chan MH, Chan PK, Griffith JF, et al. Steroid-induced osteonecrosis in severe acute respiratory syndrome: a retrospective analysis of biochemical markers of bone metabolism and corticosteroid therapy. Pathology 2006;38:229–35.
100. Wang S, Wei M, Han Y, et al. Roles of TNF-alpha gene polymorphisms in the occurrence and progress of SARS-CoV infection: a case-control study. BMC Infect Dis 2008;8:27.
101. Lau EM, Chan FW, Hui DS, et al. Reduced bone mineral density in male severe acute respiratory syndrome (SARS) patients in Hong Kong. Bone 2005;37:420–4.
102. Leow MK, Kwek DS, Ng AW, et al. Hypocortisolism in survivors of severe acute respiratory syndrome (SARS). Clin Endocrinol (Oxf) 2005;63:197–202.
103. Chan HL, Kwan AC, To KF, et al. Clinical significance of hepatic derangement in severe acute respiratory syndrome. World J Gastroenterol 2005;11:2148–53.
104. Yang Z, Xu M, Yi JQ, et al. Clinical characteristics and mechanisms of liver damage in patients with severe acute respiratory syndrome. Hepatobiliary Pancreat Dis Int 2005;4:60–3.
105. Davydow DS, Desai SV, Needham DM, et al. Psychiatric morbidity in survivors of the acute respiratory distress syndrome: a systematic review. Psychosom Med 2008;70:512–9.
106. Hawryluck L, Gold WL, Robinson S, et al. SARS control and psychological effects of quarantine, Toronto, Canada. Emerg Infect Dis 2004;10:1206–12.
107. Styra R, Hawryluck L, Robinson S, et al. Impact on health care workers employed in high-risk areas during the Toronto SARS outbreak. J Psychosom Res 2008;64:177–83.
108. Ko SF, Lee TY, Huang CC, et al. Severe acute respiratory syndrome: prognostic implications of chest radiographic findings in 52 patients. Radiology 2004;233:173–81.
109. Wong KT, Antonia GE, Hui DS, et al. Severe acute respiratory syndrome: thin-section computed tomography features, temporal changes, and clinicoradiologic correlation during the convalescent period. J Comput Assist Tomogr 2004;28:790–5.
110. Emmanuel JV, Pua U, Wansaicheong GK, et al. Radiographic features of SARS in paediatric patients: a review of cases in Singapore. Ann Acad Med Singapore 2006;35:340–4.
111. Schmidt M, Brixner V, Ruster B, et al. NAT screening of blood donors for severe acute respiratory syndrome coronavirus can potentially prevent transfusion associated transmissions. Transfusion 2004;44:470–5.
112. Tang P, Louie M, Richardson SE, et al. Interpretation of diagnostic laboratory tests for severe acute respiratory syndrome: the Toronto experience. CMAJ 2004;170:47–54.
113. Tsao KC, Chen GW, Huang CG, et al. False positive antibody results against human T-cell lymphotropic virus in patients with severe acute respiratory syndrome. J Med Virol 2005;77:331–6.
114. Chan PK, To WK, Ng KC, et al. Laboratory diagnosis of SARS. Emerg Infect Dis 2004;10:825–31.
115. Keightley MC, Sillekens P, Schippers W, et al. Real-time NASBA detection of SARS-associated coronavirus and comparison with real-time reverse transcription-PCR. J Med Virol 2005;77:602–8.
116. Chan KH, Poon LL, Cheng VC, et al. Detection of SARS coronavirus in patients with suspected SARS. Emerg Infect Dis 2004;10:294–9.
117. Hung IF, Cheng VC, Wu AK, et al. Viral loads in clinical specimens and SARS manifestations. Emerg Infect Dis 2004;10:1550–7.

118. Pang RT, Poon TC, Chan KC, et al. Serum proteomic fingerprints of adult patients with severe acute respiratory syndrome. Clin Chem 2006;52: 421–9.
119. Yip TT, Chan JW, Cho WC, et al. Protein chip array profiling analysis in patients with severe acute respiratory syndrome identified serum amyloid a protein as a biomarker potentially useful in monitoring the extent of pneumonia. Clin Chem 2005;51:47–55.
120. Ohnishi K, Sakaguchi M, Kaji T, et al. Immunological detection of severe acute respiratory syndrome coronavirus by monoclonal antibodies. Jpn J Infect Dis 2005;58:88–94.
121. Xu X, Gao X. Immunological responses against SARS-coronavirus infections in humans. Cell Mol Immunol 2004;1:119–22.
122. Li L, Gu J, Shi X, et al. Biosafety level 3 laboratory for autopsies of patients with severe acute respiratory syndrome: principles, practices, and prospects. Clin Infect Dis 2005;41:815–21.
123. Sandrock C, Stollenwerk N. Acute febrile respiratory illness in the ICU: reducing disease transmission. Chest 2008;133:1221–31.
124. Tsai YH, Wan GH, Wu YK, et al. Airborne severe acute respiratory syndrome coronavirus concentrations in a negative-pressure isolation room. Infect Control Hosp Epidemiol 2006;27:523–5.
125. Gao W, Tamin A, Soloff A, et al. Effects of a SARS-associated coronavirus vaccine in monkeys. Lancet 2003;362:1895–6.
126. Chen Z, Zhang L, Qin C, et al. Recombinant modified vaccinia virus Ankara expressing the spike glycoprotein of severe acute respiratory syndrome coronavirus induces protective neutralizing antibodies primarily targeting the receptor binding region. J Virol 2005;79:2678–88.
127. Bai B, Lu X, Meng J, et al. Vaccination of mice with recombinant baculovirus expressing spike or nucleocapsid protein of SARS-like coronavirus generates humoral and cellular immune responses. Mol Immunol 2008;45:868–75.
128. Faber M, Lamirande EW, Roberts A, et al. A single immunization with a rhabdovirus-based vector expressing severe acute respiratory syndrome coronavirus (SARS-CoV) S protein results in the production of high levels of SARS-CoV-neutralizing antibodies. J Gen Virol 2005;86:1435–40.
129. Woo PC, Lau SK, Tsoi HW, et al. SARS coronavirus spike polypeptide DNA vaccine priming with recombinant spike polypeptide from *Escherichia coli* as booster induces high titer of neutralizing antibody against SARS coronavirus. Vaccine 2005;23:4959–68.
130. See RH, Zakhartchouk AN, Petric M, et al. Comparative evaluation of two severe acute respiratory syndrome (SARS) vaccine candidates in mice challenged with SARS coronavirus. J Gen Virol 2006;87:641–50.
131. Hu S, Wang QH, Wang XJ, et al. Expression of recombinant spike protein of SARS-coronavirus in vaccinia virus and analysis of its immunogenicity. Bing Du Xue Bao 2007;23:287–91.
132. DiNapoli JM, Kotelkin A, Yang L, et al. Newcastle disease virus, a host range-restricted virus, as a vaccine vector for intranasal immunization against emerging pathogens. Proc Natl Acad Sci U S A 2007;104:9788–93.
133. Tsunetsugu-Yokota Y, Ato M, Takahashi Y, et al. Formalin-treated UV-inactivated SARS coronavirus vaccine retains its immunogenicity and promotes Th2-type immune responses. Jpn J Infect Dis 2007;60:106–12.
134. Luo F, Feng Y, Liu M, et al. Type IVB pilus operon promoter controlling expression of the severe acute respiratory syndrome-associated coronavirus

nucleocapsid gene in *Salmonella enterica* serovar Typhi elicits full immune response by intranasal vaccination. Clin Vaccine Immunol 2007;14:990–7.

135. Ranpirnase: amphibian ribonuclease A, P-30 protein-alfacell. Drugs R D 2007;8: 120–4.
136. Lee JS, Poo H, Han DP, et al. Mucosal immunization with surface-displayed severe acute respiratory syndrome coronavirus spike protein on *Lactobacillus casei* induces neutralizing antibodies in mice. J Virol 2006;80:4079–87.
137. Bukreyev A, Lamirande EW, Buchholz UJ, et al. Mucosal immunization of African green monkeys (*Cercopithecus aethiops*) with an attenuated parainfluenza virus expressing the SARS coronavirus spike protein for the prevention of SARS. Lancet 2004;363:2122–7.
138. Sui J, Li W, Roberts A, et al. Evaluation of human monoclonal 80R for immunoprophylaxis of severe acute respiratory syndrome by an animal study, epitope mapping, and analysis of spike variants. J Virol 2005;79:5900–6.
139. Imai Y, Kuba K, Penninger JM. Angiotensin-converting enzyme 2 in acute respiratory distress syndrome. Cell Mol Life Sci 2007;64:2006–12.
140. Zhu Z, Chakraborti S, He Y, et al. Potent cross-reactive neutralization of SARS coronavirus isolates by human monoclonal antibodies. Proc Natl Acad Sci U S A 2007;104:12123–8.
141. ter Meulen J, van den Brink EN, Poon LL, et al. Human monoclonal antibody combination against SARS coronavirus: synergy and coverage of escape mutants. PLoS Med 2006;3:e237.
142. Yang ZY, Werner HC, Kong WP, et al. Evasion of antibody neutralization in emerging severe acute respiratory syndrome coronaviruses. Proc Natl Acad Sci U S A 2005;102:797–801.
143. Fu CY, Huang H, Wang XM, et al. Preparation and evaluation of anti-SARS coronavirus IgY from yolks of immunized SPF chickens. J Virol Methods 2006; 133:112–5.
144. Barnard DL, Day CW, Bailey K, et al. Evaluation of immunomodulators, interferons and known *in vitro* SARS-coV inhibitors for inhibition of SARS-coV replication in BALB/c mice. Antivir Chem Chemother 2006;17:275–84.
145. Lau AC, So LK, Miu FP, et al. Outcome of coronavirus-associated severe acute respiratory syndrome using a standard treatment protocol. Respirology 2004;9: 173–82.
146. Tai DY. Pharmacologic treatment of SARS: current knowledge and recommendations. Ann Acad Med Singapore 2007;36:438–43.
147. Saijo M, Morikawa S, Fukushi S, et al. Inhibitory effect of mizoribine and ribavirin on the replication of severe acute respiratory syndrome (SARS)-associated coronavirus. Antiviral Res 2005;66:159–63.
148. Chiou HE, Liu CL, Buttrey MJ, et al. Adverse effects of ribavirin and outcome in severe acute respiratory syndrome: experience in two medical centers. Chest 2005;128:263–72.
149. Amici C, Di Coro A, Ciucci A, et al. Indomethacin has a potent antiviral activity against SARS coronavirus. Antivir Ther 2006;11:1021–30.
150. Wu CJ, Jan JT, Chen CM, et al. Inhibition of severe acute respiratory syndrome coronavirus replication by niclosamide. Antimicrobial Agents Chemother 2004; 48:2693–6.
151. Tan ELC, Ooi EE, Lin C-Y, et al. Inhibition of SARS coronavirus infection *in vitro* with clinically approved antiviral drugs. Emerg Infect Dis 2004;10:581–6.
152. Chu CM, Cheng VC, Hung IF, et al. Role of lopinavir/rotonavir in the treatment of SARS: initial virological and clinical findings. Thorax 2004;59:252–6.

153. Chan KS, Lai ST, Chu CM, et al. Treatment of severe acute respiratory syndrome with lopinavir/ritonavir: a multicentre retrospective matched cohort study. Hong Kong Med J 2003;9:399–406.
154. Golda A, Pyrc K. Recent antiviral strategies against human coronavirus-related respiratory illnesses. Curr Opin Pulm Med 2008;14:248–53.
155. Ikejiri M, Saijo M, Morikawa S, et al. Synthesis and biological evaluation of nucleoside analogues having 6-chloropurine as anti-SARS-CoV agents. Bioorg Med Chem Lett 2007;17:2470–3.
156. Xu Y, Jia Z, Zhou L, et al. Evaluation of the safety, immunogenicity and pharmacokinetics of equine anti-SARS-CoV F(ab′)(2) in macaque. Int Immunopharmacol 2007;7:1834–40.
157. Tong TR. SARS coronavirus anti-infectives. Recent Pat Antiinfect Drug Discov 2006;1:297–308.
158. Kuhn JH, Li W, Radoshitzky SR, et al. Severe acute respiratory syndrome coronavirus entry as a target of antiviral therapies. Antivir Ther 2007;12:639–50.
159. De Clercq E. Potential antivirals and antiviral strategies against SARS coronavirus infections. Expert Rev Anti Infect Ther 2006;4:291–302.
160. Jackwood MW. The relationship of severe acute respiratory syndrome coronavirus with avian and other coronaviruses. Avian Dis 2006;50:315–20.
161. Ren W, Li W, Yu M, et al. Full-length genome sequences of two SARS-like coronaviruses in horseshoe bats and genetic variation analysis. J Gen Virol 2006;87:3355–9.
162. Booth CM, Stewart TE. Severe acute respiratory syndrome and critical care medicine: the Toronto experience. Crit Care Med 2005;31(Suppl 1):S53–60.

Swine Influenza (H1N1) Pneumonia: Clinical Considerations

Burke A. Cunha, MD, MACP[a,b,*]

KEYWORDS

- Pandemic influenza • CPK • Relative lymphopenia
- Thrombocytopenia • CA-MRSA CAP

HISTORY

Influenza is a viral zoonosis of birds and mammals that has probably existed since antiquity. In antiquity, populations were small and less concentrated, limiting influenza potential. As animals became domesticated and lived in close proximity to human populations, populations concentrated in urban centers, setting the stage for the introduction of zoonotic influenza into the human population. Influenza can maintain itself in rural populations because of ongoing changes in immunity mediated by influenza viral antigenic drift and shift. Because influenza immunity is strain-specific, influenza may be maintained and may result in epidemics in large, closed urban populations. Attack rates of influenza are relatively high but mortality is relatively eg ~ 1 % low. Influenza mortality is highest in the very young, the very old, and the immunosuppressed. Influenza (human seasonal) has the potential for rapid spread and may involve large populations. Even though the mortality associated with epidemics is relatively low, the total number of fatalities involved may be huge. In the 1918–1919 influenza A (H1N1) pandemic, the mortality rate was 1%, but because massive numbers of people were infected, there were 50 million fatalities.[1–3]

Clinical descriptions of influenza were first clearly described by Caus in 1551. The English physician described a "sweating disease" characterized by fever, headache, and myalgias that killed some patients rapidly but lasted only a few days in those that survived. Although the English sweating sickness might have been due to influenza, the findings were nonspecific and did not resemble the first recognized influenza epidemic, which occurred in Germany, England, and Italy in 1173. Subsequent influenza epidemics occurred in France and Italy in 1323 and 1387. Villaini and Segui were the first to use the term "una influenza," referring to some "celestial influence" that was thought to be responsible for the infection. The French described influenza

[a] Infectious Disease Division, Winthrop-University Hospital, 259 First Street, Mineola, Long Island, NY 11501, USA
[b] State University of New York School of Medicine, Stony Brook, NY, USA
* Infectious Disease Division, Winthrop-University Hospital, Mineola, NY 11501.

Infect Dis Clin N Am 24 (2010) 203–228
doi:10.1016/j.idc.2009.10.001
id.theclinics.com
0891-5520/10/$ – see front matter

as the grip, because patients appeared to be gripped or seized by influenza. Thousands of people were affected by these early epidemics but the first pandemic spread through Europe in 1510. In 1679, Sydenem provided the first accurate clinical description of influenza. In 1933, Smith isolated influenza A virus. Three years later, Burnette was the first to culture the influenza virus in embryonated eggs. In 1941, Hearst was the first to describe the hemagglutination reactions of influenza. Frances, in 1939, was the first to isolate influenza B and later in 1950, Taylor was the first to isolate influenza C.[2–4]

The great influenza pandemic of 1918 to 1919 was due to an H1N1 strain. In 1997, and again recently, outbreaks of avian influenza (H5N1) virus have occurred, affecting humans as well as poultry. Since 1997, avian influenza (H5N1) emerged in terms of lethality with a high mortality rate ie, 60% among young healthy adults, and has as yet unrealized pandemic potential. Avian influenza (H5N1) strain resembles the 1918 to 1919 pandemic strain. Fortunately, avian influenza (H5N1) outbreaks over the past decade have been limited with minimal person-to-person spread. However, avian influenza (H5N1), like the influenza A (H1N1) strain of 1918 to 1919, has pandemic potential if the virus mutates, permitting efficient person-to-person transmission. The influenza A (H1N1) pandemic of 1918 to 1919 was remarkable in many respects. The pandemic was unprecedented in its mortality and virulence, and was accompanied by 2 unusual sequelae, namely, encephalitis and postinfluenza Parkinson disease.[5–7] The 1918 to 1919 influenza A (H1N1) pandemic was noteworthy in that the death rate was highest in young healthy adults.[6,8–10] The majority of the early deaths in young healthy individuals were due to influenza pneumonia alone and not simultaneous/subsequent bacterial pneumonia.[4,11–16]

The swine influenza A (H1N1) pandemic began in 2009.[17] Swine influenza (H1N1) is a novel influenza A virus comprising a reassortment of 4 distinct genetic elements, namely, swine, human, avian, and Eurasian swine genetic components, which combine into a single influenza virus, swine influenza (H1N1). The swine influenza (H1N1) pandemic rapidly spread from Mexico to the United States and the world in the spring of 2009. The initial spread from Mexico was via tourists/travelers returning home from Mexico. Foci of swine influenza (H1N1) strains became established across wide geographic areas.[17–20] As with other influenza A pandemics, the initial "herald wave" (in the late spring/summer) involved large numbers of individuals with relatively few deaths. Lethal swine influenza (H1N1) pneumonia affected primarily young and healthy adults. The epidemiologic hallmark of pandemic influenza is its, "pandemic signature," ie, most early mortalities are among young healthy adults. Human seasonal influenza affects primarily the very young, elderly, and those with comorbidities. Repeated passages through hosts, usually results in increased viral virulence. Excluding the effect of the (H1N1) vaccine, there is concern that subsequent waves of swine influenza (H1N1) may be more lethal than the first.[8,11,21]

MICROBIOLOGY

Members of the family *Orthomyxoviridae* have a segmented negative strand RNA genome. In the *Orthomyxoviridae* family are the influenza A, B, and C viruses. The single-stranded RNA influenza viruses differ in the length of their RNA segments, that is, influenza A and B have 8 RNA segments whereas influenza C has 7 segments. Influenza A, B, and C viruses are spherical and covered by a lipid envelope from host cell membrane. Influenza B and C have no subtypes. Subtypes are characteristic of the influenza A virus. Influenza A viruses are classified on the basis of their surface glycoproteins of the hemagglutinin (HA) and neuraminidase agglutinating (NA) proteins. Influenza A viruses have 16 different HA and 9 different NA subtypes.

However, only 3 HA subtypes and 2 NA subtypes have been implicated in human influenza epidemics. The 3 HA subtypes in human outbreaks are H1, H2, and H3, and the 2 NA subtypes are N1 and N2. The surface HA proteins are HA glycoproteins in a rod-shaped spike with a hydrophobic carboxy terminal based in the viral envelope. The hydrophobic end of the rod-shaped spike projects from the virus and is the binding site for sialic acid residues in host receptor cells. The HA surface glycoprotein is responsible for viral adherence to the host cell, whereas the HA glycoprotein is responsible for attachment of the virus and penetration of the influenza A virus into the host cell. The NA surface glycoprotein is mushroom-shaped and is also implanted in the lipid envelope at the amino acid end of the glycoprotein. NA glycoprotein cleaves terminal sialic acid residues, which are responsible for release of virus from infected host cells and spread of the influenza virus to other cells in the respiratory tract. Influenza viruses also have M2 proteins, which are important in uncoding the virus. M2 proteins, which are the matrix proteins, are present only in influenza A viruses and appear on the surface of infected host cells. M1 proteins are surface structural proteins important in viral budding.[22–24]

Influenza A and B viruses bind to sialic acid receptors on the host cell surface and begin the infectious process. Human influenza viruses attach preferentially to the α2, 6 linkage to galactose containing oligosaccharides. In contrast, avian influenza viruses preferentially bind to α23 linkages. Influenza C viruses bind to 9-*O*-acetyl-*N*-acetylneuraminic acid receptors. Influenza A viruses are widely distributed in nature. Avian species are the primary reservoir for all 16 HA and 9 NA influenza A subtypes. Other natural hosts of influenza A viruses are humans, horses, and swine. Human influenza viruses replicate in respiratory epithelial cells, whereas avian influenza A virus is replicated in respiratory and gastrointestinal epithelial cells.[22–25]

Swine influenza is an influenza A virus that consists of distinctive genetic influenza A elements from swine, human, avian, and Eurasian swine strains of influenza (H1N1). The swine influenza (H1N1) pandemic was totally unpredicted. As with the "herald waves" of previous influenza A pandemics, large numbers of people were infected but relatively few died. The virulence of avian influenza (H5N1) remains worrisome.[21] To date, avian influenza (H5N1) has been highly lethal in relatively small numbers of patients. It is thought that avian influenza (H5N1) is relatively inefficient in bird-to-human and human-to-human transmission, thus far limiting its human pandemic potential. With the swine influenza (H1N1) pandemic, although mortality rates are low, the potential for pandemic spread has been demonstrated during the spring/summer initial "herald wave". Lethal, swine influenza (H1N1) affects primarily young healthy adults.[5,6,22–25]

EPIDEMIOLOGY

Influenza viruses are spread by airborne aerosols/droplets from infected individuals while speaking, coughing, or sneezing. Fomites are also implicated in the transmission of influenza. Nonhuman influenza infections are spread from respiratory/gastrointestinal infections of the host animal.[2,3,26] Influenza viruses remain viable at cool temperatures under conditions of low humidity on nonporous surfaces.

Influenza viruses may be detected in the general population throughout the year, but peak in the winter months. In the northern hemisphere, peak human seasonal influenza season is in February whereas in the southern hemisphere, where winter months occur between May and August, flu usually peaks in June or July. Epidemics of influenza A are characterized by a sudden increase in acute respiratory illnesses. In epidemics, usually influenza A or influenza B predominates, although both influenza A and B may occur together in epidemics. Avian influenza (H5N1) may be transmitted from direct contact with infected birds or humans.[2,5,22,23]

Influenza has a short incubation period of approximately 2 days (range, 1–5 days). During the initial phase of the illness, there are high concentrations of influenza virus in respiratory secretions responsible for its spread via airborne transmission. One of the characteristics of influenza viruses is their changing antigenicity. Minor changes in surface glycoproteins resulting from stepwise point mutations in HA/NA glycoproteins are called "antigenic drift." Sequential amino acid changes occurring over a period of years resulting in HA/NA glycoprotein changes occur every 2 to 3 years and are termed "antigenic shift." Influenza epidemics occur every 6 to 10 years and are due to antigenic shifts exposing the population to strains to which it has not been exposed previously. For this reason, pandemic influenza A has a high attack rate in individuals of all age groups who are not susceptible, particularly children. Unlike epidemics of influenza that occur during the winter months, pandemic influenza may occur at any time and spread rapidly from country to country, facilitated by travel. The twentieth century has experienced 3 influenza pandemics, 2 of which have emerged from China. The highest late excess fatalities occur are among the elderly, who succumb to influenza because of comorbid conditions/bacterial complications, whereas early deaths among young healthy patients are most often due to severe influenza pneumonia alone.[5,22–26]

Influenza has also been responsible for nosocomial outbreaks. Nosocomial influenza is usually due to influenza A and, less commonly, influenza B strains. In contrast to community-acquired infections, nosocomial outbreaks are brief, lasting 1 to 3 weeks versus months in community-acquired outbreaks. Health care workers may be important in initiating or spreading influenza in nursing homes, chronic care facilities, or hospitals. Nosocomial influenza has occurred in immunized hosts, suggesting that there is suboptimal protection in elderly nursing home residents.[23–26]

Swine influenza (H1N1) is spread primarily via aerosols/droplets and to a lesser extent via hand-to-face transmission. Avian (H5N1) and swine influenza (H1N1) may be transmitted in aircraft (unrecirculated cabin air) via aerosol/droplet transmission. Because swine influenza (H1N1), like avian influenza (H5N1), is often accompanied by gastrointestinal symptoms (ie, diarrhea), there may be potential for viral spread from feces. As with seasonal human influenza A, swine influenza (H1N1) may be spread nosocomially.[27]

CLINICAL PRESENTATION

Mild to moderate influenza is clinically indistinguishable from illnesses caused by other respiratory viruses that present as influenzalike illnesses (ILIs). Peak incidence of influenza historically is in February in the northern hemisphere, but the influenza season may start earlier and last into early spring. Avian influenza (H5N1) has a nonseasonal distribution, and swine influenza (H1N1) has occurred in summer and winter. Excluding pandemics and epidemics, influenza is a relatively mild 3-day illness, that is, a mild respiratory infection with a high attack rate and low mortality. Pandemic influenza also has a high attack rate, but due to highly virulent strains has a high mortality.[22–25,28]

In adults, severe influenza A has a distinctive clinical presentation, which is not easily confused with other causes of viral pneumonia.[23,29,30] Like severe acute respiratory syndrome (SARS), hantavirus pulmonary syndrome (HPS), and adenovirus, severe influenza A pneumonia begins abruptly, but influenza A patients often can recall the exact time of onset of the illness. Severe human seasonal influenza A is accompanied by fever higher than 39°C/102°F and chills, accompanied by severe myalgias and dry cough with or without hemoptysis. Purulent sputum suggests superimposed bacterial community-acquired pneumonia (CAP) due to MSSA/CA-MRSA. Another noteworthy feature of human seasonal influenza is severe debilitating fatigue rapidly making victims bedridden. Prostration is profound and is accompanied by headache and prominent myalgias. Some infections present with myalgias, but the myalgias of influenza are peculiarly severe and are localized to the neck and back. Retro-orbital pain is common, and conjunctival suffusion may be present in severe seasonal human influenza A. Conjunctival suffusion may be present in avian influenza (H5N1) but is uncommon with swine influenza (H1N1). The clinical constellation of an ILI with fever higher than 39°C/102°F and severe myalgias especially of the neck/back, with profound prostration, clinically differentiates severe influenza A in adults from ILIs (**Table 1**).[22–25,28,30]

The clinical presentation of avian influenza (H5N1) resembles severe human influenza A in adults and affects primarily young healthy adults, whereas nonepidemic pandemic/epidemic human influenza A primarily affects the very young, elderly, and debilitated. Pandemic influenza A affects primarily young healthy adults (ie, "pandemic signature") rather than the very young, elderly, and immunocompromised. Swine influenza (H1N1) has demonstrated its "pandemic signature," that is, most fatal cases have occurred in young healthy adults.[28,31]

Several nonspecific laboratory test abnormalities are associated with human influenza A in adults. The severity of human influenza A is related to the degree/duration of leukopenia and relative lymphopenia.[31,32] The nonspecific laboratory test hallmark of influenza A (human, avian, and swine) is otherwise unexplained relative lymphopenia. Relative lymphopenia is an inconsistent feature of swine influenza (H1N1) in children; lymphocytosis is more common. In adults, relative lymphopenia is usually accompanied by thrombocytopenia. In adults with human and avian (H5N1) influenza, leukopenia if present may be an indicator of severity. Leukopenia in swine influenza (H1N1) when present usually occurs with relative lymphopenia and thrombocytopenia.[33] Atypical lymphocytes are not a usual feature of swine influenza (H1N1) in adults but may be present in children.

From a radiographic perspective, influenza (human, avian, swine) has no distinctive features. Initially, the chest radiograph (CXR) shows no or minimal infiltrates. Later, (>48 hours) bilateral patchy interstitial infiltrates appear as influenza pneumonia progresses. The presence of focal segmental/lobar infiltrates on the admission CXR of adults with influenza indicates simultaneous bacterial CAP, due to *Staphylococcus aureus* (MSSA/CA-MRSA) CAP.[30] Patients with influenza/ILI and simultaneous *S aureus* CAP present with purulent sputum, high spiking fevers, often with cyanosis/hypotension. *S aureus* CAP, whether due to methicillin-sensitive *S aureus* (MSSA) or methicillin-resistant *S aureus* (MRSA), presents in the same way clinically and on CXR. The CXR of *S aureus* (MSSA/MRSA) CAP in patients with influenza pneumonia are characterized by rapid cavitation in 72 hours or less. In adults, *S aureus* (MSSA/MRSA) CAP occurs only in patients with influenza/ILI (**Table 2**).[30,31,34–38]

Gastrointestinal symptoms (ie, nausea, vomiting, or diarrhea) are more common with avian and swine influenza (H1N1) than with human influenza. Serum aspartate and alanine transaminases (AST/ALT) are often mildly/transiently elevated in avian (H5N1) and swine influenza (H1N1). Another key laboratory finding in swine influenza (H1N1) patients is an elevated creatine phosphokinase (CPK). Some patients with highly elevated CPKs may also have rhabdomyolysis. Seasonal human influenza A and avian influenza A (H5N1) may have mild to moderate elevations of the serum lactate dehydrogenase (LDH). Whereas certain nonspecific laboratory abnormalities are typical of swine influenza (H1N1), for example, otherwise unexplained relative

Table 1
Winthrop-University Hospital Infectious Disease Division's point system for diagnosing severe influenza A in adults (modified)

Symptoms[a]	Point Score	Signs[a]	Point Score	Laboratory Tests[a]	Point Score
Hyperacute onset	+3	Fever (>39°C/102°F)	+2	Leukocytosis[c]	–5
Severe prostration	+5	Dry cough	+1	Leukopenia	+3
Generalized muscle aches	+3	Conjunctival suffusion	+5	Relative lymphopenia	+3
Retro-orbital pain	+5	Hemoptysis	+3	Thrombocytopenia	+3
Severe back of neck/lumbar aches	+5	Localized rales[b]	–3	Chest radiograph	
		Cyanosis	+5	No/minimal infiltrates (<48 hours)	+3
				Bilateral patchy infiltrates[b] (>48 hours)	+5
				Focal/segmental infiltrates[b]	–5
Likelihood of severe influenza A					
Total points	>20 = Severe influenza A highly probable 10–20 = Mild/moderate influenza A likely <10 = Influenza A unlikely				

[a] Otherwise unexplained, acute, and related to influenza.
[b] Unless with bacterial CAP.
[c] Leukocytosis without relative lymphopenia and thrombocytopenia.

Adapted from Cunha BA. The clinical diagnosis of severe viral influenza A. Infection 2008;36:92–3; Cunha BA. Pneumonia essentials. 3rd edition. Sudbury (MA): Jones & Bartlett; 2010.

Table 2
Clinical presentations and diagnostic features of severe influenza A pneumonia

	Influenza Pneumonia	Influenza with *Simultaneous* Bacterial CAP	Influenza Followed by *Sequential* Bacterial CAP
Usual pathogen	Influenza A[a]	Influenza A ***with*** *Staphylococcus aureus* (MSSA/CA-MRSA) CAP	Influenza A ***followed by*** *Streptococcus pneumoniae* or *Haemophilus influenzae* CAP
Presentation of CAP	Subacute/acute	Acute	Influenza then an interval of clinical improvement (5–7 days) followed by CAP
Symptoms	Severe myalgias (neck/back) Debilatating fatigue Retro-orbital pain Dry cough (± mild hemoptysis) Shortness of breath ± pleuritic chest pain	Same as influenza A *plus* hemoptysis, productive cough/ purulent sputum ± pleuritic chest pain	After 5–7 days following influenza, new fevers and productive cough/ purulent sputum ± pleuritic chest pain
Signs	Fever Conjunctival suffusion Dyspnea (± cyanosis) No rales	Same as influenza *plus* localized rales ± consolidation	Localized rales ± consolidation
Laboratory tests	Hypoxemia (A-a gradient >35) Relative lymphopenia Thrombocytopenia ± Leukopenia Sputum: WBC with normal/or no flora	Same as influenza *plus* Leukocytosis Sputum: WBCs with Gram + cocci (in clusters)	Minimal/no hypoxemia (A-a gradient <35) Leukocytosis Sputum: WBCs with Gram + cocci (*in pairs*) or GNBs
Chest radiograph	No infiltrates (early) Bilateral patchy interstitial infiltrates (later) No/small pleural effusion(s)	Focal segmental/lobar infiltrates *with* rapid cavitation <72 h	Focal segmental/lobar infiltrates *without* cavitation ± consolidation ± pleural effusion
Mortality	+++	++++	+

Abbreviations: A-a, alveolar arterial gradient; CAP, community-acquired pneumonia; GNBs, gram-negative bacilli; MRSA, methicillin-resistant *S aureus*; MSSA, methicillin-sensitive *S aureus*; WBC, white blood cell count.
[a] Uncomplicated influenza is a 3-day illness.
Data from Cunha BA. Pneumonia essentials. 3rd edition. Sudbury (MA): Jones & Bartlett; 2010.

lymphopenia, thrombocytopenia, mildly elevated AST/ALT, and elevated CPKs, other findings argue against the diagnosis, for example, elevated serum ferritin levels, hypophosphatemia, elevated cold agglutinin titers, and so forth.[30–32,34] In influenza (human, avian, swine) pneumonia, hypoxemia is a reflection of the severity of influenza in the interstitium of the lungs. Viral involvement of the lung interstitium may result in an oxygen diffusion defect manifested as hypoxemia and an increased A-a gradient. The greater the degree/duration of hypoxemia (A-a gradient >35), the more severe and potentially fatal is influenza (human, avian, swine) pneumonia.[30,31]

As with avian influenza (H5N1), hospitalized adults with swine influenza (H1N1) pneumonia rarely present with or subsequently develop bacterial pneumonia CAP.[33,36] During the 1957 to 1958 Asian influenza A pandemic, some patients presented with influenza A pneumonia and simultaneous *S aureus* CAP. Still others, especially the elderly, later developed *Streptococcus pneumoniae* or *Haemophilus influenzae* CAP 1 to 2 weeks into their recovery. As with avian influenza (H5N1), young healthy adults with swine influenza (H1N1) pneumonia, have only rarely presented with superimposed *S aureus* (MSSA/CA-MRSA) CAP. Adult swine influenza (H1N1), like avian influenza (H5N1) pneumonia simultaneous or subsequent bacterial CAP remains relatively rare.[36–40]

DIFFERENTIAL DIAGNOSIS

The differential diagnosis of severe viral CAPs in normal hosts includes cytomegalovirus (CMV), and adenovirus, and in compromised hosts RSV and CMV. Viral pneumonias presenting as severe CAPs have a similar radiological appearance, that is, no/minimal infiltrates early (<48 hours), followed later (>48 hours) by bilateral diffuse patchy interstitial infiltrates. Adult influenza A pneumonia (human, avian, swine) as well as other severe viral CAPs are accompanied by variable degrees of hypoxemia and a high A-a gradient >35. Bacterial CAP rarely, if ever, complicates severe CMV or adenoviral CAP.[30]

In general, viral pneumonias are not accompanied by pleuritic chest pain because pathophysiologically they are interstitial and not pleurally based but influenza A may be accompanied by bilateral "pleuritic" chest pain. The "pleuritic chest pain" of influenza A pneumonia is due to direct viral involvement of the intercostal muscles mimicking pleuritic chest pain. The pleuritic chest pain of bacterial CAPs is unilateral and related to the location of the underlying infiltrate.[30] Influenza/ILI complicated by simultaneous CA-MRSA/MSSA CAP is characterized by a necrotizing pneumonia with rapidly cavitating infiltrates on CXR with or without pleuritic chest pain. MSSA/CA-MRSA (PVL+ strains) with influenza/ILI is often accompanied by cyanosis/hypotension (see **Table 2**).[36–40]

Swine influenza (H1N1) resembles avian influenza (H5N1) in its predilection for young healthy adults.[39–50] The epidemiologic clue to avian influenza (H5N1) is recent close contact with infected poultry or people in Europe or Asia. The diagnosis of avian influenza (H5/N1) may be missed if the hemagglutinin inhibition (HI) test is used to diagnose influenza A because this test is insensitive to avian hemagglutinins.[30,39] The diagnosis of avian influenza (H5N1) is by hemagglutinin-specific reverse transcription-polymerase chain reaction (RT-PCR) for avian influenza (H5N1).

The other illness that does not clinically resemble influenza A is SARS. Unlike adult human seasonal influenza A, loose stools/diarrhea occurs in some and the illness lasts longer than 3 days. In contrast to influenza/avian influenza, the white blood cell (WBC) count and platelet counts in SARS are usually normal but may be slightly decreased. Relative lymphopenia is present, as are mild increases in the serum transaminases (AST/ALT). Like seasonal human influenza A, elevations of the CPK and LDH are not uncommon. Diagnosis of SARS is by specific serology or viral isolation.[30,51]

The clinical clue to SARS is the recent contact history with infected poultry or someone with SARS from Europe or Asia. Unlike seasonal human influenza A, SARS is a biphasic infection. At onset, fever decreases after a few days and the patient improves, but unlike seasonal human influenza A, fever recurs in a few days when the patient re-presents with signs and symptoms of viral pneumonia ie, CXR shows bilateral patchy interstitial infiltrates. Like avian influenza (H5N1), SARS has not been complicated by bacterial CAP.[30,50,51]

In the differential diagnosis of influenza/ILIs, HPS should be considered if there has been close contact usually after about 2 weeks postexposure to a rodent.[52] Like SARS, HPS is a biphasic illness, that is, the initial phase is the febrile phase, followed by the cardiopulmonary phase. Later, HPS patients progress through an oliguric/diuretic phase and finally to a convalescent phase. The distinguishing clinical feature of HPS is noncardiogenic pulmonary edema. HPS is not a 3-day illness like influenza. In HPS leukocytosis (up to 90,000/mm^3) rather than leukopenia is the rule. The nonspecific laboratory hallmark of HPS is the presence of immunoblasts.[30,52] Diagnosis of HPS is by IgM enzyme-linked immunosorbent assay or RT-PCR (**Table 3**).

CLINICAL DIAGNOSIS

Sporadic seasonal human influenza A cases may occur throughout the year, but influenza activity in the northern hemisphere peaks in February (November–March), and in the southern hemisphere in July (May–September). Influenza occurring during the peak influenza season is often more severe than that which occurs sporadically throughout the year.[22–25]

In adults with swine influenza (H1N1), pneumonia presents in adults as an ILI with a temperature higher than 39°C (102°F) accompanied by prominent myalgias; these are the key clinical findings. Many patients also have headache, sore throat, or dry cough, with or without loose stools/diarrhea. Conjunctival suffusion is rare. The onset of swine influenza (H1N1) pneumonia is often abrupt but a preceeding ILI prodrome is common. Mild cases of swine influenza (H1N1) are indistinguishable from ILIs. Adult patients who require hospitalization have characteristic clinical nonspecific laboratory abnormalities.[17–20]

In adults hospitalized with swine influenza (H1N1) pneumonia, otherwise unexplained relative lymphopenia is uniformly present.[34] However, clinicians must be careful to not ascribe relative lymphopenia in patients to swine influenza (H1N1) pneumonia until the patient's medical history is reviewed for other disorders associated with relative lymphopenia. Besides human seasonal and avian influenza other infectious causes of relative lymphopenia include CMV, human herpesvirus (HHV)-6, HHV-8, human immunodeficiency virus (HIV), miliary tuberculosis (TB), Legionnaire's disease, typhoid fever, Q fever, brucellosis, SARS, malaria, babesiosis, Rocky Mountain spotted fever (RMSF), histoplasmosis, dengue fever, Chickungunya fever, ehrlichiosis, parvovirus B19, HPS, West Nile encephalitis (WNE), and viral hepatitis (early). Noninfectious causes of relative lymphopenia include cytotoxic drugs, steroids, sarcoidosis, systemic lupus erythematosus (SLE), lymphoma, rheumatoid arthritis (RA), radiation therapy, Wiskott-Aldrich syndrome, Whipple's disease, severe combined immunodeficiency disease (SCID), common variable immune deficiency (CVID), Di George's syndrome, Nezelof's syndrome, intestinal lymphangiectasia, constrictive pericarditis, tricuspid regurgitation, Kawasaki's disease, idiopathic CD_4 cytopenia, Wegener's granulomatosis, acute/chronic renal failure, hemodialysis; myasthenia gravis, celiac disease, alcoholic cirrhosis, coronary bypass, congestive heart failure (CHF), acute pancreatitis, and carcinomas.[30]

Relative lymphopenia with swine influenza (H1N1) pneumonia may be profound and prolonged. The degree/duration of relative lymphopenia also has prognostic implications. Typically, an increase in the percentage of lymphocytes precedes clinical

Table 3
Differential diagnosis of severe influenza/influenza like illnesses

Clinical Features	Influenza (Human Seasonal/Swine)	Avian Influenza (H5N1)	SARS	HPS
Epidemiology	2 d	<7 d	5 d	4 d
Incubation period (mean)	(1–4 d)	(2–5 d)	(2–10 d)	(2–15 d)
Recent exposure				
Influenza	+	–	+	–
Birds	–	+	+	–
Rodents	–	–	–	+
Asian travel	–	+	+	–
Symptoms				
Biphasic illness	–	+	±	–
Fever/chills	+	+	+	+
Profound weakness	+	–	–	+
Headache/muscle aches	+	+	+	+
Dry cough	+	+	–	+
Sore throat	+	+	–	–
Runny nose	+	±	–	–
Hemoptysis	±	±	–	–
SOB → early	+	+	–	–
→ late	±	±	+	+
Substernal discomfort/burning	±	–	–	±
Pleuritic chest pain	±	–	–	+
Loose stools/diarrhea	±	+	±	+
Abdominal pain	–	–	–	+
Signs				
Fever >39°C/102°F	+	+	±	±
Conjunctival suffusion	+	+	+	–
Injected oropharynx	+	+	–	+[a]
Laboratory tests[f]				
Leukopenia	±*	+	–	+[d]
Relative lymphopenia	+	+	+	–
Atypical lymphocytes	–	–	–	–
Immunoblasts	–	–	–	+
Thrombocytopenia	±	±	±	+
Mildly elevated serum transaminases (AST/ALT)	±	+	+	+
Elevated LDH	–	+	+	+
Elevated CPK	+	+	+	+
CXR				
Minimal/no infiltrates (early)	+	+	+	+
Bilateral patchy infiltrates (late)	+	+	+	+[e]
Focal segmental/lobar infiltrates	–[b]	–[b]	+[c]	–

Abbreviations: CPK, creatinine phosphokinase; CXR, Chest radiograph; HPS, hantavirus pulmonary syndrome; LDH, lactate dehydrogenase; SARS, severe acute respiratory syndrome; SOB, shortness of breath.

* Usually normal WBC count.
[a] With exudates.
[b] Unless bacterial CAP.
[c] Infiltrates often ovoid or round.
[d] Leukocytosis later with hemoconcentration and increase in severity.
[e] Noncardiogenic pulmonary edema.
[f] HI test for influenza A negative in avian influenza (H5N1); use PCR to diagnose avian influenza (H5N1).
Data from Cunha BA. Pneumonia essentials. 3rd edition. Sudbury (MA): Jones & Bartlett; 2010.

improvement.[30] Atypical lymphocytes are present in a variety of viral illnesses but are not usually present in adults with influenza A or avian influenza (H5N1). Also, atypical lymphocytes are not a feature of adult swine influenza (H1N1) but may be present in children with swine influenza (H1N1).[30] With swine influenza (H1N1) pneumonia, thrombocytopenia does not occur as an isolated entity but accompanies/follows relative lymphopenia. Leukocytosis, rather than leukopenia, is the rule in hospitalized adults with swine influenza (H1N1) pneumonia. When leukopenia is present, it occurs together with the relative lymphopenia or thrombocytopenia. Also, as with severe seasonal human influenza A, leukopenia may rarely be an isolated finding in fatal cases of swine influenza (H1N1) pneumonia in adults (**Figs. 1–4**).[30,53]

Another important nonspecific laboratory clue in adult influenza (human, swine, and avian) are elevated CPKs. Severe swine influenza (H1N1) pneumonia, like seasonal human influenza A and avian influenza (H5N1) pneumonia, may be accompanied by high elevations of CPK, with or without rhabdomyolysis. Highly elevated cold agglutinin titers are not a feature of swine influenza (H1N1) pneumonia in adults, and their presence should suggest another diagnosis, for example, *Mycoplasma pneumoniae* CAP. In adults with swine influenza (H1N1) pneumonia, serum transaminases (AST/ALT) are often transiently mildly/moderately elevated. Highly elevated serum ferritin levels or hypophosphatemia are not features of swine influenza (H1N1) pneumonia and should suggest an alternate diagnosis, for example, Legionnaire's disease. In adults, a quick way to differentiate ILIs from swine influenza (H1N1) pneumonia is a fever higher than 39°C/102°F accompanied by severe myalgias with otherwise unexplained relative lymphopenia thrombocytopenia, elevated serum transaminases (AST/ALT) or an elevated CPK.[30,53]

A diagnostic weighted point score system was developed at Winthrop-University Hospital by the Infectious Disease Division during the "herald wave" of swine influenza (H1N1) pandemic to clinically differentiate admitted adults with swine influenza (H1N1) pneumonia from ILIs and other patients with cardiac/pulmonary symptoms. While the diagnostic point score system was accurate and useful early in the pandemic, a more simplified/rapid approach was developed; the swine influenza diagnostic triad. The

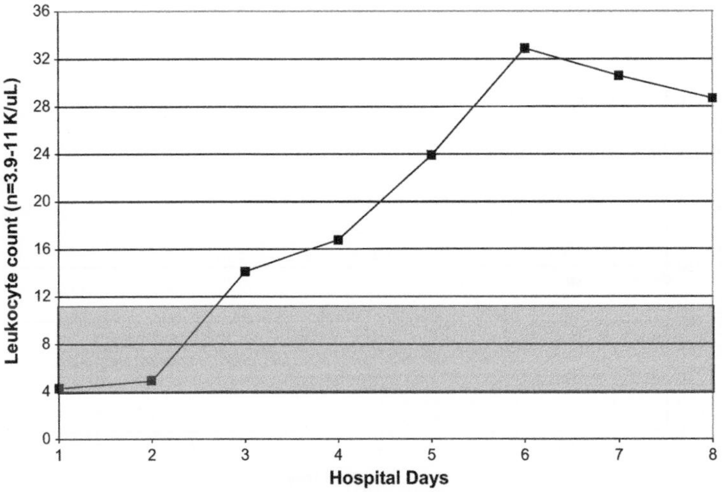

Fig. 1. Serial WBC counts in a case of fatal swine influenza (H1N1) pneumonia. (*From* Cunha BA, Syed U, Mikail N. Rapid clinical diagnosis in fatal swine influenza (H1N1) pneumonia in adult with negative rapid influenza diagnostic tests (RIDTs): diagnostic swine influenza triad. Heart & Lung 2010;39:78–86; with permission.)

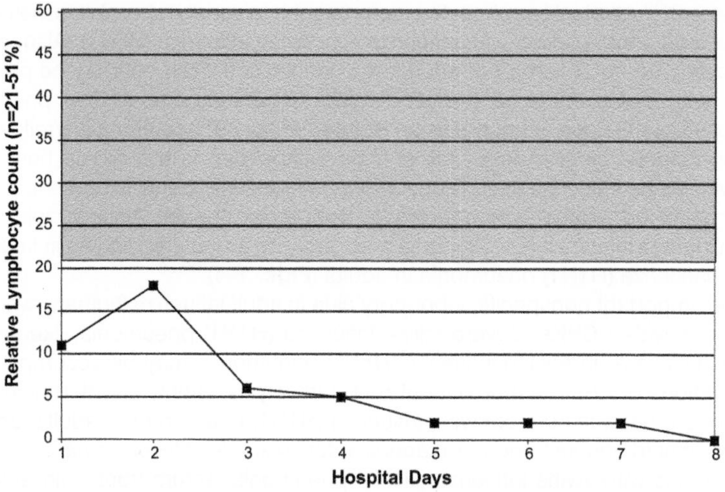

Fig. 2. Relative lymphopenia in a case of fatal swine influenza (H1N1) pneumonia. (*From* Cunha BA, Syed U, Mickail N, et al. Rapid clinical diagnosis in fatal swine influenza (H1N1) pneumonia in an adult with negative rapid influenza diagnostic tests (RIDTs): Diagnostic swine influenza triad. Heart Lung 2010;39:78–86: with permission.)

Winthrop-University Hospital Infectious Disease Division's diagnostic triad was then used as the basis for making a probable clinical diagnosis of swine influenza (H1N1) in rapid influenza diagnostic tests (RIDT)-negative hospitalized adults, to determine which patients should be on influenza precautions and treated with oseltamivir (**Table 4**, **Box 1**).[54]

Also, a key component in the Winthrop-University Hospital Infectious Disease Division's diagnostic swine influenza triad for the diagnosis of hospitalized adults with

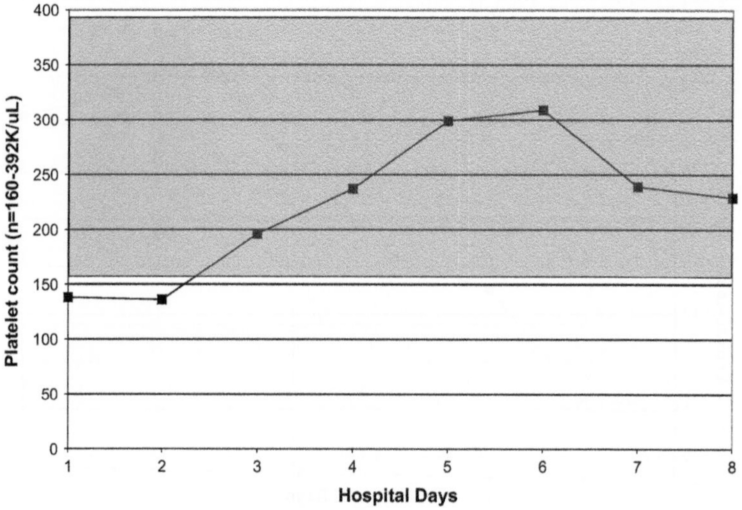

Fig. 3. Serial platelet counts in a case of fatal swine influenza (H1N1) pneumonia. (*From* Cunha BA, Syed U, Mickail N, et al. Rapid clinical diagnosis in fatal swine influenza (H1N1) pneumonia in an adult with negative rapid influenza diagnostic tests (RIDTs): Diagnostic swine influenza triad. Heart Lung 2010;39:78–86: with permission.)

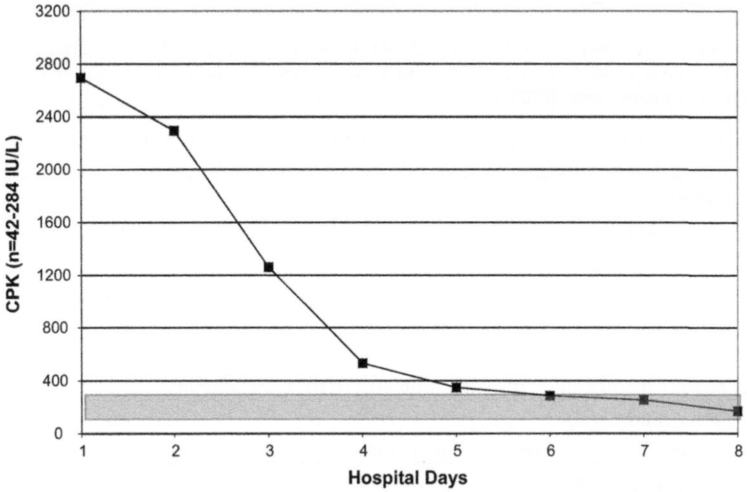

Fig. 4. Serial CPK in a case of fatal swine influenza (H1N1) pneumonia. (*From* Cunha BA, Syed U, Mickail N, et al. Rapid clinical diagnosis in fatal swine influenza (H1N1) pneumonia in an adult with negative rapid influenza diagnostic tests (RIDTs): Diagnostic swine influenza triad. Heart Lung 2010;39:78–86; with permission.)

swine influenza (H1N1) pneumonia was dry cough, fever, and a CXR without focal segmental/lobar infiltrates.[30,53] Adult patients presenting with an ILI, fever, and shortness of breath with an admission CXR with focal segmental/lobar infiltrates invariably had an alternate diagnosis, namely, CHF, asthma, acute exacerbation of chronic bronchitis (AECB), preexisting lung disease, or bacterial CAP. In an adult hospitalized with an ILI without the diagnostic swine influenza triad, focal segmental/lobar infiltrate on the admission CXR effectively rules out the diagnosis of swine influenza (H1N1) pneumonia.[33]

As the result of the experience in the 1957 to 1958 Asian influenza pandemic, there has been concern about the potential for simultaneous or sequential bacterial CAPs with pandemic influenza A. Patients presenting with human influenza A and CXR infiltrates that rapidly cavitate (within <72 hours) should suggest MSSA/CA-MRSA CAP superimposed underlying influenza/ILI. This presentation has been reported in the literature sporadically with seasonal human influenza A during the past few years.[55–58] In adults, seasonal human influenza A pneumonia may also be complicated by subsequent bacterial CAP after a period of improvement (usually 5–7 days). Adults with human seasonal influenza A improve, then may re-present with new onset of fever and new focal segmental/lobar infiltrates on CXR. The pathogen in this setting is either *S pneumoniae* or *H influenzae,* not *S aureus* (MSSA/CA-MRSA). Adults with influenza A pneumonia presenting simultaneous MSSA/CA-MRSA CAP are critically ill, with high spiking fevers, cyanosis, and hypotension and a fatal outcome is not uncommon. However, most admitted adult patients with severe influenza A pneumonia have not been complicated by simultaneous or subsequent bacterial CAP.

In the recent avian influenza (H5N1) pneumonia experience in Europe and Asia, this has also been the case, that is, severe or fatal cases have not been complicated by simultaneous or subsequent bacterial CAP.[41–50] Deaths from severe avian influenza (H5N1) pneumonia have been due to severe hypoxemia, which is also the case with most fatal cases of seasonal human influenza A. In the "herald wave" of recent pandemic, the majority of swine influenza (H1N1) pneumonia deaths occurred

Table 4
Swine influenza (H1N1) pneumonia: Winthrop-University Hospital Infectious Disease Division's clinical weighted diagnostic point score system for adults and negative rapid influenza diagnostic tests (RIDTs)

Adults with an ILI with dry cough, fever >39°C/102°F and a CXR with no focal/segmental lobar infiltrates and negative RIDTs[a]:	
Key clinical finding:	
• Severe myalgias	+5
• Relative lymphopenia[b,c]	+5
• Elevated CPK (otherwise unexplained)[c]	+3
• Elevated serum transaminases (AST/ALT)[c]	+2
• Thrombocytopenia[c]	+5
Argues *against* the diagnosis of swine influenza (H1N1) pneumonia:	
• Relative bradycardia	−5
• Leukopenia without relative lymphopenia or thrombocytopenia[c]	−2
• Atypical lymphocytes	−1
• Highly elevated serum ferritin levels (>2 × n)[c]	−5
• Hypophosphatemia[c]	−3
Swine influenza Diagnostic Point Score totals:	Maximum score: 20
Probable swine influenza (H1N1) pneumonia	>15
Possible swine influenza (H1N1) pneumonia	10–15
Unlikely swine influenza (H1N1) pneumonia	<10

[a] Diagnostic tests negative for all other viral CAP pathogens (CMV, SARS, HPS, RSV metapneumoviruses, parainfluenza viruses, adnoviruses).
[b] Other causes of relative lymphopenia: *Infectious causes*: CMV, HHV-6, HHV-8, HIV, military TB, Legionella, typhoid fever, Q fever, brucellosis, SARS, malaria, babesiosis, influenza, avian influenza, RMSF, histoplasmosis, dengue fever, Chickungunya fever, ehrlichiosis, parvovirus B19, HPS, WNE, viral hepatitis (early); *Noninfectious causes*: cytotoxic drugs, steroids, sarcoidosis, SLE, lymphoma, RA, radiation therapy, Wiskott-Aldrich syndrome, Whipple disease, severe combine immunodeficiency disease (SCID), common variable immune deficiency (CVID), Di George's syndrome, Nezelof's syndrome, intestinal lymphangiectasia, constrictive pericarditis, tricuspid regurgitation, Kawasaki's disease, idiopathic CD_4 cytopenia, Wegener's granulomatosis, acute/chronic renal failure, hemodialysis; myasthenia gravis, celiac disease, alcoholic cirrhosis, coronary bypass, CHF, acute pancreatitis, carcinomas (terminal).
[c] Otherwise unexplained.
Data from Cunha BA, Syed U, Stroll S, et al. Winthrop-University Hospital Infectious Disease Division's swine influenza (H1N1) pneumonia diagnostic weighted point score system for hospitalized adults with influenza-like illnesses (ILIs) and negative rapid influenza diagnostic tests (RIDTs). Heart Lung 2009;38:534–8.

primarily in young healthy adults without comorbidities.[56] The cause of death in most fatal swine influenza (H1N1) pneumonia cases has been due to severe hypoxemia and not due to simultaneous/subsequent bacterial CAP.[35–40]

The admission CXR is of critical importance in evaluating swine influenza (H1N1) pneumonia. Because CAP coinfections are rare, the presence of a focal segmental/lobar infiltrates should suggest another diagnosis, for example, bacterial CAP. In hospitalized adults with swine influenza (H1N1) pneumonia, the admission CXR typically is clear without infiltrates or shows an accentuation of basilar markings/atelectasis which may be unilateral or bilateral. On CXR in severe cases, within 48 hours there is rapid progression to bilateral patchy interstitial infiltrates. Unilateral or bilateral small pleural effusions are not uncommon. Adult hospitalized patients with swine influenza (H1N1) pneumonia who present with, or rapidly develop bilateral patchy

Box 1
Swine influenza (H1N1) pneumonia: case definitions in hospitalized adults

Definite swine influenza (H1N1) pneumonia (laboratory criteria)

ILI with dry cough, temperature higher than 39°C/102°F and a CXR with no focal/segmental lobar infiltrates *plus one or more of these positive tests:*

- Rapid influenza A test
- Respiratory fluorescent antibody (FA) viral panel
- RT-PCR for swine influenza (H1N1)

Probable swine influenza (H1N1) pneumonia (clinical criteria)

ILI with temperature higher than 39°C/102°F with severe myalgias and a CXR with no focal/segmental lobar infiltrates *with negative influenza tests* (see above)[a] *plus this diagnostic triad:* (any 3)

- Relative lymphopenia[b]
- Thrombocytopenia[b]
- Elevated serum transaminases[b]
- Elevated CPKs[b]

[a] Diagnostic tests negative for other viral CAP pathogens (CMV, SARS, HPS, RSV metapneumoviruses, parainfluenza viruses, adenoviruses).
[b] Otherwise unexplained.
Data from Cunha BA, Syed U, Stroll S, et al. Winthrop-University Hospital Infectious Disease Division's swine influenza (H1N1) pneumonia diagnostic weighted point score system for hospitalized adults with influenza-like illnesses (ILIs) and negative rapid influenza diagnostic tests (RIDTs). Heart Lung 2009;38:534–8.

interstitial infiltrates, may also have small pleural effusions. Consolidation is unusual and if present it occurs, later in patients on ventilatory support. Cavitation is not a feature of swine influenza (H1N1) pneumonia in adults.[33]

The Winthrop-University Hospital Infectious Disease Division's diagnostic swine influenza triad has been useful for the rapid clinical presumptive diagnosis of swine influenza (H1N1) pneumonia in hospitalized adults with negative RIDTs and a negative CXR, that is, accentuated basilar markings/atelectasis, but not focal segmental/lobar infiltrates, and differentiates swine influenza (H1N1) pneumonia from ILIs as well as bacterial pneumonias.[33,54]

Mimics of Swine Influenza (H1N1) Pneumonia

During "herald wave" of the swine influenza (H1N1) pandemic, an unexplained increase in Legionnaire's disease occurred before the usual late summer/early fall peak incidence of legionella CAP. This may be analogous to the increased incidence/severity of acute bacterial appendicitis during human influenza A/B outbreaks. Regardless of the mechanism, clinicians should be alert for Legionnaire's disease mimicing swine influenza (H1N1) pneumonia.

In adults the best non-specific laboratory test markers helpful in differentiating Legionnaire's disease from swine influenza (H1N1) pneumonia are the presence of focal segmental/lobar infiltrates on CXR, relative bradycardia, hypophosphatemia, and highly elevated ferritin levels. Serum procalcitonin levels (PCT) are not elevated in swine influenza (H1N1) pneumonia, but are elevated in Legionnaire's disease. The other atypical CAP that may be mimic Legionnaire's disease or swine influenza

(H1N1) pneumonia is Q fever. Q fever CAP has many of the features of Legionnaire's disease, namely, elevated serum ferritin levels, mildly increased serum transaminases (AST/ALT), and relative bradycardia. However, Q fever CAP is often accompanied by splenomegaly, which is not a feature of Legionnaire's disease or swine influenza (H1N1) pneumonia. As with *M pneumoniae*, elevated cold agglutinins may occur with Q fever CAP but are not a feature of Legionnaire's disease or swine influenza (H1N1) pneumonia. Relative lymphopenia is common with Legionnaire's disease, Q fever, and swine influenza (H1N1) pneumonia, but leukopenia and thrombocytopenia are not laboratory markers of either Legionnaire's disease or Q fever CAP.[30,33,55]

LABORATORY DIAGNOSIS

Influenza virus is present in respiratory secretions early in the illness. Nasopharyngeal swabs or washings may be used for viral isolation. In general, higher concentrations of virus are found in nasal secretions than in oropharyngeal secretions. During influenza A epidemics, oropharyngeal secretions contain higher concentrations of influenza virions than nasal secretions. In alveolar macrophages, influenza A viruses produce cytopathogenic effects (CPEs), but are nonspecific and difficult to detect. CPEs due to influenza A are apparent in approximately 50% of cultures within 3 days of inoculation and in approximately 90% within 5 days. Identification of cells showing CPE may be verified using immunofluorescent technique or type/subtype specific antisera. The most common rapid method of influenza laboratory diagnosis is by FA techniques. For FA testing for respiratory viruses, nasopharyngeal aspirates are preferred to swabs. FA influenza assays identify viral antigens in infected respiratory epithelial cells.[22–25]

During the "herald wave" of the swine influenza (H1N1) pandemic in New York, it was realized that there were problems with screening tests, that is, RIDTs. It was hoped that rapid screening tests for influenza A would detect swine influenza (H1N1), an influenza A virus. Rapid influenza A test positivity was usually predictive of RT-PCR positivity for swine influenza (H1N1). It was quickly realized that negative rapid influenza A testing did not rule out swine influenza (H1N1). False negative rapid influenza A testing for swine influenza (H1N1) was 30%. Respiratory FA viral testing detects influenza A, influenza B, metapneumoviruses, RSVs, parainfluenza viruses, and adenoviruses. Unfortunately, respiratory FA viral testing did not correlate with either rapid influenza A testing or RT-PCR testing. Although the definitive test for swine influenza (H1N1) diagnosis remains RT-PCR, during the pandemic, RT-PCR testing was restricted. Restricted RT-PCR testing resulted in tremendous difficulties in making/ruling out the diagnosis of swine influenza (H1N1) and in initiating/discontinuing influenza precautions.[53–55,59]

Because of restricted swine influenza (H1N1) RT-PCR testing, clinical criteria were developed for patients presenting with ILIs who had a negative rapid influenza A test. By combining key clinical and nonspecific laboratory features, a clinical diagnosis of probable swine influenza was developed at Winthrop-University Hospital by the Infectious Disease Division. This permitted an operational clinical approach to placing admitted adult patients on influenza precautions/treatment, and was also useful in differentiating swine influenza (H1N1) from its mimics.[54] (see **Box 1**, **Figs. 1–4**, **Tables 3–5**).

THERAPY

Until relatively recently, there were no effective anti-influenza antivirals. Amantadine and rimantadine has been used for influenza prophylaxis/therapy and act by interfering with the attachment of the virus to uninfected hosts' respiratory epithelial cells. The current anti-influenza antivirals currently available are zanamivir and oseltamivir.

Both of these antivirals decrease the duration/severity of illness. Oseltamivir is administered orally but zanamivir is administered via an inhaler, which is problematic for some patients.[30] Unfortunately, there is now widespread resistance to oseltamivir, greatly diminishing the therapeutic options in influenza and avian influenza (H5N1). At present, oseltamivir remains effective against most strains of swine influenza (H1N1). Oseltamivir is usually given for 5 days, but in severe cases, therapy has been given for 10 days. For severely ill hospitalized patients with swine influenza (H1N1) pneumonia unable to take oral medications, eg, oseltamivir, peramivir is available from the CDC for IV administration. In severe cases of influenza A, amantadine may have some role because of its effect on dilatation of the distal bronchioles. By increasing distal bronchiolar aeration, oxygenation may be improved, which may be critical in severe influenza A.[60–67]

COMPLICATIONS AND PROGNOSIS

The prognosis of influenza A is related primarily to strain virulence. Most patients with mild to moderate influenza A recover without specific anti-influenza therapy. However, influenza A may be severe, and may be fatal in the very young and the elderly with impaired cardiopulmonary function. With pandemic influenza A, the prognosis depends on the virulence of the strain and may be fatal in young, healthy adults. Such has clearly been the case in the recent avian influenza (H5N1) epidemic in Asia whose fatalities, as in the 1918 to 1919 pandemic, were due in the main to influenza pneumonia and was frequently fatal without bacterial superinfection. Severe influenza A pneumonia with superimposed *S aureus* CAP have the worst prognosis. Others who initially present with influenza may later be complicated by subsequent bacterial pneumonia due to *S pneumoniae* or *H influenzae*, and have the same prognosis as noninfluenza patients with *S pneumoniae* or *H influenzae* CAP.

There is a late excess mortality with influenza A, that occurs after the acute episode eg, elderly patients with borderline cardiopulmonary function succumb to heart failure or acute myocardial infarction from the hypoxemia/stress of swine influenza (H1N1) pneumonia. In severe cases of respiratory failure/ARDS, extracorporeal membrane oxygenation (ECMO) has been lifesaving in some.[68] Although influenza is a 3-day illness, postinfluenza fatigue may last for weeks or months. In influenza, prognosis is worse in those patients who develop encephalitis. Following the 1918 to 1919 influenza pandemic, some patients developed Parkinson disease decades later. The prognosis in influenza depends on several factors including the virulence of the strain, the age/immune status of the host, cardiopulmonary function, and complications, for example, encephalitis or bacterial CAP.[1,2,16] The most important intervention in adults with severe swine influenza (H1N1) pneumonia is prolonged ventilatory support. Because these patients are not complicated by simultaneous or subsequent bacterial CAP, empiric antimicrobial therapy seems to be unnecessary in swine influenza (H1N1) pneumonia. The degree and duration of relative lymphopenia/leukopenia as well as the severity and duration of hypoxemia are key prognostic indicators. An improvement in relative lymphopenia and a decrease in oxygen (FIO_2) are predictive of recovery.

SUMMARY AND HISTORICAL PERSPECTIVE

There are differences of opinion on the cause of early deaths in influenza pandemics. Most early deaths in young healthy individuals in the 1918–1919 pandemic seemed to be caused by influenza A pneumonia alone. Based on autopsy specimen cultures, which are notoriously unreliable, some believe the high mortality rate of the

Table 5
Winthrop-University Hospital Infectious Disease Division's swine influenza (H1N1) pneumonia diagnostic weighted point system in adults with negative rapid influenza diagnostic tests (RIDTs)

Clinical Features	Point Scores	Swine Influenza (H1N1) Laboratory Diagnosed	Swine Influenza (H1N1) Clinically Diagnosed	ILIs not Swine Influenza (H1N1)	CMV CAP	Q Fever CAP	Legionella CAP
Adults with an ILI with dry cough, fever >39°C/102°F and a CXR with no focal/segmental lobar infiltrates[a]							
• Severe myalgias	+5	+5	+5	0	0	0	0
• Relative lymphopenia (otherwise unexplained[b])	+5	+5	+5	0	+5	+5	+5
• Elevated CPK (otherwise unexplained)	+3	+3	+3	0	0	0	+5
• Elevated serum transaminases (otherwise unexplained)	+2	+2	+2	0	+2	+2	+2
• Thrombocytopenia (otherwise unexplained)	+5	+5	+5	0	+5	+2	0
Argues *against* the diagnosis of (H1N1):							
• Relative bradycardia (otherwise unexplained)	−5	0	0	0	0	0	−5
• Leukopenia (otherwise unexplained)	−2	0	0	0	0	0	0
• Atypical lymphocytes	−1	0	0	0	0	0	0
• Highly elevated serum ferritin levels (>2 × n)	−5	0	0	0	0	0	−5
• Hypophosphatemia	−3	0	0	0	0	0	−3
Swine influenza Diagnostic Point Score totals:	Total score:	20	20	0	12	9	−1
Probable swine influenza (H1N1) pneumonia = >15 Possible swine influenza (H1N1) pneumonia = 10–15 Unlikely swine influenza (H1N1) pneumonia = <10							

Abbreviation: ILIs, Influenzalike illnesses.

[a] Q fever and legionnaire's disease CAPs usually have focal segmental/labor infiltrates.

[b] Other causes of relative lymphopenia: *Infectious causes*: CMV, HHV-6, HHV-8, HIV, military TB, Legionella, typhoid fever, Q fever, brucellosis, SARS, malaria, babesiosis, influenza, avian influenza, RMSF, histoplasmosis, dengue fever, Chickungunya fever, ehrlichiosis, parvovirus B19, HPS, WNE, viral hepatitis (early); *Noninfectious causes*: cytotoxic drugs, steroids, sarcoidosis, SLE, lymphoma, RA, radiation therapy, Wiskott-Aldrich syndrome, Whipple disease, severe combine immunodeficiency disease (SCID), common variable immune deficiency (CVID), Di George syndrome, Nezelof syndrome, intestinal lymphangiectasia, constrictive pericarditis, tricuspid regurgitation, Kawasaki disease, idiopathic CD_4 cytopenia, Wegener granulomatosis, acute/chronic renal failure, hemodialysis; myasthenia gravis, celiac disease, alcoholic cirrhosis, coronary bypass, CHF, acute pancreatitis, carcinomas (terminal).

Data from Cunha BA, Syed U, Stroll S, et al. Winthrop-University Hospital infectious disease division's swine influenza (H1N1) pneumonia diagnostic weighted point score system for adults with Influenza Like Illnesses (ILIs) and negative Rapid Influenza Diagnostic Tests (RIDTs). Heart Lung 2009;38:534–8.

Table 6
Lessons learned during the "herald wave" of the swine influenza (H1N1) pandemic in spring/summer of 2009 at Winthrop-University Hospital

Laboratory Diagnosis: Rapid Influenza and RT-PCR Testing	Clinical Diagnosis: Winthrop-University Hospital Infectious Disease Division's Diagnostic Swine Influenza (H1N1) Triad	Infection Control Considerations

• Rapid influenza A test positivity correlated fairly well with RT-PCR positivity
• 30% of rapid influenza A tests for swine flu were falsely negative
• Some admitted adult patients with influenzalike illnesses (ILIs) with negative rapid influenza A tests were not placed on influenza precautions resulting in extensive contact investigations of patients/visitors by Infection Control and of exposed employees by the Employee Health Service
• A laboratory diagnosis of swine influenza was made by RT-PCR but testing was restricted
• Another problem with RT-PCR testing was that the results were not quickly available. Causing major Infectious Disease and Infection Control problems
• By the end of July, CDC acknowledged definite/probable case definition because of restricted RT-PCR testing
	• Rapid influenza testing was often not done in the ED in patients with ILIs because they had "pneumonia." Educational efforts were done to inform physicians that admitted adults with swine influenza (H1N1) had swine influenza (H1N1) pneumonia
	• Chest radiographs were critical in identifying bacterial CAPs and mimics of swine influenza (H1N1) in admitted adults with ILIs with fevers >102°F
	• Because of Infectious Disease and Infection Control problems with admitted adults who had ILIs with negative rapid influenza A testing (RIDTs) in the ED, the Infectious Disease Division developed clinical criteria to clinically diagnose probable swine influenza (H1N1) pneumonia (see **Table 4**)
	• In adults admitted with ILIs and negative rapid influenza A tests (RIDTs), the most important findings of swine influenza (H1N1) and predictive of RT-PCR positivity were:
	  • Dry cough
	  • Temperature >39°C/102°F
	  • Severe myalgias
	  • CXR with no focal segmental/lobar infiltrates
	  • Relative lymphopenia
	  • Thrombocytopenia
	  • Elevated CPK
	  • Elevated AST/ALT
		• At the peak of the pandemic, sufficient negative pressure rooms were not always available
		• Lack of adequate negative pressure single rooms delayed the transfer of nonintubated adults with swine influenza in the intensive care unit (ICU) to floors (to decrease mobile ICU congestion to free up beds for additional swine influenza patients)
		• It was difficult to determine which of the possible/probable swine influenza (H1N1) patients should have influenza precautions discontinued
		• N95 masks were used for health care personnel obtaining respiratory samples for swine influenza testing and for those involved in intubating possible/probable swine influenza (H1N1) patients
		• Some of our personnel were not fit tested for N95 masks or failed the fit test. These health care workers could use the PAPR hood
		• The supply of N95 respirators was quickly exhausted and, of necessity, surgical masks had to be used
		• There were problems with visitors who did not always observe influenza precautions. Security escorted one visitor at a time to/from swine influenza (H1N1) patient rooms
		• Bilingual signs advising people to stay out of the hospital, including the coffee shop/lobby, worked well
		• Hand sanitizing dispensers were used but visitors were frequently observed coughing without covering in the lobby and coffee shop as well as in front of the signs themselves!
		• Most health care workers and the public did not fully appreciate that swine influenza (H1N1) is primarily transmitted via aerosols/droplets as well as hand/face transmission
		• EHS furloughed or prophylaxed HCWS exposed to swine influenza (H1N1). This worked well minimizing the loss of medical personnel taking care of patients with and without swine influenza (H1N1)

Abbreviation: ILI, influenzalike illness.

Table 7
Clinical summary of lessons learned during the "herald wave" of the swine influenza (H1N1) pandemic

Diagnostic Difficulties		Infection Control Problems	Severity Indicators
Laboratory Diagnostic Difficulties RIDTs • Rapid influenza A tests false negative ≥30% • Respiratory fluorescent antibody (FA) viral tests did not improve diagnostic yield over the rapid influenza A tests, and did not always correlate with RT-PCR H1N1 results RT-PCR • RT-PCR was done in rapid influenza A negative patients to confirm/rule out the laboratory diagnosis of swine influenza • RT-PCR testing was usually restricted causing major problems with initially/ diagnosing influenza precautions • Later when RT-PCR became available, commonly, RT-PCR results were reported after 5–7 days • In some cases of clinically certain swine influenza, the RT-PCR was negative • Possible explanations include: - poor specimen sample - oropharyngeal secretions may be negative for RT-PCR swine influenza (H1N1) with *lung specimens* that are positive	Clinical Diagnostic Difficulties • Definite (laboratory) diagnosis • Diagnosis was problematic (see laboratory diagnosis above) in admitted patients, differentiating ILI from swine influenza (H1N1) pneumonia • Clinical diagnosis rested on ruling out: • Bacterial CAPs, eg, Legionnaires' disease • Viral CAPs, eg, CMV, RSV, metapneumovirus • Cardiopulmonary disorders, eg, exacerbation of CAD, CHF, AECB • Probable (clinical) diagnosis Based on key clinical features in admitted adults with ILIs • Dry cough • temperature >102°F • Severe myalgias Based on non-specific laboratory tests[a] • Relative lymphopenia • Thrombocytopenia • Leukopenia (if with relative lymphopenia/ thrombocytopenia) • Elevated CPKs • CXR • clear/accentuated basilar lung marking • Bilateral patchy interstitial infiltrates/ARDS • Small unilateral/bilateral pleural effusion • No focal segmental/lobar (cavitary/ non-cavitary) infiltrates	Influenza Precautions (Droplet and Contact) • Many patients not placed on influenza precautions because of negative RIDTs • Patients later determined to have probable/definite swine influenza (H1N1) were eventually placed on precautions resulting in extensive/labor intensive contact investigation of exposed health care workers, patients and visitors Duration of Precautions • Duration of H1N1 shedding in respiratory secretions remains unclear • After oseltamivir therapy, H1N1 shedding in respiratory secretions terminated by day #3	Laboratory Test Indicators • Degree/duration of relative lymphopenia • Leukopenia (with relative lymphopenia/ thrombocytopenia) • Profound/prolonged hypoxemia (A-a gradient >35) Demographic Indicators • Pregnancy • Obesity/diabetes mellitus • Young healthy adults (not the very young, elderly)

Swine Influenza (H1N1) Prophylaxis	Swine Influenza (H1N1) Therapy	Mimics of Swine Influenza (H1N1) Pneumonia	Complications of Swine Influenza (H1N1)
Prophylaxis • Oseltamivir seemed to be effective • Resistance strains (rare but of concern)	Therapy Antiviral Interventions • Oseltamivir seemed effective in mild/moderately ill patients • Peramivir was useful in those unable to take/failed oseltamivir Interventions to Improve Oxygenation • Amantadine seemed to improve oxygenation in some • Ventilator support the single most important lifesaving intervention • In those unable to be oxygenated by ventilator, extracorporeal membrane oxygenation (ECMO) was life saving in some patients	Adults • Influenza A (human seasonal) • Avian influenza (H5N1) • Legionnaires' disease • Adenoviruses • Cytomegalovirus (CMV) Children • Respiratory syncytial virus (RSV) • Metapneumovirus • Influenza B	Pulmonary • Viral pneumonia due to swine influenza (H1N1) • Respiratory failure • ARDs • Bacterial co-infections remained the exception rather than the rule • Main problem is the limited literature reporting "bacterial co-infections" was recognizing organisms from respiratory secretions/lung specimens represented colonization not infection (without appropriate clinical correlation) • Highest potential co-infections rates reported only 0–4% • Highest rates reported 24% in those given CAP antibiotics suggested many/most of these isolates representing colonization rather than true infection • Excluding the above single report, antibiotics for bacterial CAP complicating swine influenza (H1N1) pneumonia appeared to be unnecessary Extrapulmonary CNS • Encephalitis was rare Cardiac • Increased evidence of acute myocardial infarction in healthy young adults • Exacerbation of existing CAD/CHF • Myocarditis Other • Unexplained increase in incidence/severe or acute appendicitis • Unexplained increase in Legionnaires' Disease during the swine influenza (H1N1) pandemic • Rhabdomyositis

[a] Otherwise unexplained.

1918–1919 influenza pandemic was due to superimposed bacterial pneumonia, for example, *S pneumoniae.* Most lung specimens from autopsies of young healthy military recruits clearly show the pathologic changes of influenza alone. Based on the pathologic comparisons of viral and bacterial pneumonia, it seems that the majority of early deaths in young healthy military recruits was due to severe hypoxemia. Late excess mortality seems to have been due to influenza precipitated decompensation in those with antecedent borderline cardiopulmonary function/reserve.

Most recently, *S aureus* was recognized as an important pathogen in the 1957– 1958 Asian influenza A pandemic. In 1957–1958 Asian influenza A pandemic, influenza presented as pneumonia alone or simultaneously with *S aureus* or subsequently with *S pneumoniae* or *H influenzae* CAP. Because the 1957–1958 influenza A pandemic clinicians had modern bacteriologic and virologic diagnostic methods, clinicians attributed the excess mortality to late bacterial CAP. The unusual severity of the 1918–1919 influenza A pandemic seems to have been related to a particularly virulent strain of influenza A (H1N1), not unlike the virulence of avian influenza (H5N1). In the recent experience with avian influenza (H5N1), it is interesting to note that despite high mortality of ~ 60% in young adults, avian influenza deaths have been due to avian influenza (H5N1) pneumonia alone and not simultaneous/subsequent bacterial CAP.[69–70]

A summary of lessons learned during the "herald wave" of the swine influenza (H1N1) pandemic is presented here in tabular form (**Tables 6** and **7**). The important take-home lessons for clinicians in the summary relate to laboratory and clinical diagnosis, infection control concerns, and empiric antibiotic use.[71–85]

REFERENCES

1. Ewald PW. Influenza. In: Evolution of infectious disease. New York: Oxford University Press; 1994. p. 10–116.
2. Crosby AW. Influenza. In: Kiple KF, editor. The Cambridge world history of human disease. New York: Cambridge University Press; 1993. p. 807–11.
3. Aufderheide AC, Rodriguez-Martin C. Influenza. In: Aufderheide AC, Rodriguez-Martin C, editors. The Cambridge encyclopedia of human paleopathology. New York: Cambridge University Press; 1998. p. 210–2.
4. Sydenham T. Influenza. In: Major RH, editor. Classic descriptions of disease. Springfield (MA): Charles C. Thomas, Publisher; 1978. p. 201–2.
5. Douglas RG Jr. Influenza in man. In: Kilbourne ED, editor. The influenza viruses and influenza. Orlando (FL): Academic Press; 1975. p. 395.
6. Cunha BA. Influenza: historical aspects of epidemics and pandemics. Infect Dis Clin North Am 2004;18:141–56.
7. Ravenholt RT, Foege WH. Before our time: 1918 influenza, encephalitis lethargica, parkinsonism. Lancet 1982;2:860–4.
8. Conner LA. The symptomatology and complications of influenza. JAMA 1919;73: 321–5.
9. Kolte IV, Skinhoj P, Keiding N, et al. The Spanish flu in Denmark. Scand J Infect Dis 2008;40:538–46.
10. Sheretz RJ, Sheretz HJ. Influenza in the preantibiotic era. Infect Dis Clin Pract 2006;14:127.
11. Winternitz MC, Wason IM, McNamara FP. The pathology of influenza. New Haven (CT): Yale University Press; 1920.
12. Wolbach SB. Comments on the pathology and bacteriology of fatal influenza cases as observed at Camp Devens, Mass. Bull Johns Hopkins Hosp 1919;30:104–5.

13. Stevens KM. The pathophysiology of influenzal pneumonia in 1918. Perspect Biol Med 1918;25:115–25.
14. Mulder J, Hers JF. Influenza. Groningen (The Netherlands): Wolters-Noordhoff; 1979.
15. Klotz O. The pathology of epidemic influenza. In: Studies on epidemic influenza, comprising clinical and laboratory investigations by members of the faculty of the school of medicine. Pittsburgh (PA): University of Pittsburgh Press; 1919. p. 255–61.
16. Andrewes FW. The bacteriology of influenza. In: Great Britain Ministry of Health. Reports on public health and medical subjects, no. 4: report on the pandemic of influenza, 1918–1919. London: His Majesty's Stationery Office; 1920. p. 110–26.
17. Centers for Disease Control and Prevention (CDC). Outbreak of swine-origin influenza A (H1N1) virus infection—Mexico, March-April 2009. MMWR Morb Mortal Wkly Rep 2009;58:467–70.
18. Centers for Disease Control and Prevention (CDC). Swine-origin influenza A (H1N1) virus infections in a school—New York City, April 2009. MMWR Morb Mortal Wkly Rep 2009;58:470–2.
19. Gallaher WR. Towards a sane and rational approach to management of Influenza H1N1 2009. Virol J 2009;6:51.
20. Rezza G. Swine-origin influenza virus A (H1N1)v: lessons learnt from the early phase of the epidemic. Eur J Public Health 2009;19:572–3.
21. Cohen J, Enserink M. Infectious disease. As swine flu circles globe, scientists grapple with basic questions. Science 2009;324:572–3.
22. Kilbourne ED, editor. The influenza viruses and influenza. Orlando (FL): Academic Press; 1975.
23. Debré R, Couvreur J. Influenza: clinical features. In: Debré R, Celers J, editors. Clinical virology: the evaluation and management of human viral infections. Philadelphia: WB Saunders; 1970. p. 507–15.
24. Nicholson KG, Webster RG, Hay AJ, editors. Textbook of influenza. Oxford (UK): Blackwell Science; 1998.
25. Van Voris LP, Young JF, Bernstein JM, et al. Influenza viruses. In: Belshe RB, editor. Textbook of human virology. Littleton (MA): PSG Publishing Company; 1984. p. 267–81.
26. Atmar RL. Influenza viruses. In: Murray PR, Baron EJ, Jorgensen JH, et al, editors. Manual of clinical microbiology. 9th edition. Washington, DC: ASM Press; 2007. p. 1340–51.
27. Hayden FG, Palese P. Influenza virus. In: Richman DD, Whitley RJ, Hayden FG, editors. Clinical virology. 3rd edition. Washington, DC: ASM Press; 2009. p. 943–76.
28. Sym D, Patel PM, El-Chaar GM. Seasonal, avain and novel H1N1 influenza: prevention and treatment modalities. Ann Pharmacother 2009;43:2001–11.
29. Harper SA, Bradley JS, Englund JA, et al. Seasonal influenza in adults and children: diagnosis, treatment, chemoprophylaxis and institutional outbreak management: clinical practice guidelines of the Infectious Diseases Society of America. Clin Infect Dis 2009;48:1003–32.
30. Cunha BA. Pneumonia essentials. 3rd edition. Sudbury (MA): Jones & Bartlett; 2010.
31. Cunha BA. The clinical diagnosis of severe viral influenza A. Infection 2008;36: 92–3.
32. Kim HM, Lee YW, Lee KJ, et al. Alveolar macrophages are indispensable for controlling influenza viruses in lungs of pigs. J Virol 2008;82:4265–74.

33. Mollura DJ, Asnis DS, Crupi RS, et al. Imaging findings in a fatal case of pandemic swine-origin influenza A (H1N1). AJR Am J Roentgenol 2009;193:1500–3.
34. Agarwal PP, Cinti S, Kazerooni EA, et al. Chest radiographic and CT findings in novel swine-origin influenza A (H1N1) virus (S-OIV) infection. AJR Am J Roentgenol 2009;193:1488–93.
35. Cunha BA. A useful clinical approach to community-acquired methicillin-resistant *Staphylococcus aureus* (CA-MRSA) infections. J Hosp Infect 2008;68:271–73.
36. Cunha BA. Methicillin-resistant *Staphylococcus aureus*: clinical manifestations and antimicrobial therapy. Clin Microbiol Infect 2005;11:33–42.
37. Tacconelli E, De Angelis G. Pneumonia due to methicillin-resistant *Staphylococcus aureus*: clinical features, diagnosis and management. Curr Opin Pulm Med 2009;15:218–48.
38. Kallen AJ, Brunkard J, Moore Z, et al. *Staphylococcus aureus* community-acquired pneumonia during the 2006 to 2007 influenza season. Ann Emerg Med 2009;53:358–65.
39. Cheng VC, Lau YK, Lee KL, et al. Fatal co-infection with swine origin influenza virus A/H1N1 and community-acquired methicillin-resistant *Staphylococcus aureus*. J Infection 2009;259:1–5.
40. Cunha BA, Syed U, Strollo S. Bacterial pneumonia rare with fatal swine influenza (H1N1) pneumonia: if chest films have no focal segmental/lobar infiltrates, empiric antibiotic therapy is unnecessary. J Chemotherapy 2010;21:584–5.
41. Hien ND, Ha NH, Van NT, et al. Human infection with highly pathogenic avian influenza virus (H5N1) in northern Vietnam, 2004–2005. Emerg Infect Dis 2009;15:19–23.
42. Writing Committee of the Second World Health Organization consultation on clinical aspects of human infection with avian influenza A (H5N1) virus. Update on avian influenza A (H5N1) virus infection in humans. N Engl J Med 2008;358:261–73.
43. Thomas JK, Noppenberger J. Avian influenza: a review. Am J Health Syst Pharm 2007;64:149–65.
44. Ozbay B, Sertogullarindan B, Tekin M, et al. Influenza-associated pneumonia in a Turkish area with endemic avian influenza. Respirology 2008;13:444–6.
45. Sandrock C, Kelly T. Clinical review: update of avian influenza A infections in humans. Crit Care 2007;11:209–18.
46. To KF, Chan PK, Chan KF, et al. Pathology of fatal human infection associated with avian influenza A H5N1 virus. J Med Virol 2001;63:242–6.
47. Tran TH, Nguyen TL, Nguyen TD, et al. Avian influenza A (H5N1) in 10 patients in Vietnam. N Engl J Med 2004;350:1179–88.
48. Uyeki TM. Human infection with highly pathogenic avian influenza A (H5N1) virus: review of clinical issues. Clin Infect Dis 2009;49:279–90.
49. Gambotto A, Barratt-Boyes SM, de Jong MD, et al. Human infection with highly pathogenic H5N1 influenza virus. Lancet 2008;371:1464–75.
50. Yuen KY, Chan PKS, Peiris M, et al. Clinical features and rapid viral diagnosis of human disease associated with avian influenza A H5N1 virus. Lancet 1998;351:467–71.
51. Rainer TH. Severe acute respiratory syndrome: clinical features, diagnosis, and management. Curr Opin Pulm Med 2004;10:159–65.
52. Rhodes LV, Huang C, Sanchez AJ, et al. Hantavirus pulmonary associated with Monongahela virus, Pennsylvania. Emerg Infect Dis 2000;6:616–21.
53. Cunha BA, Pherez FM, Strollo S. Swine influenza H1N1: diagnostic dilemma early in the pandemic. Scand J of Infect 2009;41:900–2.

54. Cunha BA, Syed U, Strollo S, et al. Winthrop-University Hospital infectious disease division's swine influenza (H1N1) pneumonia diagnostic weighted point score system for adults with Influenza Like Illnesses (ILIs) and negative Rapid Influenza Diagnostic Tests (RIDTs). Heart Lung 2009;38:534–8.
55. Cunha BA, Pherez FM, Schoch PE. The diagnostic importance of relative lymphopenia as a marker of swine influenza (H1N1) in adults. Clin Infect Dis 2009;49: 1454–6.
56. Louria DB, Blumenfeld HL, Ellis JT, et al. Studies on influenza in the pandemic of 1957–1958. Pulmonary complications of influenza. J Clin Invest 1959;38:213–65.
57. Robertson L, Caley JP, Moore J. Importance of *Staphylococcus aureus* in pneumonia in the 1957 epidemic of influenza A. Lancet 1958;2:233–6.
58. Petersdorf RG, Fusco JJ, Harter DH, et al. Pulmonary infections complicating Asian influenza. Arch Intern Med 1959;103:262–72.
59. Vasoo S, Stevens J, Singh K. Rapid antigen tests for diagnosis of pandemic (Swine) influenzae A/H1N1. Clin Infect Dis 2009;49:1090–3.
60. Cunha BA. Amantadine may be lifesaving in severe influenza A. Clin Infect Dis 2006;43:1574–5.
61. Centers for Disease Control and Prevention (CDC). Update: drug susceptibility of swine-origin influenza A (H1N1) viruses, April 2009. MMWR Morb Mortal Wkly Rep 2009;58:433–5.
62. Influenza Project Team. Oseltamivir resistance in human seasonal influenza viruses (A/H1N1) in EU and EFTA countries: an update. Euro Surveill 2008;13:8032.
63. Kawai N, Ikematsu H, Iwaki N, et al. A change in the effectiveness of amantadine for the treatment of influenza over the 2003–2004, 2004–2005, and 2005–2006 influenza seasons in Japan. J Infect Chemother 2007;13:314–9.
64. Meijer A, Lackenby A, Hungnes O, et al. Oseltamivir-resistant influenza virus A (H1N1), Europe, 2007-08 season. Emerg Infect Dis 2009;15:552–60.
65. Van der Vries E, van den Berg B, Schutten M. Fatal oseltamivir-resistant influenza virus infection. N Engl J Med 2008;359:1074–6.
66. Couzin-Frankel J. Swine flu outbreak. What role for antiviral drugs? Science 2009; 324:705.
67. Hurt AC, Selleck P, Komadina N, et al. Susceptibility of highly pathogenic A (H5N1)Avian influenza viruses to the neuraminidase inhibitors and adamantanes. Antiviral Res 2007;73:228–31.
68. Davies A, Jones D, Bailey M, et al. Extracorporeal Membrane oxygenation for 2009 influenza A (H1N1) acute respiratory distress syndrome. JAMA 2009;302: 1888–95.
69. Andreasen V, Viboud C, Simonsen L. Epidemiologic characterization of the 1918 influenza pandemic summer wave in Copenhagen: implications for pandemic control strategies. J Infect Dis 2008;197:270–8.
70. Steel J, Palese P. The 1918 Influenza pandemic: lessons from the past raise questions for the future. In: Klenk HD, Matrosovich MN, Stech J, editors. Avian Influenza. Monogr Virol, vol 27. Basel: Karger; 2008. p. 272–86.
71. Cunha BA, Thekkel V, Cohan C. Swine influenza (H1N1): contact investigation burden because of failure to institute influenza precautions with negative rapid influenza A diagnostic test results. Infect Control Hosp Epidemiol 2010;31:102–4.
72. Cunha BA, Thekkel V, Krilov L. Nosocomial swine influenza (H1N1) pneumonia: lessons learned from an illustrative case. J Hosp Infect 2009; 72, in press.
73. Charlier C, Enouf V, Lanternier F, et al. Kinetics of nasopharyngeal shedding of novel H1N1 (swine-like) influenza A virus in an immunocompetent adult under oseltamivir therapy. Clin Microbiol Infect 2009;15:1189–91.

74. Dominguez-Cherit G, Lapinsky SE, Macias AE, et al. Critically ill patients with 2009 influenza A (H1N1) in Mexico. JAMA 2009;302:1872–9.
75. MMWR. Bacterial coinfections in lung tissue specimens from fatal cases of 2009 pandemic influenza A (H1N1)—United States, May–August 2009, 77.
76. MMWR. Hospitalized patients with novel influenza A (H1N1) infection—California, April–May, 2009. MMWR Morb Mortal Wkly Rep 2009;58:536–41.
77. Kumar A, Zarychanski R, Pinto R, et al. Critically ill patients with 2009 influenza A (H1N1) in Canada. JAMA 2009;302:1880–7.
78. MMWR. Intensive-care patients with severe novel influenza A (H1N1) virus infection—Michigan, June 2009. MMWR Morb Mortal Wkly Rep 2009;58:749–52.
79. Bin C, Xingwang L, Yeulong S, et al. Clinical & epidemiologic characteristics of 3 early cases of influenza A pandemic (H1N1) 2009 virus infection, People's Republic of China, 2009. Emerging Infect Dis 2009;15:1418–22.
80. Cunha BA. Swine influenza (H1N1) pneumonia: bacterial airway colonization common but fatalities due to bacterial pneumonia remain relatively rare. J Clin Virol 2009. [Epub ahead of print].
81. Barlow GD, on behalf of the BSAC Council. Swine flu and antibiotics. J Antimicrob Chemother 2009;10:1–6.
82. Mauad I, Hajjar LA, Callegari CA, et al. Lung pathology in fatal novel human influenza A (H1N1) infection. Am J Respir Crit Care Med 2009. [Epub ahead of print].
83. Cunha BA, Klein NC, Strollo S, et al. Legionnaire's disease mimicking swine influenza (H1N1) pneumonia. Heart & Lung 2010;39, in press.
84. Klein N, Chak A, Chengot A, et al. Case report: a fatal case of severe H1N1 influenza A (Swine flu) pneumonia in an HIV positive patient. Emerg Infect Dis 2010; 16:149–50.
85. Cunha BA, Syed U, Mikail N. Rapid clinical diagnosis in fatal swine influenza (H1N1) pneumonia in adult with negative rapid influenza diagnostic tests (RIDTs): diagnostic swine influenza triad. Heart & Lung 2010;39:78–86.

Specific Diagnostic Tests for Atypical Respiratory Tract Pathogens

René te Witt, BSc*, Willem B. van Leeuwen, PhD,
Alex van Belkum, PhD

KEYWORDS

• *Mycoplasma pneumoniae* • *Legionella pneumophila*
• *Chlamydophila pneumoniae* • Diagnostic tests

The term "atypical pneumonia" most commonly refers to pneumonia caused by *Chlamydophila pneumoniae*, *Mycoplasma pneumoniae*, or *Legionella* species. Although *Bordetella pertussis/parapertussis*, *Franscissella tularensis*, and several respiratory parasites, fungi, and viruses are also part of the spectrum of causative agents, these organisms will not be discussed further in this article. *C pneumoniae*, *M pneumoniae*, and *Legionella* spp are increasingly recognized as frequent and important pathogens in (acute) respiratory tract infections (RTI), such as community-acquired pneumonia (CAP) and exacerbations of chronic bronchitis.[1,2]

For the detection of these pathogens, serology is still considered the gold standard.[2] However, serologic results are often unreliable and usually available too late to have an impact on patient management. Optimal serologic testing for individual patient care depends on the age of the patient, timing of serum collection, whether paired (acute and convalescent) sera are obtained, availability of appropriate equipment, and experience of the laboratory personnel. The latest developments in diagnostic strategies include the application of Nucleic Acid Amplification Techniques (NAATs), such as Nucleic Acid Sequence-Based Amplification (NASBA), (real-time) Polymerase Chain Reaction (PCR), Strand Displacement Amplification (SDA), Multi Ligation-dependent Probe Amplification (MLPA), and others in the detection of an extended number of agents responsible for RTI. Advantages of real-time PCR over traditional PCR include a more rapid turnaround time and the complete lack of post-amplification analysis. Results can be obtained within the same day of specimen receipt, allowing appropriate focusing of therapy and reduction of unnecessary antibiotic therapy in RTI.[3,4]

Department of Medical Microbiology and Infectious Diseases, Unit Research and Development, Erasmus MC, 's-Gravendijkwal 230, 3015 CE, Rotterdam, The Netherlands
* Corresponding author.
E-mail address: r.tewitt@erasmusmc.nl (R. te Witt).

Infect Dis Clin N Am 24 (2010) 229–248
doi:10.1016/j.idc.2009.10.013 **id.theclinics.com**
0891-5520/10/$ – see front matter

Viruses cause a large proportion of RTI and are responsible for extensive morbidity and mortality. The availability and use of these new molecular diagnostic tools in virology has contributed tremendously to a better understanding of the viral etiology of RTI. This, however, depends on the populations studied, the geographic location, and seasonality. Next to the increasing importance of viral agents, the role of the bacterial pathogens *C pneumoniae*, *M pneumoniae,* and *Legionella* spp in RTI is becoming more clear.[5–7] Novel diagnostic tests are more frequently presented and these also cover bacterial agents of RTI.[8]

The overall diagnostic approach for these bacterial pathogens is depicted in **Table 1** and will be described in separate sections in this article. The quality of different types of specimens commonly collected to detect pathogens causing RTI and different processing routes have been compared, and are important features in the diagnostic setting. These will also be discussed in forthcoming sections.

Depending on the technological and financial possibilities, a microbiological laboratory should optimize its diagnostic strategy by applying a combination of classical and/or real-time amplification tests for the detection of viruses and the atypical bacterial agents. When implementing such a strategy, a balance between performance criteria (sensitivity, specificity) and convenience criteria (clinical utility, turnaround time, and costs) will have to be defined. In the end, this should result in the optimization of clinical patient management. This article reviews the microbiological tests that are currently available for the detection of *M pneumoniae, C pneumoniae,* and *Legionella* spp; their clinical performance; and their future in the clinical microbiology laboratory.

Collaborative, large scale, multicenter, retrospective, and prospective studies will facilitate optimal validation of new NAATs on the basis of large collections of diverse clinical samples.

MYCOPLASMA PNEUMONIAE

Historically, serology has been the most common laboratory method for the diagnosis of *M pneumoniae* infections. An infection is defined as a fourfold increase in antibody titer in acute and convalescent sera and is still considered the "gold standard" for reliably defining infection.[9] Although culture and PCR are also used, nonclinical persistence of the viable organism or dead cells for variable periods of time following acute infection remains a challenge in the assessment of the significance of a positive culture or PCR assay result.

Culture

The time required for microbiological culturing, ranging from a few days to 3 weeks, renders cultivation impractical for patient management. Hence, culture expertise is not widely available, except in specialized research and reference laboratories.

Serologic Testing

M pneumoniae has both lipid and protein antigens that can induce antibody responses that can be detected after about 1 week of infection, peaking at 3 to 6 weeks, followed by a gradual decline. This response facilitates several different types of serologic assays, based on these different antigens and technologies. Serology is a useful epidemiologic tool in circumstances where the likelihood of RTI caused by *M pneumoniae* is high, but it is not optimally suited for direct management of individual patients. Its main disadvantage is the need for both acute and convalescent paired sera collected 2 to 4 weeks apart from each other that should be tested simultaneously

Table 1
Diagnostic approaches for the detection of bacterial atypical RTI pathogens

Pathogen	Clinical Sample	"New" Test	Gold Standard
Legionella spp	Urine	Antigen test	
	Respiratory samples	NAAT	Culture
	Serum		IgG/IgM
C pneumoniae	Respiratory samples	NAAT	Culture
	Serum		IgG/IgM
M pneumoniae	Respiratory samples	NAAT	Culture
	Serum		IgG/IgM

Abbreviations: NAAT, Nucleic Acid Amplification Technique; RTI, respiratory tract infection.

for IgM and IgG to confirm seroconversion indicative for infection. In a recent study, it was demonstrated that the percentage of persons with acute infection who demonstrate a positive IgG response in the acute phase was less than 50%.[10] This low sensitivity could be explained by the presence of specific IgG from previous infections or slow IgG increase in the individuals tested. However, when convalescent sera were tested, the number of IgG-positive specimens increased to 82%. A single measurement of IgM might indicate an acute infection if the test is performed at least 7 days after onset, but the test could be false negative if the test is performed before. This same study revealed that only 14 (52%) of 27 acute-phase sera tested positive by various IgM assays; however, this number increased to 39 (88%) when convalescent sera were tested. IgM antibodies can persist for several weeks to months. Another study showed that the IgM ImmunoCard (Meridian Bioscience, Cincinnati, OH) had a sensitivity of only 32% for the detection of acute *M pneumoniae* infection in seropositive children suffering from pneumonia.[11] Again, the sensitivity increased to 89% when paired sera were analyzed. These findings suggest that diagnosis of RTI should not be based on a single IgM measurement in a patient's serum, as was suggested in several other studies.[12,13] It is important to realize and to emphasize that the antibody response may also be delayed in some infections or can even be absent if the patient is immunosuppressed or immunodeficient.

M pneumonia is a mucosal pathogen, and for that reason, IgA is produced in an early state of the infection. Measurement of serum IgA either alone or in combination with IgM may therefore be an alternative for the diagnosis of an acute infection. Unfortunately, very few commercial assays include reagents for IgA detection. The limited number of studies that involved detection of IgA generally documented improved detection of acute infection, especially in adults.[14–16] However, one study measured IgG, IgM, and IgA antibodies in healthy blood donors and in patients with various infections caused by microorganisms other than *M pneumoniae*, using various commercial enzyme immuno assays (EIA).[15] It was documented that 23% of the blood donors and 54% of the patients with various non-*Mycoplasma* infections were positive for IgA, raising doubts about its value to accurately diagnose a current *M pneumoniae* infection. Talkington and colleagues[10] showed that single-use EIAs were better able to identify seropositive samples than several plate-type EIAs. However, plate-type EIAs may be more efficient and cost effective in laboratories that need high throughput.

Molecular Testing

Owing to the relative insensitivity and prolonged time needed for the detection of *M pneumoniae* by culture, the need for paired acute and convalescent sera collected

2 to 4 weeks apart for optimal serologic diagnosis and other problems inherent to serologic assays as described before, PCR gained considerable interest very soon after its introduction in the late 1980s. The first reports of PCR suited for detection of *M pneumoniae* appeared in 1989.[17,18] Since then, more than 200 papers describing the use of classical PCR for detection of *M pneumoniae* in human infections were published. Gene targets used in various PCR protocols for *M pneumoniae* detection include the ATPase operon, the P1 adhesin, 16S rRNA gene, the elongation factor Tu coding gene (*tuf* gene) and the repetitive element repMP1 (**Table 2**).[17–21] The sensitivity of PCR is very high, theoretically corresponding to a single organism. However, its major advantage is the exclusive gain of time.

Several real-time PCR assays have also been described.[21–27] Comparison of (real-time) PCR with culture and/or serology has yielded various results that are not always concordant. As would be expected, molecular-based assays often demonstrate superior sensitivity for detection of acute infection over serology and culture,[13,23,28] although this is not always the case.[25,29] Positive PCR results in culture-negative persons without evidence of respiratory tract disease suggest inadequate assay specificity, persistence of the organism after infection, or asymptomatic carriage. Quantitative studies may be required before we can draw final conclusions on the usefulness and clinical applicability. Positive PCR results in seronegative patients could be the result of an inadequate immune response to earlier successful antibiotic treatment or sampling before specific antibody response. Negative PCR results in culture-proven or seropositive patients might be caused by the presence of inhibitors or technical problems with the assay and its target gene. If antibiotics have been administered, PCR results may be negative even though serology is positive.

Because *M pneumoniae* is only one of a variety of fastidious and/or slow-growing pathogenic microorganisms responsible for RTI with clinically similar manifestations,

Table 2
Original references on NAAT for atypical RTI pathogens

Gene Target	Authors	References
M pneumoniae		
ATPase operon	Bernet et al	18
P1 adhesin	Jensen et al	17
16S rDNA	van Kuppeveld et al	19
tuf	Luneberg et al	20
repMP1	Dumke et al	21
Legionella spp		
16S rDNA	Jonas et al	93
23S-5S	Herpers et al	101
5S rDNA	Kessler et al	103
mip	Lindsay et al	106
C pneumoniae		
ompA	Kaltenboeck et al	122
pstI	Campbell et al	126
pmp4	Mygind et al	128
16S rDNA	Gaydos et al	129

Abbreviations: NAAT, Nucleic Acid Amplification Technique; RTI, respiratory tract infection.

there has been considerable interest and effort to develop multiplex PCR assays for single-step detection of multiple causative agents. Most assays now include gene targets for *M pneumoniae, C pneumoniae, L pneumophila,* and, occasionally, other organisms.[26,30–40] Still, monoplex assays seem to have higher sensitivity and specificity than multiplex assays.[41]

NASBA, which is a technique based on isothermal RNA amplification, has also been applied for the detection of *M pneumoniae* in clinical samples.[42] Initial studies have shown that the performance of NASBA is comparable to PCR in terms of sensitivity. A multiplex NASBA assay targeting *M pneumoniae, C pneumoniae,* and *L pneumophila* has also been described.[43] Other techniques such as multiplex reverse-transcription PCR have been described recently[44] and will be developed further over the years to come.[45]

In 2002 and 2004, the diagnostic performance of laboratories for the molecular detection of *M pneumoniae* was investigated.[41] For these two quality control exercises with a 2-year interval, specimens were spiked with *M pneumoniae*. In 2002, only 2 of 12 participants obtained 100% correct results, 2 of 12 produced false positive results and 10 of 12 had between 0 of 9 and 8 of 9 correct positive results. In 2004, correct results were obtained in 15 of 18 participating laboratories and no false positive results were reported. Multiplex PCR and NASBA formats scored fewer samples positive than the monoplex reactions. This shows that the quality of the molecular tests is improving and that one should carefully consider whether single tests or multiplex tests will be used.

Diagnostic Efficacy in Different Clinical Samples

Clinical samples suitable for *M pneumoniae* PCR include nasopharyngeal and oropharyngeal secretions, sputa, bronchoalveolar lavages (BALs), and throat swabs. Many patients with *M pneumoniae* infection do not produce significant amounts of sputum; especially children fail to do so. Michelow and colleagues[29] evaluated nasopharyngeal and oropharyngeal samples obtained from children with serologically proven *M pneumoniae* pneumonia and reported that either specimen type was equally effective for bacterial detection by PCR. Still, combining results from both clinical sites provided the most significant diagnostic yield. One group of investigators found sputa to be superior sources over nasopharyngeal aspirates and throat swabs in young adults with serologically proven *M pneumoniae* infection[46]; however, others found no difference in the detection efficiency of *M pneumoniae* using PCR in the various anatomic sites.[47] Gnarpe and colleagues[48] compared nasopharyngeal swabs and oropharyngeal swabs for the detection of *M pneumoniae* by PCR. A total of seven patients were seropositive for *M pneumoniae* and, of these, six were positive from oropharyngeal swabs and only two were positive from nasopharyngeal swabs. Another study compared nasopharyngeal swabs to oropharyngeal swabs in children and found no significant difference in the detection of *M pneumoniae* by PCR.[47] The authors did note that nasopharyngeal swabs were more likely to be problematic than oropharyngeal swabs because of the presence of PCR inhibitors or lack of respiratory epithelial material. Honda and colleagues[49] applied capillary PCR to sputum, BALs, and oropharyngeal swabs. The highest rate of detection was shown for oropharyngeal swabs.

Loens and colleagues[43,50] combined the results of two studies on LRTIs. From 25 patients both an oropharyngeal swab and a sputum were available for NAAT analysis and culture. In both studies, sputa were the preferred specimens. Raty and colleagues[46] collected sputum, a nasopharyngeal aspirate, and an oropharyngeal swab from 32 young military employees suffering from pneumonia during an

M pneumoniae outbreak and applied PCR. This study also concluded that sputum is the best sample to detect *M pneumoniae*. Dorigo-Zetsma and colleagues[51] confirmed this finding. Care should be taken when applying NAAT to sputum samples because inhibitors occur frequently in sputum and this may be difficult to eliminate.[52]

In conclusion, if a sputum sample is available, this might be the most optimal specimen for *M pneumoniae* detection by culture and NAAT. A nasopharyngeal swab, nasopharyngeal aspirate, or oropharyngeal swab might be the second best option for analysis by NAAT.

LEGIONELLA SPP

Legionella pneumophila was identified as an important causative agent of severe RTI. The first cases of Legionnaires' disease or Legionellosis were discovered among attendants of an American Legion convention in Philadelphia in 1976.[53] Pontiac fever is caused by the same bacterium. This produces milder respiratory illness without pneumonia.

Legionella spp are waterborne bacterial species that can be found in tap water to which the first outbreak was attributed, but also in water from cooling towers, air-conditioning, ventilators, and humidifiers.[54]

Culture

Culture-based isolation of *Legionella* spp from body fluids is still considered the gold standard for the diagnosis of Legionellosis. Culture requires special enriched media, adequate processing of specimens, and technical expertise. Several days are required to obtain a positive result, with most *Legionella* spp colonies being detected within 4 to 7 days. *Legionella* species other than *L pneumophila* may grow at a slower rate and may, therefore, be detectable only after 10 days of incubation.[55,56] Some *Legionella* spp have unusual colony morphology and may be easily overlooked. The standard medium to culture *Legionella* is buffered charcoal yeast extract (BCYE) agar supplemented with α-ketoglutarate, with or without selective antimicrobial agents. The antibiotics most commonly added are polymyxin to control commensal flora, anisomycin against yeasts, and cefamandole or vancomycin against gram-positive bacteria.[57]

Serologic Testing

Indirect immunofluorescence assay (IFA) was used to detect antibodies in patients from the Philadelphia outbreak, which turned out to be instrumental in determining the cause of the illness. Since then, a number of serologic tests have been developed and evaluated.[58–68] Of the various antibody detection methods that are available, IFA and enzyme-linked immunosorbent assays (ELISA) are the most commonly used. Nowadays, many laboratories prefer ELISA over IFA testing, because they are less subjective, more accurate than IFA testing, and have the potential for automated high-throughput performance. The reported sensitivities vary from 41% to 94%.[56] A recent study showed sensitivities of 64%, 61%, and 44% for ELISA, IFA, and rapid microagglutination assays, respectively.[69] In ELISA, half of the patients showed a seroconversion in IgM and the other half showed a seroconversion in IgG. Other studies have shown that the early immune response primarily involves IgM and that IgM tests must be included for optimal sensitivity.[70–73] Seroconversion may take several weeks, which is a major limitation of serologic testing. In most cases, a fourfold increase in antibody titer is detected within 3 to 4 weeks, but in some cases this may take more than 10 weeks.[74] Obviously, this severely compromises the timeline of serologic testing. Acute-phase IFA antibody titers of greater than or equal to 256 during pneumonia were once considered sufficient for a presumptive diagnosis, but this has been shown to be unreliable, given the high prevalence of *Legionella* antibody positivity in persons without clinical evidence for Legionellosis.[75] Another disadvantage of serologic testing is its incapability to accurately detect all *Legionella* species and serogroups. In addition, a diagnosis by a fourfold IgG or IgM titer increase can only be made retrospectively and cannot support patient management. Therefore, there is an urgent need for additional tests for *Legionella* diagnosis in the early stage of disease.

Antigen Detection

The detection of *Legionella* antigen in urine was developed shortly after the first outbreak in Philadelphia.[76] *Legionella* antigen can be detected in urine as early as 24 hours after onset of symptoms and antigen shedding persists for days to weeks. The detected antigen is a component of the lipopolysaccharide portion of the *Legionella* cell wall.[77,78] The urinary antigen tests combine reasonable sensitivity (80%–95%) and high specificity (95%–100%) with very rapid results.[79,80] Nowadays, it is the most commonly used laboratory test for *Legionella* diagnosis.[81,82] In Europe, the proportion of cases diagnosed by urinary antigen detection has increased rapidly from 15% in 1995, 33% in 1998, 74% in 2004, to more than 90% in 2006.[83]

Commercial kits that use both radioimmunoassay (RAI) and EIA methodologies have been available for several years and have similar performance characteristics.[55] Agglutination assays have also been introduced, but these have not yet provided an acceptable level of sensitivity and specificity.[84] In addition, immunochromatographic assays (IA) have been developed that have similar sensitivity and specificity as compared with EIA.[85] The majority of IA is most sensitive for the detection of the Pontiac monoclonal antibody type of *L pneumophila* serogroup 1 (up to 90%), less sensitive for other monoclonal antibody types of *L pneumophila* serogroup 1 (to 60%), and poorly sensitive (to 5%) for other *L pneumophila* serogroups and other *Legionella* species.[86,87] An important feature of these assays is its high specificity (>99%).

The sensitivity of urinary antigen detection appears to be associated with the clinical severity of the disease.[88] Yzerman and colleagues[88] tested two enzyme immunoassays, Binax Legionella Urinary Antigen EIA (Binax, Portland, ME) and Biotest Legionella Urine Antigen EIA (Biotest, Dreieich, Germany) and one immunochromatographic assay, Binax NOW Urinary Antigen Test (Binax), using urine samples from outbreak related Legionellosis patients. For patients with mild Legionellosis, the test sensitivities ranged from 40% to 53%, whereas for patients with severe Legionellosis, the sensitivities reached 88% to 100%. These findings have implications for the diagnostic process in patients with mild pneumonia and suggest that patients with mild pneumonia may be underdiagnosed if only the urine antigen test is used. The use of concentrated urine samples increased sensitivity without a decreasing the specificity. Since this concentration step is timely and laborious, some laboratories only use this approach in case of equivocal results or strong clinical indication.

Another association between test sensitivity and certain defined subpopulations has been described by Helbig and colleagues.[85] The clinical utility of *Legionella* urinary antigen assays for the diagnosis of Legionnaire's disease has been assessed by using samples from 317 culture-proven cases. The sensitivities of the Binax EIA and Biotest EIA urinary tests were found to be 94% and 94% for travel-associated infection and 87% and 76% for community-acquired infection, but only 44% and 46% for nosocomially acquired infection.

Several new immunochromatographic urinary antigen tests for the detection of *L pneumophila* serogroup 1 have been developed.[79,89] The Binax NOW urinary antigen test, in concordance with the findings of previous studies, has excellent sensitivity and specificity. The performance of some new tests is below the acceptable level for diagnostic assays (**Table 3**).[89]

Molecular Testing

The first assay designed to detect the DNA of *L pneumophila*, was based on RIA in which a radiolabeled ribosomal probe specific for all strains of *Legionella* spp was applied. Researchers reported a varying sensitivity and specificity for this assay.[90,91] The use of this probe for the detection of Legionellosis at one hospital resulted in 13

Table 3
Performance of urinary antigen detection tests

	Sensitivity			
Urinary Antigen Test	**NCU**	**CU**	**Specificity**	**References**
SAS Legionella test (SA Scientific, San Antonio, TX)	82.9%	NT	99.0%	79
Binax NOW urinary antigen test (Binax, Portland, ME)	91.4%	NT	100.0%	79
Binax Legionella urinary antigen EIA (Binax, Portland, ME)	97.1%	NT	NT	80
Biotest Legionella urine antigen EIA (Biotest, Dreieich, Germany)	91.4%	NT	NT	80
Binax NOW urinary antigen test (Binax, Portland, ME)	94.3%	NT	NT	80
Binax Legionella urinary antigen EIA (Binax, Portland, ME)	86.5%	NT	NT	85
Biotest Legionella urine antigen EIA (Biotest, Dreieich, Germany)	76.0%	NT	NT	85
Biotest EIA (Biotest, Dreieich, Germany)	94.6%	NT	100.0%	86
Bartels EIA (Bartels Inc, Trinity Biotech Company, Wicklow, Ireland)	74.1%	91.5%	100.0%	87
Biotest Legionella urine antigen EIA (Biotest, Dreieich, Germany)	51.7%	91.5%	100.0%	87
Biotest Legionella urine antigen EIA (Biotest, Dreieich, Germany)	71.0%	74.0%	NT	88
Binax Legionella urinary antigen EIA (Binax, Portland, Maine)	69.0%	79.0%	NT	88
Binax NOW urinary antigen test (Binax, Portland, ME)	72.0%	81.0%	NT	88
Rapid U Legionella antigen test (Diamondial, Sees, France)	71.2%	NT	96.6%	89
SD Bioline Legionella urinary antigen test (Standard Diagnostics Inc, Kyonggi-do, Korea)	31.5%	NT	98.9%	89
Binax NOW urinary antigen test (Binax, Portland, ME)	91.8%	NT	100.0%	89

Abbreviations: CU, concentrated urine; NCU, non-concentrated urine; NT, not tested.

false positive cases and the assay was removed from the market soon after it falsely recorded this pseudo outbreak.[92]

Legionella PCR is available in an increasing number of laboratories that use a variety of in-house or commercial assays. Diagnostic PCR assays target specific *Legionella pneumophila* DNA regions within 16S rRNA genes,[93–100] the 23S-5S spacer,[101] 5S rDNA,[102,103] or the macrophage inhibitor potentiator (*mip*) gene.[104–107] The application of PCR to nonrespiratory samples seems particularly attractive for patients who do not produce sputum. *Legionella* DNA can be detected in urine, serum, and leukocyte samples obtained from patients with Legionellosis, with sensitivities ranging from 30% to 86%.[102,108–110] The sensitivity of the detection of *Legionella* DNA in serum is relatively low (50%–60%) in Legionellosis patients, but was shown to be higher (70%–90%) in patients with more severe disease.[108,109] When testing samples from the lower respiratory tract (bronchoalveolar lavage), PCR has repeatedly shown to have a sensitivity equal to or higher than culture.[99,100,111] Indeed, PCR has been considered by some authors to be the test of choice for patients who produce sputum.[111] However, a number of false positive results have been reported, both with commercially available tests and with in-house tests.[55,99] A problem with the interpretation of these false positive results is the question of whether these are truly false positive or whether it was the reference method that failed. It is difficult to solve this issue and, at present, there is only one study available where the authors determined the exact sensitivity and specificity of *Legionella* PCR in patients with pneumonia of unknown etiology.[112] Diederen and colleagues[112] demonstrated that variation of DNA targets influence the test performance. PCR designed on the detection of 16S RNA had a sensitivity and specificity of 86% and 95%; as for PCR designed to detect the *mip* gene, this was 92% and 98%, respectively. In conclusion, laboratory workers and clinicians must be cautious when interpreting results and should not hesitate to question the results, especially when these results are unexpected based on clinical presentation and local epidemiology. Only one study describes a multicenter comparison of molecular methods for detection of *Legionella* spp.[113] The authors compared the methods of nine laboratories for 12 sputum samples with *L pneumophila* or *Legionella longbeachae* and conclude that PCR targeting the *mip* gene is *L pneumophila* specific and 16S rRNA gene amplification is genus specific.

Relevance of Sample Type

Legionella spp can be isolated from a variety of sample types, although sputum and bronchoalveolar lavages are the samples of choice. Sputum samples are generally considered to be optimal for isolation of *L pneumophila* in patients with RTI. Culture results depend on the severity of illness, with the lowest result (15%–25%) for mild pneumonia and the highest result (>90%) for severe pneumonia.[111] A major limitation of culturing the pathogen from sputum is the fact that fewer than 50% of *Legionella* patients produce sufficient amounts of sputum.[111,114] Most patients with Legionellosis produce nonpurulent sputum. Obviously, laboratories that reject sputum samples containing limited mucosal polymorphonuclear leukocytes may reject potential positive samples. Ingram and Plouffe[115] demonstrated that up to 84% of *L pneumophila*–positive samples would have been discarded by using sputum purulence screens and they recommended acceptance of all aspects of sputum suspected for *Legionella* culture. Estimated sensitivities of sputum culture range from less than 10% to 80% and vary between individual laboratories.[55,111]

In conclusion, urinary antigen detection is currently the most helpful rapid test for the diagnosis of *Legionella* infection. The use of rapid urinary antigen tests reduces mortality and avoids unnecessary or inappropriate use of antibiotics in patients with

CAP. However, combining test results from more than one sampling site appears to improve the diagnostic accuracy. Especially in this diagnostic segment, molecular testing may play an important (future) role.

CHLAMYDOPHILA PNEUMONIAE
Culture

For *C pneumoniae*, culture on cell lines has traditionally been considered as a reference and standard diagnostic method. However, because of the important limitations in the cultivation of *C pneumoniae* (technical complexity, limited viability of the bacteria, slow growth, and variable diagnostic success), performance of culture remains restricted to specialized laboratories. Hence, the use of culture as a diagnostic tool is suboptimal and not often recommended. Still, the most common method for diagnosis of *C pneumoniae* infection is serology. Assays available for detection of *C pneumoniae*–specific antibodies include Micro Immuno Fluorescence (MIF) tests, ELISAs, and EIAs, each of which exists in a variety of in-house and commercial variations.

Recommendations by the Centers for Disease Control and Prevention (CDC) and the practical guidelines of the Infectious Disease Society of America (IDSA) defined the main criteria for the diagnosis of acute *C pneumoniae* infection as a single IgM titer of greater than or equal to 1:64 or a fourfold increase in the IgG titer in acute serum and convalescent serum, measured 4 weeks apart from each other. The use of single IgG or IgA titers is discouraged because of the relatively high overall seroprevalence in healthy populations.[116] However, several studies deviated widely from these guidelines and there are several inherent limitations to the serodiagnosis of *C pneumoniae* infection.[117–121]

Serologic Testing

Serologic testing at best offers a retrospective diagnosis. In primary infections, IgM antibodies appear 2 to 3 weeks and IgG antibodies appear 6 to 8 weeks after infection, whereas in reinfections, IgM may be absent or of low titer and IgG appears earlier, within 2 to 3 weeks after infection.

The MIF assay has been repeatedly demonstrated to be insensitive and it showed a poor correlation with the detection of *C pneumoniae* by culture or PCR, particularly in children. Only 1% to 3% of culture-positive children in a study by Hammerschlag[122] met the serologic criteria for acute infection. Wellinghausen and colleagues[119] reported that 17 patients with CAP had seronegative results with MIF.

Generally, the specificity of serologic testing may be suboptimal as well. Serologic evidence of acute infection was found in 19% of healthy adults who had negative results by culture and PCR.[122] This lack of specificity may result from serologic cross-reactivity with other *Chlamydia* species, as well as *Mycoplasma* spp or *Bartonella* spp. In addition, other limitations of the MIF test relate to a lack of standardized reagents, technical complexity, and subjective end point determination, all of which result in significant intra- and interlaboratory variation of test performance. One study evaluated the interlaboratory reliability of the MIF test for measurement of *C pneumoniae*–specific IgA and IgG titers for 392 serum samples, using reagents and antigens obtained from a common source. The investigators observed agreement between IgA and IgG titers to be as low as 55% and 38%, respectively.[123]

EIAs may overcome some of the limitations of the MIF test by being more objective in the interpretation of the results and less technically demanding. Hermann and colleagues[124] compared seven commercial EIAs or ELISAs with four MIF assays for detection of specific IgG antibodies. The authors used serum samples from 80 healthy subjects and reported sensitivities and specificities ranging from 42% to 100% and from 88% to 100%, respectively. The SeroCP ELISA Savyon Diagnostic and Quant EIA (Savyon, Ashdod, Israel) showed the best sensitivities, 96% and 92%, respectively, followed by the Vircell ELISA (Viva Diagnostica, Köln-Hürth, Germany) and the Labsystems EIA (Labsystems, Helsinki, Finland), which each had a sensitivity of about 75%.

Molecular Testing

For reasons of the previously mentioned issues with culture and serology, PCR can be an interesting alternative for diagnosis of *C pneumoniae* infections. The first reports of PCR application for the detection of *C pneumoniae* appeared in 1990 and 1992.[125,126] Since then, more than 250 studies describing the use of PCR for detection of *C pneumoniae* in human infections have been published. Gene targets used in various types of PCR for *C pneumoniae* include the *ompA* gene,[127] *pstI*,[126] *pmp4*,[128] and 16S rDNA.[129] Real-time PCR assays have also been described.[128,130–134] Multicenter studies that use a large and diverse repertoire of clinical specimens and compare data independently are likely to provide important insights into the performance of new assays. Two such studies describing multicenter comparisons of the performance of various NAAT tests for detection of *C pneumoniae* in respiratory specimens have been published. Both studies revealed significant variations of test performance from laboratory to laboratory. Chernesky and colleagues[135] compared a *C pneumoniae* PCR kit from Abbot (Abbott Laboratories, North Chicago, IL) with five conventional PCR assays, using specimens spiked with pre-extracted DNA. Loens and colleagues[41] used spiked respiratory specimens to compare the performance of several in-house PCR assays. Correct results were produced in 12 of 16 and 13 of 18 tests in 2002 and 2004, respectively. Both of these studies revealed significant intercenter discordance of detection rates, using different or even the same tests. Both multiplex PCR and NASBA formats scored a smaller number of positive samples than the monoplex tests.

Relevance of Sample Type

The choice of a specimen from the respiratory tract has an impact on the sensitivity of *C pneumoniae* isolation and detection by culture and PCR. In a study in which the authors enrolled 260 previously healthy children (3–12 years), it was shown that the nasopharynx may be superior to the throat as a source of materials to be used for isolation of *C pneumoniae*. Of 34 children from whom *C pneumoniae* was isolated, nasopharyngeal swabs were positive for all children, but oropharyngeal swabs were positive for only 50% of the same group.[136] During a *C pneumoniae* outbreak, Boman and colleagues[137] collected sputum, oropharyngeal swabs, and nasopharyngeal swabs from 116 patients presenting an RTI. When the authors compared the performances of PCR, culture, and antigen detection for samples from three different niches in 61 patients for whom all samples were available, 20 patients were positive for *C pneumoniae*, for whom 7 nasopharyngeal swabs, 10 oropharyngeal swabs, and 20 sputum samples were considered to be true positives. Sensitivities of PCR, culture, and antigen detection by EIA for sputum samples were 95%, 100%, and 80%, respectively. Sensitivities for the other types of specimen sampling sites were much lower (25%–50%). The clinical relevance of sputum for the detection of *C pneumoniae* was confirmed by Kuoppa and colleagues.[131] In this study, a sputum sample, a nasopharynx aspirate, and an oropharyngeal swab from 35 patients suspected of having a *C pneumonia* infection were examined by PCR. Most samples had *C pneumoniae* DNA copies below 1×10^4 genome copies/mL, but most of the sputum samples contained higher inoculant of *C pneumoniae* DNA, with an average of 8.6×10^5 copies/mL. However, these results are in contrast with those obtained by Verkooyen and colleagues,[138] who examined sputum, nasopharyngeal swabs, oropharyngeal swabs, and throat wash specimens by PCR and culture from 156 hospitalized CAP patients. The highest sensitivity in this study was obtained by applying PCR on nasopharyngeal swabs (51.3%). Surprisingly, none of the sputum samples tested was positive.

Gnarpe and colleagues[48] compared PCR results for *C pneumoniae* from nasopharyngeal swabs and oropharyngeal swabs in 66 patients presenting with RTI. Of a total of 18 patients positive for *C pneumoniae*, in 15 patients the oropharyngeal swab was the only positive specimen, whereas for 3 patients both the oropharyngeal swab and the nasopharyngeal swab yielded a positive PCR result. In conclusion, sputum may be the preferred specimen for detection of *C pneumoniae* by NAAT.

SUMMARY

Historically, atypical agents of RTI were merely detected on the basis of microbiological culture. Without exception, sensitivity and specificity of such cultures did not meet criteria of excellence. Hence, a variety of antigen- or antibody-mediated tests was developed. Unfortunately, none of these individual tests was in itself sufficient to reliably identify the causative infectious agents. Also, the more recent availability of a variety of NAATs did not (yet) solve this problem. In today's clinical microbiology laboratories no widely accepted gold standard for the detection of *M pneumoniae, C pneumoniae,* and *Legionella* spp is available. Technicians and physicians have to rely on a combination of test results that, together with clinical presentation of the patient, may lead to a presumptive identification of a causative agent at best. Although great diagnostic improvements have been made over the past 20 years, no final tool is as yet available. Future biomarker discovery is still required before the ultimate test for the diagnosis of atypical RTI agents will become available.

REFERENCES

1. File TM Jr, Tan JS, Plouffe JF. The role of atypical pathogens: *Mycoplasma pneumoniae, Chlamydia pneumoniae*, and *Legionella pneumophila* in respiratory infection. Infect Dis Clin North Am 1998;12(3):569–92, vii.
2. Blasi F. Atypical pathogens and respiratory tract infections. Eur Respir J 2004; 24(1):171–81.
3. Charles PG. Early diagnosis of lower respiratory tract infections (point-of-care tests). Curr Opin Pulm Med 2008;14(3):176–82.
4. Nicolau DP. Treatment with appropriate antibiotic therapy in community-acquired respiratory tract infections. Am J Manag Care 2004;10(Suppl 12): S381–8.
5. Boersma WG, Daniels JM, Lowenberg A, et al. Reliability of radiographic findings and the relation to etiologic agents in community-acquired pneumonia. Respir Med 2006;100(5):926–32.
6. Oosterheert JJ, Bonten MJ, Schneider MM, et al. Predicted effects on antibiotic use following the introduction of British or North American guidelines for community-acquired pneumonia in The Netherlands. Clin Microbiol Infect 2005;11(12): 992–8.
7. van der Eerden MM, Vlaspolder F, de Graaff CS, et al. Comparison between pathogen directed antibiotic treatment and empirical broad spectrum antibiotic

treatment in patients with community acquired pneumonia: a prospective randomised study. Thorax 2005;60(8):672–8.
8. Reijans M, Dingemans G, Klaassen CH, et al. RespiFinder: a new multiparameter test to differentially identify fifteen respiratory viruses. J Clin Microbiol 2008;46(4):1232–40.
9. Gavranich JB, Chang AB. Antibiotics for community acquired lower respiratory tract infections (LRTI) secondary to *Mycoplasma pneumoniae* in children. Cochrane Database Syst Rev 2005;(3):CD004875.
10. Talkington DF, Shott S, Fallon MT, et al. Analysis of eight commercial enzyme immunoassay tests for detection of antibodies to *Mycoplasma pneumoniae* in human serum. Clin Diagn Lab Immunol 2004;11(5):862–7.
11. Ozaki T, Nishimura N, Ahn J, et al. Utility of a rapid diagnosis kit for *Mycoplasma pneumoniae* pneumonia in children, and the antimicrobial susceptibility of the isolates. J Infect Chemother 2007;13(4):204–7.
12. Nir-Paz R, Michael-Gayego A, Ron M, et al. Evaluation of eight commercial tests for *Mycoplasma pneumoniae* antibodies in the absence of acute infection. Clin Microbiol Infect 2006;12(7):685–8.
13. Beersma MF, Dirven K, van Dam AP, et al. Evaluation of 12 commercial tests and the complement fixation test for *Mycoplasma pneumoniae*-specific immunoglobulin G (IgG) and IgM antibodies, with PCR used as the "gold standard". J Clin Microbiol 2005;43(5):2277–85.
14. Yoo SJ, Oh HJ, Shin BM. Evaluation of four commercial IgG- and IgM-specific enzyme immunoassays for detecting *Mycoplasma pneumoniae* antibody: comparison with particle agglutination assay. J Korean Med Sci 2007;22(5):795–801.
15. Csango PA, Pedersen JE, Hess RD. Comparison of four *Mycoplasma pneumoniae* IgM-, IgG- and IgA-specific enzyme immunoassays in blood donors and patients. Clin Microbiol Infect 2004;10(12):1094–8.
16. Souliou E, Almasri M, Papa A, et al. Laboratory diagnosis of *Mycoplasma pneumoniae* respiratory tract infections in children. Eur J Clin Microbiol Infect Dis 2007;26(7):513–5.
17. Jensen JS, Sondergard-Andersen J, Uldum SA, et al. Detection of *Mycoplasma pneumoniae* in simulated clinical samples by polymerase chain reaction. Brief report. APMIS 1989;97(11):1046–8.
18. Bernet C, Garret M, de Barbeyrac B, et al. Detection of *Mycoplasma pneumoniae* by using the polymerase chain reaction. J Clin Microbiol 1989;27(11):2492–6.
19. van Kuppeveld FJ, Johansson KE, Galama JM, et al. 16S rRNA based polymerase chain reaction compared with culture and serological methods for diagnosis of *Mycoplasma pneumoniae* infection. Eur J Clin Microbiol Infect Dis 1994;13(5):401–5.
20. Luneberg E, Jensen JS, Frosch M. Detection of *Mycoplasma pneumoniae* by polymerase chain reaction and nonradioactive hybridization in microtiter plates. J Clin Microbiol 1993;31(5):1088–94.
21. Dumke R, Schurwanz N, Lenz M, et al. Sensitive detection of *Mycoplasma pneumoniae* in human respiratory tract samples by optimized real-time PCR approach. J Clin Microbiol 2007;45(8):2726–30.
22. Hardegger D, Nadal D, Bossart W, et al. Rapid detection of *Mycoplasma pneumoniae* in clinical samples by real-time PCR. J Microbiol Methods 2000;41(1):45–51.
23. Templeton KE, Scheltinga SA, Graffelman AW, et al. Comparison and evaluation of real-time PCR, real-time nucleic acid sequence-based amplification, conventional PCR, and serology for diagnosis of *Mycoplasma pneumoniae*. J Clin Microbiol 2003;41(9):4366–71.

24. Ursi D, Dirven K, Loens K, et al. Detection of *Mycoplasma pneumoniae* in respiratory samples by real-time PCR using an inhibition control. J Microbiol Methods 2003;55(1):149–53.
25. Pitcher D, Chalker VJ, Sheppard C, et al. Real-time detection of *Mycoplasma pneumoniae* in respiratory samples with an internal processing control. J Med Microbiol 2006;55(Pt 2):149–55.
26. Morozumi M, Ito A, Murayama SY, et al. Assessment of real-time PCR for diagnosis of *Mycoplasma pneumoniae* pneumonia in pediatric patients. Can J Microbiol 2006;52(2):125–9.
27. Di Marco E, Cangemi G, Filippetti M, et al. Development and clinical validation of a real-time PCR using a uni-molecular Scorpion-based probe for the detection of *Mycoplasma pneumoniae* in clinical isolates. New Microbiol 2007;30(4):415–21.
28. Nilsson AC, Bjorkman P, Persson K. Polymerase chain reaction is superior to serology for the diagnosis of acute *Mycoplasma pneumoniae* infection and reveals a high rate of persistent infection. BMC Microbiol 2008;8:93.
29. Michelow IC, Olsen K, Lozano J, et al. Diagnostic utility and clinical significance of naso- and oropharyngeal samples used in a PCR assay to diagnose *Mycoplasma pneumoniae* infection in children with community-acquired pneumonia. J Clin Microbiol 2004;42(7):3339–41.
30. Tong CY, Donnelly C, Harvey G, et al. Multiplex polymerase chain reaction for the simultaneous detection of *Mycoplasma pneumoniae, Chlamydia pneumoniae,* and *Chlamydia psittaci* in respiratory samples. J Clin Pathol 1999;52(4):257–63.
31. Corsaro D, Valassina M, Venditti D, et al. Multiplex PCR for rapid and differential diagnosis of *Mycoplasma pneumoniae* and *Chlamydia pneumoniae* in respiratory infections. Diagn Microbiol Infect Dis 1999;35(2):105–8.
32. Grondahl B, Puppe W, Hoppe A, et al. Rapid identification of nine microorganisms causing acute respiratory tract infections by single-tube multiplex reverse transcription-PCR: feasibility study. J Clin Microbiol 1999;37(1):1–7.
33. Welti M, Jaton K, Altwegg M, et al. Development of a multiplex real-time quantitative PCR assay to detect *Chlamydia pneumoniae, Legionella pneumophila* and *Mycoplasma pneumoniae* in respiratory tract secretions. Diagn Microbiol Infect Dis 2003;45(2):85–95.
34. Ginevra C, Barranger C, Ros A, et al. Development and evaluation of Chlamylege, a new commercial test allowing simultaneous detection and identification of *Legionella, Chlamydophila pneumoniae,* and *Mycoplasma pneumoniae* in clinical respiratory specimens by multiplex PCR. J Clin Microbiol 2005;43(7): 3247–54.
35. Khanna M, Fan J, Pehler-Harrington K, et al. The pneumoplex assays, a multiplex PCR-enzyme hybridization assay that allows simultaneous detection of five organisms, *Mycoplasma pneumoniae, Chlamydia* (Chlamydophila) *pneumoniae, Legionella pneumophila, Legionella micdadei,* and *Bordetella pertussis,* and its real-time counterpart. J Clin Microbiol 2005;43(2):565–71.
36. McDonough EA, Barrozo CP, Russell KL, et al. A multiplex PCR for detection of *Mycoplasma pneumoniae, Chlamydophila pneumoniae, Legionella pneumophila,* and *Bordetella pertussis* in clinical specimens. Mol Cell Probes 2005;19(5): 314–22.
37. Raggam RB, Leitner E, Berg J, et al. Single-run, parallel detection of DNA from three pneumonia-producing bacteria by real-time polymerase chain reaction. J Mol Diagn 2005;7(1):133–8.
38. Stralin K, Backman A, Holmberg H, et al. Design of a multiplex PCR for *Streptococcus pneumoniae, Haemophilus influenzae, Mycoplasma pneumoniae*

and *Chlamydophila pneumoniae* to be used on sputum samples. APMIS 2005; 113(2):99–111.
39. Geertsen R, Kaeppeli F, Sterk-Kuzmanovic N, et al. A multiplex PCR assay for the detection of respiratory bacteria in nasopharyngeal smears from children with acute respiratory disease. Scand J Infect Dis 2007;39(9):769–74.
40. Wang Y, Kong F, Yang Y, et al. A multiplex PCR-based reverse line blot hybridization (mPCR/RLB) assay for detection of bacterial respiratory pathogens in children with pneumonia. Pediatr Pulmonol 2008;43(2):150–9.
41. Loens K, Beck T, Ursi D, et al. Two quality control exercises involving nucleic acid amplification methods for detection of *Mycoplasma pneumoniae* and *Chlamydophila pneumoniae* and carried out 2 years apart (in 2002 and 2004). J Clin Microbiol 2006;44(3):899–908.
42. Loens K, Ieven M, Ursi D, et al. Detection of *Mycoplasma pneumoniae* by real-time nucleic acid sequence-based amplification. J Clin Microbiol 2003;41(9):4448–50.
43. Loens K, Beck T, Ursi D, et al. Development of real-time multiplex nucleic acid sequence-based amplification for detection of *Mycoplasma pneumoniae, Chlamydophila pneumoniae*, and *Legionella* spp. in respiratory specimens. J Clin Microbiol 2008;46(1):185–91.
44. Kumar S, Wang L, Fan J, et al. Detection of 11 common viral and bacterial pathogens causing community-acquired pneumonia or sepsis in asymptomatic patients by using a multiplex reverse transcription-PCR assay with manual (enzyme hybridization) or automated (electronic microarray) detection. J Clin Microbiol 2008;46(9):3063–72.
45. Atkinson TP, Balish MF, Waites KB. Epidemiology, clinical manifestations, pathogenesis and laboratory detection of *Mycoplasma pneumoniae* infections. FEMS Microbiol Rev 2008;32:956–73.
46. Raty R, Ronkko E, Kleemola M. Sample type is crucial to the diagnosis of *Mycoplasma pneumoniae* pneumonia by PCR. J Med Microbiol 2005;54(Pt 3):287–91.
47. Reznikov M, Blackmore TK, Finlay-Jones JJ, et al. Comparison of nasopharyngeal aspirates and throat swab specimens in a polymerase chain reaction-based test for *Mycoplasma pneumoniae*. Eur J Clin Microbiol Infect Dis 1995; 14(1):58–61.
48. Gnarpe J, Lundback A, Gnarpe H, et al. Comparison of nasopharyngeal and throat swabs for the detection of *Chlamydia pneumoniae* and *Mycoplasma pneumoniae* by polymerase chain reaction. Scand J Infect Dis Suppl 1997; 104:11–2.
49. Honda J, Yano T, Kusaba M, et al. Clinical use of capillary PCR to diagnose *Mycoplasma pneumonia*. J Clin Microbiol 2000;38(4):1382–4.
50. Loens K, Beck T, Ursi D, et al. Evaluation of different nucleic acid amplification techniques for the detection of *M. pneumoniae, C. pneumoniae* and *Legionella* spp. in respiratory specimens from patients with community-acquired pneumonia. J Microbiol Methods 2008;73(3):257–62.
51. Dorigo-Zetsma JW, Verkooyen RP, van Helden HP, et al. Molecular detection of *Mycoplasma pneumoniae* in adults with community-acquired pneumonia requiring hospitalization. J Clin Microbiol 2001;39(3):1184–6.
52. Loens K, Ursi D, Goossens H, et al. Molecular diagnosis of *Mycoplasma pneumoniae* respiratory tract infections. J Clin Microbiol 2003;41(11):4915–23.
53. Fraser DW, Tsai TR, Orenstein W, et al. Legionnaires' disease: description of an epidemic of pneumonia. N Engl J Med 1977;297(22):1189–97.
54. Winn WC Jr. Legionnaires disease: historical perspective. Clin Microbiol Rev 1988;1(1):60–81.

55. Fields BS, Benson RF, Besser RE. *Legionella* and Legionnaires' disease: 25 years of investigation. Clin Microbiol Rev 2002;15(3):506–26.
56. Den Boer JW, Yzerman EP. Diagnosis of *Legionella* infection in Legionnaires' disease. Eur J Clin Microbiol Infect Dis 2004;23(12):871–8.
57. Doern GV. Detection of selected fastidious bacteria. Clin Infect Dis 2000;30(1): 166–73.
58. Lennette DA, Lennette ET, Wentworth BB, et al. Serology of Legionnaires disease: comparison of indirect fluorescent antibody, immune adherence hemagglutination, and indirect hemagglutination tests. J Clin Microbiol 1979; 10(6):876–9.
59. Holliday MG. The diagnosis of Legionnaires' disease by counter immunoelectrophoresis. J Clin Pathol 1980;33(12):1174–8.
60. Yonke CA, Stiefel HE, Wilson DL, et al. Evaluation of an indirect hemagglutination test for *Legionella pneumophila* serogroups 1 to 4. J Clin Microbiol 1981; 13(6):1040–5.
61. Soriano F, Aguilar L, Gomez Garces JL. Simple immunodiffusion test for detecting antibodies against *Legionella pneumophila* serotype 1. J Clin Microbiol 1982;15(2):330–1.
62. Wreghitt TG, Nagington J, Gray J. An ELISA test for the detection of antibodies to *Legionella pneumophila*. J Clin Pathol 1982;35(6):657–60.
63. Thompson TA, Wilkinson HW. Evaluation of a solid-phase immunofluorescence assay for detection of antibodies to *Legionella pneumophila*. J Clin Microbiol 1982;16(1):202–4.
64. Harrison TG, Taylor AG. A rapid microagglutination test for the diagnosis of *Legionella pneumophila* (serogroup 1) infection. J Clin Pathol 1982;35(9):1028–31.
65. Elder EM, Brown A, Remington JS, et al. Microenzyme-linked immunosorbent assay for detection of immunoglobulin G and immunoglobulin M antibodies to *Legionella pneumophila*. J Clin Microbiol 1983;17(1):112–21.
66. Herbrink P, Meenhorst PL, Groothuis DG, et al. Detection of antibodies against *Legionella pneumophila* serogroups 1 to 6 and the Leiden-1 strain by micro ELISA and immunofluorescence assay. J Clin Pathol 1983;36(11):1246–52.
67. Sampson JS, Wilkinson HW, Tsang VC, et al. Kinetic-dependent enzyme-linked immunosorbent assay for detection of antibodies to *Legionella pneumophila*. J Clin Microbiol 1983;18(6):1340–4.
68. Barka N, Tomasi JP, Stadtsbaeder S. ELISA using whole *Legionella pneumophila* cell as antigen. Comparison between monovalent and polyvalent antigens for the serodiagnosis of human legionellosis. J Immunol Methods 1986;93(1):77–81.
69. Yzerman EP, den Boer JW, Lettinga KD, et al. Sensitivity of three serum antibody tests in a large outbreak of Legionnaires' disease in The Netherlands. J Med Microbiol 2006;55(Pt 5):561–6.
70. Hartigan DA. Comparison of specific immunoglobulin G, M and agglutinating antibodies against *Legionella pneumophila*. Scand J Infect Dis 1981;13(4):269–72.
71. Zimmerman SE, French ML, Allen SD, et al. Immunoglobulin M antibody titers in the diagnosis of Legionnaires disease. J Clin Microbiol 1982;16(6):1007–11.
72. De Ory F, Echevarria JM, Pelaz C, et al. Detection of specific IgM antibody in the investigation of an outbreak of pneumonia due to *Legionella pneumophila* serogroup 1. Clin Microbiol Infect 2000;6(2):64–9.
73. Rojas A, Navarro MD, Fornes FE, et al. Value of serological testing for diagnosis of legionellosis in outbreak patients. J Clin Microbiol 2005;43(8):4022–5.
74. Monforte R, Estruch R, Vidal J, et al. Delayed seroconversion in Legionnaire's disease. Lancet 1988;2(8609):513.

75. Plouffe JF, File TM Jr, Breiman RF, et al. Reevaluation of the definition of Legionnaires' disease: use of the urinary antigen assay. Community Based Pneumonia Incidence Study Group. Clin Infect Dis 1995;20(5):1286–91.
76. Berdal BP, Farshy CE, Feeley JC. Detection of *Legionella pneumonophila* antigen in urine by enzyme-linked immunospecific assay. J Clin Microbiol 1979;9(5):575–8.
77. Kohler RB, Zimmerman SE, Wilson E, et al. Rapid radioimmunoassay diagnosis of Legionnaires' disease: detection and partial characterization of urinary antigen. Ann Intern Med 1981;94(5):601–5.
78. Williams A, Lever MS. Characterisation of *Legionella pneumophila* antigen in urine of guinea pigs and humans with Legionnaires' disease. J Infect 1995; 30(1):13–6.
79. Diederen BM, Peeters MF. Evaluation of the SAS Legionella test, a new immunochromatographic assay for the detection of *Legionella pneumophila* serogroup 1 antigen in urine. Clin Microbiol Infect 2007;13(1):86–8.
80. Koide M, Higa F, Tateyama M, et al. Detection of *Legionella* species in clinical samples: comparison of polymerase chain reaction and urinary antigen detection kits. Infection 2006;34(5):264–8.
81. Joseph CA. Legionnaires' disease in Europe 2000–2002. Epidemiol Infect 2004; 132(3):417–24.
82. Formica N, Yates M, Beers M, et al. The impact of diagnosis by *Legionella* urinary antigen test on the epidemiology and outcomes of Legionnaires' disease. Epidemiol Infect 2001;127(2):275–80.
83. Diederen BM. *Legionella* spp. and Legionnaires' disease. J Infect 2008;56(1): 1–12.
84. Leland DS, Kohler RB. Evaluation of the L-CLONE *Legionella pneumophila* serogroup 1 urine antigen latex test. J Clin Microbiol 1991;29(10):2220–3.
85. Helbig JH, Uldum SA, Bernander S, et al. Clinical utility of urinary antigen detection for diagnosis of community-acquired, travel-associated, and nosocomial legionnaires' disease. J Clin Microbiol 2003;41(2):838–40.
86. Harrison T, Uldum S, Alexiou-Daniel S, et al. A multicenter evaluation of the Biotest *Legionella* urinary antigen EIA. Clin Microbiol Infect 1998;4(7):359–65.
87. Dominguez J, Gali N, Blanco S, et al. Assessment of a new test to detect *Legionella* urinary antigen for the diagnosis of Legionnaires' Disease. Diagn Microbiol Infect Dis 2001;41(4):199–203.
88. Yzerman EP, den Boer JW, Lettinga KD, et al. Sensitivity of three urinary antigen tests associated with clinical severity in a large outbreak of Legionnaires' disease in The Netherlands. J Clin Microbiol 2002;40(9):3232–6.
89. Diederen BM, Peeters MF. Evaluation of two new immunochromatographic assays (Rapid U *Legionella* antigen test and SD Bioline Legionella antigen test) for detection of *Legionella pneumophila* serogroup 1 antigen in urine. J Clin Microbiol 2006;44(8):2991–3.
90. Doebbeling BN, Bale MJ, Koontz FP, et al. Prospective evaluation of the Gen-Probe assay for detection of legionellae in respiratory specimens. Eur J Clin Microbiol Infect Dis 1988;7(6):748–52.
91. Wilkinson HW, Sampson JS, Plikaytis BB. Evaluation of a commercial gene probe for identification of *Legionella* cultures. J Clin Microbiol 1986;23(2): 217–20.
92. Laussucq S, Schuster D, Alexander WJ, et al. False-positive DNA probe test for *Legionella* species associated with a cluster of respiratory illnesses. J Clin Microbiol 1988;26(8):1442–4.

93. Jonas D, Rosenbaum A, Weyrich S, et al. Enzyme-linked immunoassay for detection of PCR-amplified DNA of legionellae in bronchoalveolar fluid. J Clin Microbiol 1995;33(5):1247–52.
94. Reischl U, Linde HJ, Lehn N, et al. Direct detection and differentiation of *Legionella* spp. and *Legionella pneumophila* in clinical specimens by dual-color real-time PCR and melting curve analysis. J Clin Microbiol 2002;40(10):3814–7.
95. Rantakokko-Jalava K, Jalava J. Development of conventional and real-time PCR assays for detection of *Legionella* DNA in respiratory specimens. J Clin Microbiol 2001;39(8):2904–10.
96. Wellinghausen N, Frost C, Marre R. Detection of legionellae in hospital water samples by quantitative real-time LightCycler PCR. Appl Environ Microbiol 2001;67(9):3985–93.
97. Stolhaug A, Bergh K. Identification and differentiation of *Legionella pneumophila* and *Legionella* spp. with real-time PCR targeting the 16S rRNA gene and species identification by mip sequencing. Appl Environ Microbiol 2006;72(9):6394–8.
98. van Der Zee A, Verbakel H, de Jong C, et al. Novel PCR-probe assay for detection of and discrimination between *Legionella pneumophila* and other *Legionella* species in clinical samples. J Clin Microbiol 2002;40(3):1124–5.
99. Cloud JL, Carroll KC, Pixton P, et al. Detection of *Legionella* species in respiratory specimens using PCR with sequencing confirmation. J Clin Microbiol 2000;38(5):1709–12.
100. Templeton KE, Scheltinga SA, Sillekens P, et al. Development and clinical evaluation of an internally controlled, single-tube multiplex real-time PCR assay for detection of *Legionella pneumophila* and other *Legionella* species. J Clin Microbiol 2003;41(9):4016–21.
101. Herpers BL, de Jongh BM, van der Zwaluw K, et al. Real-time PCR assay targets the 23S-5S spacer for direct detection and differentiation of *Legionella* spp. and *Legionella pneumophila*. J Clin Microbiol 2003;41(10):4815–6.
102. Murdoch DR, Walford EJ, Jennings LC, et al. Use of the polymerase chain reaction to detect Legionella DNA in urine and serum samples from patients with pneumonia. Clin Infect Dis 1996;23(3):475–80.
103. Kessler HH, Reinthaler FF, Pschaid A, et al. Rapid detection of *Legionella* species in bronchoalveolar lavage fluids with the EnviroAmp Legionella PCR amplification and detection kit. J Clin Microbiol 1993;31(12):3325–8.
104. Ratcliff RM, Lanser JA, Manning PA, et al. Sequence-based classification scheme for the genus *Legionella* targeting the *mip* gene. J Clin Microbiol 1998;36(6):1560–7.
105. Koide M, Saito A. Diagnosis of *Legionella pneumophila* infection by polymerase chain reaction. Clin Infect Dis 1995;21(1):199–201.
106. Lindsay DS, Abraham WH, Fallon RJ. Detection of *mip* gene by PCR for diagnosis of Legionnaires' disease. J Clin Microbiol 1994;32(12):3068–9.
107. Wilson DA, Yen-Lieberman B, Reischl U, et al. Detection of *Legionella pneumophila* by real-time PCR for the *mip* gene. J Clin Microbiol 2003;41(7):3327–30.
108. Diederen BM, de Jong CM, Marmouk F, et al. Evaluation of real-time PCR for the early detection of *Legionella pneumophila* DNA in serum samples. J Med Microbiol 2007;56(Pt 1):94–101.
109. Diederen BM, Bruin JP, den Boer JW, et al. Sensitivity of *Legionella pneumophila* DNA detection in serum samples in relation to disease severity. J Med Microbiol 2007;56(Pt 9):1255.

110. Helbig JH, Engelstadter T, Maiwald M, et al. Diagnostic relevance of the detection of Legionella DNA in urine samples by the polymerase chain reaction. Eur J Clin Microbiol Infect Dis 1999;18(10):716–22.
111. Murdoch DR. Diagnosis of *Legionella* infection. Clin Infect Dis 2003;36(1):64–9.
112. Diederen BM, Kluytmans JA, Vandenbroucke-Grauls CM, et al. Utility of real-time PCR for diagnosis of Legionnaires' disease in routine clinical practice. J Clin Microbiol 2008;46(2):671–7.
113. Bencini MA, van den Brule AJ, Claas EC, et al. Multicenter comparison of molecular methods for detection of *Legionella* spp. in sputum samples. J Clin Microbiol 2007;45(10):3390–2.
114. Sopena N, Sabria-Leal M, Pedro-Botet ML, et al. Comparative study of the clinical presentation of *Legionella pneumonia* and other community-acquired pneumonias. Chest 1998;113(5):1195–200.
115. Ingram JG, Plouffe JF. Danger of sputum purulence screens in culture of *Legionella* species. J Clin Microbiol 1994;32(1):209–10.
116. Tuuminen T, Varjo S, Ingman H, et al. Prevalence of *Chlamydia pneumoniae* and *Mycoplasma pneumoniae* immunoglobulin G and A antibodies in a healthy Finnish population as analyzed by quantitative enzyme immunoassays. Clin Diagn Lab Immunol 2000;7(5):734–8.
117. Liu G, Talkington DF, Fields BS, et al. *Chlamydia pneumoniae* and *Mycoplasma pneumoniae* in young children from China with community-acquired pneumonia. Diagn Microbiol Infect Dis 2005;52(1):7–14.
118. Oosterheert JJ, van Loon AM, Schuurman R, et al. Impact of rapid detection of viral and atypical bacterial pathogens by real-time polymerase chain reaction for patients with lower respiratory tract infection. Clin Infect Dis 2005;41(10):1438–44.
119. Wellinghausen N, Straube E, Freidank H, et al. Low prevalence of *Chlamydia pneumoniae* in adults with community-acquired pneumonia. Int J Med Microbiol 2006;296(7):485–91.
120. Lauderdale TL, Chang FY, Ben RJ, et al. Etiology of community acquired pneumonia among adult patients requiring hospitalization in Taiwan. Respir Med 2005;99(9):1079–86.
121. Michelow IC, Olsen K, Lozano J, et al. Epidemiology and clinical characteristics of community-acquired pneumonia in hospitalized children. Pediatrics 2004;113(4):701–7.
122. Hammerschlag MR. *Chlamydia pneumoniae* and the lung. Eur Respir J 2000;16(5):1001–7.
123. Littman AJ, Jackson LA, White E, et al. Interlaboratory reliability of microimmunofluorescence test for measurement of *Chlamydia pneumoniae*-specific immunoglobulin A and G antibody titers. Clin Diagn Lab Immunol 2004;11(3):615–7.
124. Hermann C, Graf K, Groh A, et al. Comparison of eleven commercial tests for *Chlamydia pneumoniae*-specific immunoglobulin G in asymptomatic healthy individuals. J Clin Microbiol 2002;40(5):1603–9.
125. Holland SM, Gaydos CA, Quinn TC. Detection and differentiation of *Chlamydia trachomatis, Chlamydia psittaci*, and *Chlamydia pneumoniae* by DNA amplification. J Infect Dis 1990;162(4):984–7.
126. Campbell LA, Perez Melgosa M, Hamilton DJ, et al. Detection of *Chlamydia pneumoniae* by polymerase chain reaction. J Clin Microbiol 1992;30(2):434–9.
127. Kaltenboeck B, Kousoulas KG, Storz J. Two-step polymerase chain reactions and restriction endonuclease analyses detect and differentiate ompA DNA of *Chlamydia* spp. J Clin Microbiol 1992;30(5):1098–104.

128. Mygind T, Birkelund S, Falk E, et al. Evaluation of real-time quantitative PCR for identification and quantification of *Chlamydia pneumoniae* by comparison with immunohistochemistry. J Microbiol Methods 2001;46(3):241–51.
129. Gaydos CA, Quinn TC, Eiden JJ. Identification of *Chlamydia pneumoniae* by DNA amplification of the 16S rRNA gene. J Clin Microbiol 1992;30(4):796–800.
130. Tondella ML, Talkington DF, Holloway BP, et al. Development and evaluation of real-time PCR-based fluorescence assays for detection of *Chlamydia pneumoniae*. J Clin Microbiol 2002;40(2):575–83.
131. Kuoppa Y, Boman J, Scott L, et al. Quantitative detection of respiratory *Chlamydia pneumoniae* infection by real-time PCR. J Clin Microbiol 2002;40(6): 2273–4.
132. Reischl U, Lehn N, Simnacher U, et al. Rapid and standardized detection of *Chlamydia pneumoniae* using LightCycler real-time fluorescence PCR. Eur J Clin Microbiol Infect Dis 2003;22(1):54–7.
133. Apfalter P, Barousch W, Nehr M, et al. Comparison of a new quantitative ompA-based real-Time PCR TaqMan assay for detection of *Chlamydia pneumoniae* DNA in respiratory specimens with four conventional PCR assays. J Clin Microbiol 2003;41(2):592–600.
134. Hardick J, Maldeis N, Theodore M, et al. Real-time PCR for *Chlamydia pneumoniae* utilizing the Roche Lightcycler and a 16S rRNA gene target. J Mol Diagn 2004;6(2):132–6.
135. Chernesky M, Smieja M, Schachter J, et al. Comparison of an industry-derived LCx *Chlamydia pneumoniae* PCR research kit to in-house assays performed in five laboratories. J Clin Microbiol 2002;40(7):2357–62.
136. Block S, Hedrick J, Hammerschlag MR, et al. *Mycoplasma pneumoniae* and *Chlamydia pneumoniae* in pediatric community-acquired pneumonia: comparative efficacy and safety of clarithromycin vs. erythromycin ethylsuccinate. Pediatr Infect Dis J 1995;14(6):471–7.
137. Boman J, Allard A, Persson K, et al. Rapid diagnosis of respiratory *Chlamydia pneumoniae* infection by nested touchdown polymerase chain reaction compared with culture and antigen detection by EIA. J Infect Dis 1997;175(6): 1523–6.
138. Verkooyen RP, Willemse D, Hiep-van Casteren SC, et al. Evaluation of PCR, culture, and serology for diagnosis of *Chlamydia pneumoniae* respiratory infections. J Clin Microbiol 1998;36(8):2301–7.

Index

Note: Page numbers of article titles are in **boldface** type.

Infect Dis Clin N Am 24 (2010) 249–255
doi:10.1016/S0891-5520(09)00110-X

N

O

P

Q

R

S

T

Printed and bound by CPI Group (UK) Ltd, Croydon, CR0 4YY
03/10/2024
01040453-0009